Trauma, War, and Violence
Public Mental Health in Socio-Cultural Context

The Plenum Series on Stress and Coping

Series Editor:
Donald Meichenbaum, *University of Waterloo, Waterloo, Ontario, Canada*

Current Volumes in the Series:

BEYOND TRAUMA
Cultural and Societal Dynamics
Edited by Rolf J. Kleber, Charles R. Figley, and Berthold P. R. Gersons

COMMUTING STRESS
Causes, Effects, and Methods of Coping
Meni Koslowsky, Avraham N. Kluger, and Mordechai Reich

CREATING A COMPREHENSIVE TRAUMA CENTER
Choices and Challenges
Mary Beth Williams and Lasse A. Nurmi

ETHNICITY, IMMIGRATION, AND PSYCHOPATHOLOGY
Edited by Ihsan Al-Issa and Michel Tousignant

INTERNATIONAL HANDBOOK OF HUMAN RESPONSE TO TRAUMA
Edited by Arieh Y. Shalev, Rachel Yehuda, and Alexander C. McFarlane

INTERNATIONAL HANDBOOK OF MULTIGENERATIONAL LEGACIES OF TRAUMA
Edited by Yael Danieli

THE MENTAL HEALTH CONSEQUENCES OF TORTURE
Edited by Ellen Gerrity, Terence M. Keane, and Farris Tuma

PSYCHOTRAUMATOLOGY
Key Papers and Core Concepts in Post-Traumatic Stress
Edited by George S. Everly, Jr. and Jeffrey M. Lating

STRESS, CULTURE, AND COMMUNITY
The Psychology and Philosophy of Stress
Stevan E. Hobfoll

TRAUMA, WAR, AND VIOLENCE
Public Mental Health in Socio-Cultural Context
Edited by Joop de Jong

TRAUMATIC STRESS
From Theory to Practice
Edited by John R. Freedy and Stevan E. Hobfoll

A Continuation Order Plan is available for this series. A continuation order will bring delivery of each new volume immediately upon publication. Volumes are billed only upon actual shipment. For further information please contact the publisher.

Trauma, War, and Violence
Public Mental Health in Socio-Cultural Context

Edited by
JOOP DE JONG
Transcultural Psychosocial Organization
Amsterdam, the Netherlands

Springer Science+Business Media, LLC

ISBN 978-1-4757-7611-9   ISBN 978-0-306-47675-4 (eBook)
DOI 10.1007/978-0-306-47675-4

2002 by Springer Science+Business Media New York
Originally published by Kluwer Academic / Plenum Publishers, New York in 2002
Softcover reprint of the hardcover 1st edition 2002
http://www.wkap.nl/

10 9 8 7 6 5 4 3 2 1

A C.I.P. record for this book is available from the Library of Congress

All rights reserved

This book is copyrighted by Kluwer Academic / Plenum Publishers; however,
the contents of the individual chapters appearing in this volume are in the public domain.
If these chapters are reproduced in any form, acknowledgment of the National Institute
of Mental Health is appreciated.

Contributors

Lewis Aptekar, San Jose State University, San Jose, California

Fatima Arar, Algerian Society of Research in Psychology and Algiers University, Algiers, Algeria

Nancy Baron, Transcultural Psychosocial Organization, Uganda, Kampala, Uganda

Chérifa Bouatta, Algerian Society of Research in Psychology and Algiers University, Algiers, Algeria

Antonella Crescenzi, Tibetan Transcultural Psychosocial Organization Mental Health Project, Dharamsala, India

Joop de Jong, Transcultural Psychosocial Organization and Vrije Universiteit, Amsterdam, the Netherlands

Maurice Eisenbruch, University of New South Wales, Sydney, Australia

Mustafa Elmasri, Algerian Society of Research in Psychology, Algiers, Algeria

Eyad el-Sarraj, Gaza Community Mental Health Programme, Gaza, Palestine

Rob Giel, Emeritus, Rijksuniversiteit Groningen, Groningen, the Netherlands

Chelliah S. Jamunanantha, District Hospital, Tellipallai, Sri Lanka

Eva Ketzer, Tibetan Transcultural Psychosocial Organization Mental Health Project, Dharamsala, India

Noureddine Khaled, Algerian Society of Research in Psychology and Algiers University, Algiers, Algeria

Jaak Le Roy, Regional Community Mental Health Center, Maastricht, the Netherlands

Bhava N. Poudyal, Center for Victims of Torture and Transcultural Psychosocial Organization, Kathmandu, Nepal

Dinesh Prasain, Center for Victims of Torture and Transcultural Psychosocial Organization, Kathmandu, Nepal

Samir Qouta, Gaza Community Mental Health Programme, Gaza, Palestine

Bhogendra Sharma, Center for Victims of Torture and Transcultural Psychosocial Organization, Kathmandu, Nepal

Mohand OuAhmed Aït Sidhoum, Algerian Society of Research in Psychology and Algiers University, Algiers, Algeria

Daya Somasundaram, University of Jaffna, Jaffna, Sri Lanka

Willem A. C. M. van de Put, HealthNet International, Amsterdam, the Netherlands

Mark van Ommeren, Transcultural Psychosocial Organization and Center for Victims of Torture, Kathmandu, Nepal

Foreword

There are currently 22 million people of concern to the office of the United Nations High Commissioner for Refugees. Many of these refugees, internally displaced people and other victims of conflict have suffered, and continue to suffer, the effects of trauma. Many have witnessed killings and many have personally experienced horros such as rape, torture and hunger.

In its 1948 Universal Declaration of Human Rights, the UN General Assembly affirmed that all human beings are born free and equal in dignity and rights. The Declaration proclaims that no one should be held in slavery or subjected to torture or to cruel, inhuman, or degrading treatment or punishment. All are held to be entitled to equal protection of the law, to move about freely, to found a family, to own a property, to express their views, and to practice their chosen religion. All are held to be entitled to the indispensable economic, social and cultural benefits in their country, including an adequate standard of living, employment, education, and health care. In the years since 1948, governments have adopted many instruments that reinforce these fundamental human rights.

Despite this, gross violations of human rights continue to be perpetrated in numerous countries. War, genocide, persecution, political repression, "ethnic cleansing", terrorism, abject poverty and other calamities continue to deprive individuals of their homes, their families, their work, their schools, their places of worship, and their access of education and health care. Millions of people are deprived of their liberty, security and dignity.

In addition to the imperative of providing protection and assistance for victims of conflict and other human rights abuses, we need to address their psychosocial needs. A traumatic event can have a devastating consequence on a person's life, as well as on the lives of those who love them. Physical injuries and death are the most obvious manifestations of trauma's impact on a person's health. But over and above its impact on physical health, a traumatic event can result in psychological as well as occupational, marital and financial problems for its survivors.

Until recently, we have concentrated disproportionately on remedying external conditions. Much less has been done at the international policy-making level to address the effects of trauma. *Trauma, War, and Violence: Public Mental Health in Socio-Cultural Context* is an important milestone on a path that is increasingly considered important among UN agencies, governments and non-governmental organizations (NGOs). The book outlines a range of options for coping with intolerable stress in conflict and post-conflict situations, both in terms of good practice and prevention. It examines the psychosocial and mental health aspects of conflict, while at the same time considering the historical, political and socio-cultural context. It also describes a series of culturally sensitive intervention models in Africa and Asia, as developed by the Transcultural Psychosocial Organization.

This is an important book. It not only helps to improve our understanding of the psychosocial and mental health aspects of war and violence, but also provides valuable insight into ways of addressing the needs of victims of trauma. It is a valuable resource for professional health workers, social workers, community health workers, relief workers, members of judicial systems, human rights organizations, UN agencies, NGOs and academic institutions.

RUUD LUBBERS
UN High Commissioner for Refugees

Preface

This book describes a variety of innovative programs to address mental health and psychosocial problems in low-income countries and conflict and post-conflict areas. Governments, non-governmental organizations, United Nations agencies and colleagues will find this book useful when setting up community mental health and psychosocial services.

This book focuses specifically on the public mental health aspects of complex humanitarian and political emergencies. These emergencies combine several features: they violate human rights; involve the use of both state and non-state terror; they often occur within a country rather then across state boundaries; they include expressions of political, economic, and socio-cultural divisions; they promote competition for power and resources and result in predatory social formations; they affect large, displaced and mostly poor populations; and they often are protracted in duration and accompanied by cycles of violence.

Since every complex emergency is characterized by a combination of these features in unique socio-cultural contexts with unique resources, each public health program must use tailored interventions to the specific needs of the population. This has several consequences for this book.

First, public mental health is an interdisciplinary field. As a result, psychiatrists, psychologists, anthropologists, epidemiologists and psychotherapists have written this book.

Second public mental health tries to address the social, cultural, historical, and political determinants of mental well-being. This is best achieved by involving many sectors of the society to cooperatively deal with the consequences of complex emergencies. Therefore, appropriate public mental health work requires input from different governmental and non-governmental sectors working in health, education, women's affairs, human rights, social welfare and rural development.

Third, survivors of wars, violence, atrocities, and human rights violations are exposed to inequities in the provision of services, which results in despair and anger that causes disruption, social instability and terror. Importantly, public mental health advocates to reduce these disparities and the stigma often attached to mental health problems. They arrange for equal care withou bias to mental or physical condition, culture, country, ethnic group, gender, age or religion.

Fourth, cultural diversity is an important theme in our multicultural and global world. Public mental health tries to identify universal characteristics while simultaneously accomodating and managing context-specific expressions of distress with available resources. Interventions used to help local populations have to be adapted to that particular culture if they are to be effective. This book, by providing space for nine programs started or supported by the Transcultural Psychosocial Organization (TPO), clarifies how public mental health can be approached within different sociocultural contexts.

JOOP DE JONG
Director, TPO

Contents

Chapter 1. Public Mental Health, Traumatic Stress and Human Rights Violations in Low-Income Countries 1

Joop T. V. M. de Jong

Chapter 2. The Cambodian Experience 93

Willem A. C. M. Van de Put and Maurice Eisenbruch

Chapter 3. Community Based Psychosocial and Mental Health Services for Southern Sudanese Refugees in Long Term Exile in Uganda 157

Nancy Baron

Chapter 4. Psychosocial Consequences of War 205

Daya Somasundaram and C. S. Jamunanantha

Chapter 5. Addressing Human Rights Violations 259

Mark van Ommeren, Bhogendra Sharma, Dinesh Prasain, and Bhava N. Poudyal

Chapter 6. Addressing the Psychosocial and Mental Health Needs of Tibetan Refugees in India 283

Eva Ketzer and Antonella Crescenzi

Chapter 7. Community Mental Health as Practiced by the Gaza Community Mental Health Programme 317

Samir Qouta and Eyad el-Sarraj

Chapter 8. Walks in Kaliti, Life in a Destitute Shelter for the Displaced 337

Lewis Aptekar and Rob Giel

Chapter 9. Terrorism, Traumatic Events and Mental Health in Algeria 367

M. A. Aït Sidhoum, F. Arar, C. Bouatta, N. Khaled, and M. Elmasri

Chapter 10. How Can Participation of the Community and Traditional Healers Improve Primary Health Care in Kinshasa, Congo? 405

Jaak Le Roy

Author Index 441

Subject Index 447

Trauma, War, and Violence
Public Mental Health in Socio-Cultural Context

1

Public Mental Health, Traumatic Stress and Human Rights Violations in Low-Income Countries

A Culturally Appropriate Model in Times of Conflict, Disaster and Peace

JOOP T. V. M. DE JONG

INTRODUCTION

In this book we provide information about a variety of public mental health programs in conflict and post-conflict situations in Africa and Asia. Massive traumatic stress and human rights violations have gained the attention from governments, non-governmental organizations (NGOs) and the United Nations. The professional literature increasingly discusses psychosocial issues, mental illness, and trauma in the context of war and culture. Yet, there is little systematic knowledge on how to address the massive psychosocial consequences of violence, armed conflicts and human rights violations.

The aim of this book is to fill this gap. The various chapters emphasize psychosocial and mental health aspects, while also providing the historical, political and sociocultural background of different conflicts. We argue that without contextual insight, it is difficult to mobilize resources and help people cope with the horrors that come from armed conflicts, human rights violations or other types of disasters.

Scope of the Problem and its Geographical Distribution

The number of refugees in the world has grown over the last decades even though it peaked in 1992 and has gradually decreased since then (see Table 1).

The number of internally displaced (IDPs) shows the same trend. Estimates of IDPs reached 25 to 30 million by the end of 1994, and has fluctuated between 20 and 25 million thereafter. The decrease after 1995 is largely due to the fact that civil wars ended in a number of countries, among them Mozambique and some states in Central America, and that 3.5 million South Africans were subtracted from the total given the political changes in their country (Cohen & Deng, 1998). By 1996 estimates declined to about 20 million, although the U.S. Committee for Refugees believed the total number to be "undoubtedly higher" (USCR, 1997).

Table 2 provides information on the groups that are of concern to UNHCR. Two and a half to five percent of the refugee population consists of unaccompanied

Table 1. Number of Refugees Worldwide Over the Last Four Decades[a]

Year	Number
1960	1,400,000
1979	13,000,000
1981	16,000,000
1992	17,600,000
1993	16,300,000
1998	13,500,000
1999	11,675,380

[a]Figures of Cohon, 1981; Westermeyer, 1989; World Refugee Survey, 1999; UNHCR, 2000. For definitions of e.g. the word 'refugee' see the glossary to this book.

Table 2. Statistical Overview of Groups of Concern to UNHCR at the end of 1999

Groups of concern	Population end of 1999
Refugees	11,675,380
Asylum Seekers	1,181,600
Returned Refugees	2,509,830
Internally Displaced	3,968,700
Returned Internally Displaced Persons	1,435,290
Various	1,486,540
GRAND TOTAL	22,257,340

Source: United Nations High Commissioner for Refugees (a).

children. In 1996 UNICEF reported that in the last 10 years, 2 million children have died in war, 4–5 million have been disabled or wounded, 12 million made homeless and 1 million orphaned or separated from parents (UNICEF, 1996).

Within the global context one can distinguish cross-border migration (e.g. from Sudan to Uganda, Ethiopia and Congo, Sierra Leone, Liberia and Guinea, and vice versa; from Bhutan to Nepal; from Tibet to India; from Rwanda and Burundi to neighboring countries), internal displacement (in e.g. Angola; Cambodia; Israel–Palestine), or a combination of both (e.g. the Balkan and the Caucasus). In addition, there is cross-continental migration (e.g. Tamils, Cambodians, Iraqi and Afghani in Europe or North America).

Many of the refugees and IDPs are destitute people from poor countries who travel within or to other impoverished countries. In Mozambique the number of internally displaced persons during the Frelimo-Renamo conflict was estimated at four million and the number of refugees at more than one million out of a total population of 14 million. Currently, Sudan has an estimated four million IDPs and 500 000 refugees on a population of 35 million. Because large displacements can destabilize host countries, aggravate regional tensions, and increase environmental degradation it is amazing that nations that have traditionally offered asylum are increasingly unwilling to open their doors to massive refugee flows (Desjarlais, Eisenberg, Good, & Kleinman, 1995).

Between the 1960s and 1990s the number of refugees and IDPs increased for a variety of reasons. The first one is war, the most devastating form of human-made violence. Since World War II, there have been 127 wars and 21.8 million war-related deaths. The Red Cross estimated a total twice as high, i.e., about 40 million people killed since World War II. All but two of these 127 wars took place in low-income countries (McFarlane & De Girolamo, 1996). The differential impact of traumatic stress on low-income countries also appears from the following figures. In the period 1967–1991, an average of 117 million people living in developing countries were affected by disasters each year, as compared to about 700,000 in developed countries (a striking ratio of 166 : 1) (International Federation of Red Cross, 1993).

The militarization of low-income countries, with a combination of low intensity warfare and high-intensity lethal weaponry, is a major cause of displacement, especially of women and children. These countries have too often been the arena for conflicts between superpowers, political systems and world religions.

A second explanation for the increasing flow of refugees is the choice of a dominant socio-economic development model, often stimulated by the Structural Adjustment Programs of International Monetary Fund (IMF) and World Bank (WB), leading to marginalization of large groups of people, which in turn had led to conflicts over access to education, health care, land or drinking water (Sen, 1997).

A third explanation for forced migration is the failure of many states to fully transform themselves into democracies either after the end of communist regimes or after colonization. Weak nation states with low levels of democracy have given rise to new power elites that are not interested in the poor or in sustainable development (Van de Goor, Rupesinghe, & Sciarone, 1996). These developments have often been accompanied by political and ethnic conflicts, which in turn have added insecurity, oppression, dehumanization, torture and other forms of human rights violations, perpetuating so-called 'complex emergencies'.

For every legally defined refugee, there are more internally displaced people who may not formally be identified or served by international organizations, but who are vulnerable to similar psychosocial problems as refugees. Some uprooted populations may be refugees one day, repatriated at another time and then internally displaced. To make the problem more complex, refugees and internally displaced people often live mixed with indigenous populations who may also suffer from violence and persecution.

In addition to the approximately 13.5 million refugees and 20 million internally displaced because of armed conflicts, there are countless other economic and environmental refugees in the world. More than 70 million people around the world have left their native countries, primarily in search of work. At least 10 million of these have fled from environmental decline, such as land degradation that has diminished agricultural and water resources (Desjarlais et al., 1995).

The regional distribution of the problem is far from even as shown in Tables 3 and 4. Table 3 reports the statistical breakdown of regions of origin of the 11.7 million refugees in 1999. Table 4 shows the most important countries producing refugees and IDPs.

One reason why these figures are subject to fluctuation is the volatility of national and international relations. This is the case in the Balkans, the Great Lakes Region of Africa and in the Horn of Africa, in South-East Asia and in the former Soviet Union. In Africa, 70% of the refugee burden is borne by 12 countries. All 16 of the least-developed African countries are affected by refugee problems (McFarlane & De Girolamo, 1996).

Traumatic Stress, Risk Factors and Protective Factors

The events precipitating the act of relocation (war, persecution, hunger, disaster, death), the process of relocation (upheaval, a long and unsafe journey on foot under mental and physical strain), and settlement in refugee camps (discomfort, uncertainty, unemployment, oppression, discrimination) take a mental and physical toll. Individuals, often in such numbers as to include families and entire communities, suffer from a range of human rights violations including torture, rape, abductions, sexual violation, war wounds, deprivation of basic needs, loss

Table 3. Statistical Summary of Refugee Population by Region at the end of 1999

Region of refugee origin	Population end of 1999
Eastern Africa	1,479,000
Middle Africa	685,050
Northern Africa	637,190
Southern Africa	700
Western Africa	831,260
AFRICA Total	3,633,200
East Asia	120,900
South-central Asia	2,919,480
South-eastern Asia	708,260
Western Asia	599,560
ASIA Total	4,994,710
Eastern Europe	25,520
Northern Europe	1,020
Southern Europe	918,300
Western Europe	10
EUROPE Total	944,850
Caribbean	6,000
Central America	51,240
South America	7,300
LATIN AMERICA AND CARIBBEAN Total	64,540
Stateless And Unknown	2,061,980
GRAND TOTAL	11,699,280

Source: United Nations High Commissioner for Refugees (b).

Table 4. Top-twelve Countries Producing Refugees and Asylum Seekers and IDPs at the end of the Nineties[a]

Refugees and asylum seekers[b]		Internally displaced	
Palestinians	3,816,000	Sudan	4,000,000
Afghanistan	2,600,000	Angola	1,000,000–1,500,000
Iraq	586,000	Colombia	1,400,000
Sierra Leone	480,000	Iraq	1,000,000
Bosnia and Herzegovina	424,000	Afghanistan	540,000–1,000,000
Somalia	421,000	Burma	500,000–1,000,000
Sudan	352,000	Turkey	400,000–1,000,000
Eritrea	323,000	Azerbaijan	576,000
Liberia	310,000	Sri Lanka	560,000
Croatia	309,000	India	520,000
Angola	302,000	Burundi	500,000
Burundi	281,000	Rwanda	500,000

[a]Sources vary widely in numbers reported (cf World Refugee Survey, 1999; USCR, 1996).
[b]In 1998 there were 387,759 asylum applicants (World Refugee Survey, 1999).

of home, loss of loved ones, and premature death. Families and communities suffer from ethnic cleansing, persecution and harassment and genocide.

The resulting long- and short-term mental health and psychosocial consequences are many and varied, as the chapters of this book will show. Like all immigrants, refugees need to cope with an unfamiliar cultural environment; with the sense of loss or deprivation of family, homeland, status, possessions, and culture (Eisenbruch, 1984). They feel rejected and confused about their new roles, values and identity, all of which influence their mental health status (Cheng & Chang 1999).

When the Universal Declaration of Human Rights was adopted and proclaimed by the General Assembly of the United Nations in 1948, mental health was not mentioned. Overall, however, the human rights declaration can be interpreted as a set of preconditions favoring public mental health. A societal context where human rights are not respected like under the conditions of war, state terrorism, dictatorship and extreme poverty, must be considered as unhealthy from a psychosocial and mental health perspective. From a healing and preventive point of view, respecting human rights is essential to a society's overall mental health. Both human rights and mental health providers need to be aware of the importance of the interrelationship and coordination between these specialties (Baron, Jensen, & de Jong, 2000).

There are specific risk factors implicated in the development of mental disorders in refugees and refugee families cutting across lines of social class and cultural identity (cf Jablensky, Marsella, Ekblad, Jansson, Levi, & Bornemann, 1994; de Jong, Komproe, Van Ommeren, El Masri, Mesfin, Khaled, Somasundaram, & Van de Put, 2001; Brewin, Andrews, & Valentine, 2000). These include the following:

- Traumatic events related to armed conflict after the age 12
- Torture
- Female gender
- Socioeconomic hardship, poverty, unemployment, low education and lack of professional skills fitting the new environment
- Problems of marginalization, discrimination, acculturation, language and communication
- Poor physical health due to poor sanitation and poor health care
- Poor nutrition
- Crowding and poor physical conditions including head trauma and other physical injuries
- Collapse of social networks resulting in anomie, alienation, and poor social support
- Traumatic events, such as death, loss, or fear of such events

- Daily hassles or life stress, youth domestic stress, conflict related events during flight
- Failure to cope after the first month after the traumatic events
- Perceived lack of control over the traumatic events
- Preexisting history of psychiatric problems of individual or family, and psychiatric comorbidity

Some of these risk factors may be used to identify those in most need of help and worthy of early intervention, while other factors can assist in determining the type of services most needed.

Risk factors, however, may be balanced by protective factors. Protective factors should be identified to assess people's resiliency. Examples of protective factors are:

- The presence of a social network, including a nuclear or extended family
- Social support and self-help groups for empowerment and sharing
- Employment or other possibilities of income generation
- Access to human right organisations
- Recreation and leisure activities
- The possibility to perform culturally prescribed rituals and ceremonies
- Political and religious inspiration as a source of comfort, meaning and a perspective for the future
- Camps with a limited size
- Coping skills, intelligence and humor

Children likely experience similar risk and protective factors as adults. Yet, children are subjected to other problems, including lack of clothes and school materials. Girls often have to contribute to household tasks, mainly because their mothers spend a great deal of time obtaining water and firewood (Pynoos, Groenjian, & Steinberg, 1998; Paardekoper, de Jong, & Hermanns, 1998). Although schools constitute effective settings to provide mental health assistance to children and their families, schools are often absent or overcrowded.

The Burden of Disease

In the emergency phase of refugee care, physical health and issues of survival take precedence. Priorities are water and sanitation, food and nutrition, shelter, and control of communicable diseases such as diarrhoeal diseases, measles, respiratory infections and malaria (MSF, 1997). Tuberculosis, intestinal parasitosis, leprosy and sexually transmitted diseases such as syphilis and AIDS are common disease themes among immigrants worldwide. During the emergency phase physical health problems are often accompanied by a variety of psychosocial and mental health problems. There are no standard responses. Levels of intensity of traumatic stress and distress experienced are not clearly related. For example, a rape, death or loss of property can cause different levels of distress depending on protective factors of individual, family and community. Some people respond without a problem to their initial displacement and have symptoms of stress later, while others have symptoms at the beginning that later disappear.

The increasing awareness of the importance of traumatic stress in (post-) conflict and (post-)disaster situations reflects a global tendency to reevaluate the impact of mental problems on peoples' lives. Over the past years, a new approach (Global Burden of Disease) to measuring health status has been developed. To measure the Global Burden of Disease an internationally standardized form of the Quality Adjusted life Year (QUALY) has been developed, called the Disability Adjusted Life Year (DALY). The DALY expresses years of life lost to premature death and years lived with a disability of specified severity and duration. This method quantifies not merely the number of deaths but also the impact of premature death and disability on a population, and combines these into a single unit of measurement of the overall 'burden of disease' on the population. One might say, *one DALY is one lost year of healthy life.* The DALY is intended to be a transparent tool to enhance dialogue on the major health challenges facing humanity. To calculate DALYs for a given condition in a population, years of life lost (YLLs) and years lived with disability of known severity and duration (YLDs) for that condition have to be estimated and then the total be summed.

The World Bank, which together with WHO developed the DALY, expects that worldwide from 1990 to 2020 the Global Burden of Disease (GBD) of neuro-psychiatric disorders such as depression, alcohol dependence, bipolar disorder and schizophrenia could increase by 50% from 10.5% of the total burden to almost 15% (Murray & Lopez, 1996). In determining changes in rank for the leading sources of disease in proportion to other health problems from 1990 to 2020, these authors project that world-wide traffic accidents will rise in importance from 9th to 3rd place, war will rise from 16th to 8th place, and violence will rise from 28th to 12th place. Major depressive disorder will be the leading cause of disability worldwide for women. Behavior-related problems such as violence, diarrhoeal diseases (due to poor hygiene practices), AIDS and other sexually transmitted diseases, AIDS related dementia complex, and motor vehicle accidents cause an additional estimated 34% of the GBD. This means that more than one-third of the GBD could potentially prevented by changes in behavior. In short, worldwide almost half of the estimated total burden of disease is attributed to mental and behavioral problems.

Mental disorders are costly because their impact includes high service utilization, high rates of utilization of other services such as social services, education or the criminal justice system. In addition, mental health problems impact on employment and productivity of the person with the disorder, but also of the family or the caregiver. The DALY figures on mental health are extremely high when compared to individual diseases such as malaria that constitutes 2.6% or cancer that constitutes 5.8% of GBD (Murray & Lopez, 1996). But despite the growing recognition of the burden of mental illness on developing countries, the 'big killers' continue to command the majority of attention and funding (cf Blue & Harpham, 1998).

DALYs in (Post-)Disaster Situations

These figures could even become more extreme. For example, the complexity of collecting data in (post-) conflict areas will probably remain a major obstacle to measure DALYs in those areas. Measuring premature death is difficult in war conditions where many people die due to combat, armed conflicts, assaults or banditries. Numbers of deceased people may be unknown, and identification of the dead may be difficult when people are buried in mass graves or when warring parties obstruct identification by forensic teams. Moreover, when massive populations show extremely high levels of demoralization, anxiety and depression, it is methodologically difficult to distinguish mental cases from non-cases in cross-cultural settings. In addition, measuring disability related to specific disorders is hard to assess when most people simultaneously suffer because of extreme poverty, malnutrition, landmine accident or war acts. This makes it hard to disentangle the relative contribution to disability of anemia, parasites, chronic infectious disease, physical handicaps, and mental disorder. Despite these obstacles to measure DALYs one would expect that all the risk factors related to conflict lead to extremely high figures of DALYs in comparison to other areas, worldwide.

Morbidity Among Adults

Fortunately, most individuals exposed to extreme events are remarkably resilient. Even after fairly severe traumatic events, the majority will cope effectively if provided with the opportunities and resources to rebuild their lives. However, sometimes traumatic stressors make excessive demands that surpass the body's and the mind's ability to adjust. This may occur in situations of chronic violence such as war and civil unrest where traumatic events expose individuals to overwhelming and continuous levels of danger and fear. Repetitive exposure to very stressful circumstances may increasingly deplete resources, so individuals and communities end up in a negative spiral of loss from which it is difficult to recover. When these experiences overwhelm coping capabilities, there may be permanent damage (Solomon, 2001). Exposure to extreme stressors may result in a variety of responses. For example, short term and common effects of trauma to the individual adult tend to involve different combination of the following experiences: normal feelings of distress, vulnerability, helplessness, despair, intense, panic-level arousal and negative emotion. In addition, the person may experience a sense of being stunned, numb, and depleted, and an altered consciousness or awareness that entails a sense of derealization and depersonalization (also referred to as dissociation).

In the immediate aftermath of extreme trauma adults may also react with a time limited but acute stress disorder. Longer term and more serious reactions range from PTSD (Friedman & Jaranson, 1994), depressive disorders (Westermeyer, 1986), substance abuse (Keehn, 1980; Westermeyer, 1985), panic disorder, generalized anxiety, phobia, antisocial and other personality disorders, psychosis (Yesavage, 1983), organic brain syndrome (especially in victims of violence), and associated medical and social problems (Corcoran, 1982; Kirmayer, 1996).

Co-morbidity is common (Davidson & Foa, 1991; de Jong, Komproe, Van Ommeren, El Masri, Mesfin, Van de Put & Somasundaram, 2001b). Several studies demonstrated that PTSD frequently coexists with one or more additional diagnoses like major depression, dysthymia, anxiety disorder (Helzer, Robins, & McEvoy, 1987; Kessler, Sonnega, Bromet, Hughes, & Nelson, 1995), alcohol or substance abuse, and personality disorders. The co-existence of somatic complaints has been noted (Mc Farlane, Atchison, Rafalowicz & Papay, 1994; Shalev, Bleich, & Ursano, 1990; Litz, Keane, Fisher, Marx, B. & Monaco, 1992). The pattern of co-morbid diagnoses may vary from one setting to another but such variations do not necessarily invalidate the PTSD concept (see further on). For example, American war veterans often experience a combination of PTSD and alcohol abuse, Israelis often experience a combination of PTSD and depression, Soviets exhibit extremely high rates of alcohol abuse (Friedman & Jaranson, 1994), while tortured Bhutanese refugees often experience a combination of PTSD and persistent pain (Van Ommeren, 2000). For programming this is an important issue because high rates of co-morbidity complicate treatment decisions concerning persons with PTSD. In addition, mental health workers must decide whether to treat the co-morbid disorders concurrently or sequentially.

Epidemiology

Of the approximately 175 epidemiological studies on the mental health consequences of wars and conflicts, only a few population-based studies are carried out among adults in the afflicted areas in low-income countries. For example, 993 Cambodian refugees were studied on the Thai-Cambodian border. Most of the participants had experienced lack of food, water, shelter, and medical care; brainwashing; forced labor; and murder of a family member or friend. On the basis of responses to questionnaires, 55% qualified for a diagnosis of depression and 15% for PTSD (Mollica, Donelan, Svang, Lavelle, Elias, Frankel, & Blendon, 1993). El Sarraj, Punamäki, Salmi, & Summerfield (1996) found prevalence rates for PTSD of 20% or more among 550 torture survivors in

Gaza. Another group studied 526 Bhutanese torture survivors and a matched control group in Nepal. A diagnosis of PTSD was significantly more common in the tortured group than in the non-tortured group. Significantly more tortured refugees had high anxiety scores and high depression scores (Shrestha, Sharma, Van Ommeren, Regmi, Makaju, Komproe, Shrestha, & de Jong, 1998).

The Multi-site Impact of Man-made Disaster study (MIM-study) was carried out by TPO among a random sample of 3047 refugees, IDPs and post-conflict survivors in Algeria, Cambodia, Ethiopia, and Gaza. Seventeen percent of the non-traumatized part of the total sample showed psychopathology against 44% of those who experienced violence. The lifetime prevalence was 29% for PTSD, 12% for depressive disorder, 25% for anxiety disorder, and 5% for somatoform disorder. Seven percent of the traumatized part of the sample showed co-morbidity for three or four disorders versus one percent of the non-traumatized population and 13% co-morbidity for two disorders among the traumatized versus 3% of the non-traumatized population. The highest prevalence figures in this study were found in the Algerian sample for PTSD (37%), depression (23%) and somatoform disorder (8%). In the non-traumatized Algerian subjects high prevalence figures were found for depression (19%) and anxiety (38%). Co-morbidity of disorders was also highest among the Algerian subjects (60%). The highest prevalence for anxiety (40%) was found in the Cambodian sample. The non-traumatized Ethiopian subjects showed the lowest prevalence figures. Co-morbidity of PTSD and anxiety had the highest prevalence in all samples (de Jong, Komproe, Van Ommeren, El Masri, Mesfin, Van de Put, & Somasundaram, 2001b).

In another paper we estimated prevalence rates of PTSD and we defined 14 stress domains for lifetime events. Logistic regression analyses were used to reveal risk factors for PTSD. The prevalence rates of PTSD were 37.4% in Algeria, 28.4% in Cambodia, 15.8% in Ethiopia and 17.8% in Gaza. Conflict related trauma after age 12 was the only risk factor for PTSD in all samples, and torture in all samples except Cambodia. Psychiatric history and current illness were risk factors in Cambodia and Ethiopia. Poor quality of housing was related with PTSD in Algeria and in Gaza. The other stress domains were only risk factors for PTSD in single countries: daily hassles (Algeria), youth domestic stress and parental alcohol abuse (Cambodia), and trauma during the flight (Ethiopia). We concluded that despite the same research procedures, a wide range of prevalence rates of PTSD was found and that PTSD was not exclusively linked to a single event. In all samples at least 3 out of 14 trauma domains were identified as risk factors for PTSD. The findings of this paper confirm the idea that trauma is essential for the onset of PTSD, but that a multiplicity of other traumatic stressors determines the extent and expression of the posttraumatic stress symptoms (de Jong, Komproe, Van Ommeren, El Masri, Mesfin, Khaled, Somasundaram, & Van de Put, 2001).

In a population of IDPs affected by war trauma in Southern Uganda 55 people who experienced trauma were compared to a matched control group of 58 who did not experience trauma. Of the traumas experienced or witnessed by the trauma group 85% included severe wounds, 56% rape, 96% murder of a family member of friend, and 72% torture. The psychopathology in the trauma group included 53% with PTSD, 62% general anxiety disorder or panic disorder with or without agoraphobia and 71% with major depressive disorder. In the control group, 5% suffered from anxiety disorder and there was no diagnosis of PTSD or depression (Muller et al., 2002).

In 1995 a randomly selected group of 49 Sudanese refugees who went into exile in Uganda one to four years earlier were tested: 25% exceeded the cut-off scores for PTSD while 58% met the criteria for major depression problems (Sieswerda et al., 2002).

Based on these few studies, it appears that, in general, PTSD rates among victims of wars and persecution vary between 15 and 50%, that rates of depressive disorder between 15 and 70%, that a majority suffer from additional psychiatric disorders, and that they are a highly traumatized population that usually faced very difficult circumstances such as war and combat experiences, torture, starvation, or witnessing killings.

Traumatic Stress Among High Risk Groups

The Plight of Families. Tens of millions of children are victims of persecution or misfortune, becoming refugees, displaced persons, child soldiers, or casualties of war. Of an estimated 33 millions refugees and displaced persons in the world, 70–80% are mothers with children (Martin, 1994). Nearly 90% of the war related deaths during the last decade occurred to non-combatants and of them more than half were children. In last dozen years more than two million children have been killed in wars, and nearly 5 million more have been disabled. In addition, 12 million children who were made homeless and another million orphaned or living without their parents (UNICEF, 1997).

Living as a refugee, both in low-income and in high-income countries, creates a causal chain of disruption of communities and families. It is often reported that women, children, and the elderly are particularly vulnerable (cf Desjarlais et al., 1995). Women have to maintain their usual social role raising their children, doing household chores, or engaging in petty trade. But their burden is increased, since usual household tasks are more difficult such as greater distances in carrying water and fuel, and more difficulties in drawing water. Additionally, they feel burdened because of their idle husbands, and they often face an increased risk of rape or physical abuse. Among the Bhutanese refugees in Nepal, men were more likely to be tortured, but tortured women had more disorders than tortured men; non-tortured women had more disorders than non-tortured men (Van Ommeren, 2000). This is not to say that men as heads of families are not also burdened. Among Sudanese refugees in Northern Uganda and refugees in the shelters surrounding Addis Ababa, we observed that men were afflicted at least as seriously as women. These men lost a major life purpose by losing their work, whether they were white-collar workers or peasants. Their sense of worth and identity was further hurt by their loss of ability to protect and care for their families. Thus, gender plays a role in identifying specific groups who are at risk.

The surviving elderly carry a heavy burden in the transmission of cultural values. During rites of passage, for example, the elderly are not seen as having the same status they once had. Sometimes this is because restrictions are imposed on them by camp authorities, or due to high costs or the long duration of the rituals they are not able to carry out their traditional roles. In several areas the transmission of values is hindered by the loss of an important segment of society because of AIDS.

The hardship of children is compounded by their dependence on parents, which in (post-) war conditions where parents may have mental or psychosocial problems, is difficult to receive. If both parents have died or are lost, as often happened in Rwanda, for example, the children may be left entirely to fend for themselves. Children also face their own mental and physical vulnerability.

Overcrowding of camps or slums is a problem in many places. For example, an increase in the size of camps for "security reasons" in Mexico, resulted in an increase in child mortality (Farias, 1994). Crude death rates among refugees and internally displaced persons soar to levels as high as 50 times the baseline crude death rate in their home areas. Most of these deaths occur among young children. During periods of displacement, the mortality rate can be as much as 60 times the expected rates (Toole & Waldman, 1993; cf Yip & Sharpe, 1993).

In addition, children are especially at risk. Aggressive and antisocial behavior disorders are frequently associated with substance abuse, and seizure disorders are common among children in these circumstances (Westermeyer, 1989; Desjarlais et al., 1995). Developmental attrition leads to the failure of reaching normal developmental landmarks, making the cumulative defect even larger. Attrition is caused by inadequate intake of nourishment vital for body and mind such as a lack of proteins, calories, or micro-nutrients. Attrition manifests itself in three ways: (1) physically, as height and weight below norms for age; (2) in school settings, as learning failures and retarded mental development; and (3) behaviorally, as psychiatric disorder and social deviance. The disadvantages to which poor children are subjected—especially when exposed to man-made disasters—start during pregnancy. Poor nutrition and limited health care during pregnancy increases the likelihood of poor outcomes. If children born after a complicated pregnancy are reared under adverse social conditions, they tend to suffer long-term retardation in cognitive development (Desjarlais et al., 1995). These children are at higher risk of developing schizophrenia later in life. Children with pellagra have a higher risk of developing dementia in adulthood.

Children need familial support and should live in communities rather than in orphanages, resettlement camps or children villages. Since fund raising for children is relatively easy, donors feel they improve their image when they donate funds for the future of children. The wars in Mozambique, Zimbabwe, Eritrea, Rwanda, Congo, Sudan, and West Africa have led to the orphaning or dislocation of thousands of children who have witnessed the bloody conflict. One of the priorities for abandoned children is family reunion. In addition to the usual ways of family tracing by means of photographs or radio messages, alternative approaches may work. For example, for about 5 years, a group of nearly 10,000 Sudanese children had been fleeing forced circumscription by either the northern Sudanese army or one of the guerrilla movements of southern Sudan. Eventually they ended up living in camps in North Kenya. Each plot in the refugee camp had a large sign of one of the southern Sudanese cities to help children find one of their family members back. Children who did not find a family member lived under the supervision of an adult who received a modest per diem for his or her work. Fifty children living in ten huts in a circle cooked their own meals, visited schools, and had leisure activities under the supervision of their tutor while leading their life among the other refugees. Children in orphanages in Mozambique often appeared withdrawn, apathetic, regressed, and fearful. At times orphanages for girls turned into a breeding place for prostitution, whereas orphanages for boys easily resulted in banditry (cf Machel, 1996).

Children are not only easy victims of the violence, but they are also actively drawn into the violence. During the drafting of the Declaration of the Rights of the Child, several low- and high-income countries opposed that the minimal age of participating in a war be increased to 18 years. In a number of African, Latin American, and Asian countries, children are forced into military training and service. Many boys are forced to serve as porters or to serve in a (rebel) army, whereas young girls are forced to serve as housemaids or are sequentially raped as so-called partners of soldiers. This was a common fate in Mozambique, and it still is for children and adolescents in West Africa and northern Uganda if they are abducted by one of the rebel movements. Insubordination, be it refusal to follow orders or an attempt to desert, can result in summary execution.

In Mozambique, many children were forced by Renamo to kill a parent or an inhabitant of their own village to make it impossible for them to return to their home village (Geffray, 1990; Vines, 1991). Killing a family member in an ancestry culture may imply psychological suicide, because the soul of the perpetrator cannot reincarnate in the family's cycle of life and death. Hence, the perpetrator' soul is condemned to remain in the nebula between life and death facing an existence as a perpetual family outcast. The soul may even become a capricious and revengeful spirit attacking the living with misfortune.

In a variety of cultures, the psychological or geographic disruption of family ties is used as a strategy to transform children into willing tools of war. Atrocities, such as cutting off ears, noses, penises and breasts in Mozambique, or cutting off limbs in Sierra Leone, equal those committed by the Lords Resistance Army in Uganda or the Khmer Rouge regime in Cambodia. All these horrors are also suffered by children.

Violence and its Influence on Child Development and Society.
The price of violence can be high both for the developing child and the society. A striking parallel can be drawn between the effects of violence on the level of society and its effects on individual children and their development. Salimovich, Lira, and Weinstein (1992) have identified three core features of persistent fears among the Chilean population: (1) a sense of personal weakness, vulnerability, and a feeling of powerlessness; (2) sensory perceptions remaining in a permanent state of alert; and (3) the impossibility of testing subjective experience against reality. Such "cultures of fear" are not only produced by (para)militia or police forces (in Latin America, but also in the former Yugoslavia, the Caucasian republics, Western Nepal and Sri Lanka), but also by cults of violence and counterviolence (e.g. in Mozambique, Uganda, Liberia, or Sierra Leone) (Allen, 1991; Jeyaraja Tambiah, 1992; Wilson, 1992; de Jong, 2000).

During and after a war, the "culture of fear" may interact with the chronic sequential war traumas and with the daily difficulties of living in a devastated area, a refugee camp, or a repressive environment. This may lead to a continuous traumatic stress syndrome showing some similarities with the ICD-10 category of complex PTSD or enduring personality change after catastrophic experience. These individual diagnoses show a striking similarity with the above mentioned core features of the culture of fear.

It should be no surprise that the consequences of violence can work their way into the practices of everyday life, because violence in a community results in reworking of the moral sensibilities and hence influences the behavior of groups and individuals. On a community level, it is tempting to hypothesize a relation between this continuous traumatic stress and the occurrence of recurrent cycles of violence as a temporarily effect but it also has long run consequences, which is what has happened in the Middle East, Southern Africa, Algeria, Latin America and the former Soviet Union. It is also tempting to postulate that the violence in Israel and Palestine or in the South African townships, for example, is to some extent a rebound phenomenon of a rebellious younger generation no longer willing to endure the humiliations. The prevailing fear and suspicion weave their way into society and affect mutual support structures, personal commitments, belief in justice, and belief in democratization and human rights.

Trauma and its Consequences Among Children. In contrast to adults, there is a wide variety of studies in children and adolescents in (post-) conflict conditions in low-income countries. Although the general phenomenology of trauma is comparable for children and adults (Pynoos & Nader, 1993), it may take different forms and symptoms at different stages. A child's ability to cope is a function of its developmental stage, and traumatic experiences may retard or accelerate development (Pynoos et al., 1998).

Mahjoub (1995) summarized knowledge about the psychosocial consequences of wars among children and adolescents. Although he believes that the long-term effects of wars on children need additional attention he says, children, as a group, appear to suffer less from wars than adults for the following reasons: (a) children forget easier; (b) they are less concerned and too young to understand the horrors; and (c) because they have more future are able to distract them from the past. Mahjoub's also believes that a traumatic syndrome among children has not yet been well defined; gender differences have not been observed; certain age groups are less vulnerable than others (e.g., until the age of 2–3 years and during the latency period), and like adults, their stress is mediated through the environment.

One of the important mediators that has a moderating and protective effect for children is family support. The role of the family and the reactions of parents have been shown in the British studies after World War II as well as in studies in kibbutzim and among Palestinians (Punamäki, 1987; Williams, 1990). Other mediators are stage of development (Pynoos et al., 1996); personality (Giel, 1998); the coping style of the child (Punamäki & Suleiman, 1990; Shisana & Celentano, 1987); the ideological commitment of the child (Baker, 1990; Punamäki, 1996); and social support (Shisana & Celentano, 1987; Halpern, 1982).

Traumatic Stress Symptoms in Different Age Groups of Children. The following section describes symptoms seen in children related to traumatic stress. The symptoms are based on clinical impressions and on empirical research and described in accordance with different developmental stages. The reactions may be limited to a couple of days or weeks or may persist over a period of months or years.

Preschool children may show frequent or continuous crying, clinging, bedwetting, and loss of bowel control, thumb and finger sucking, frequent nightmares and night terrors, as well as unusual fear of actual or imagined objects.

Children of early school age may display similar behavior and be overtly unhappy, nervous, restless, irritable, and fearful. Self-stimulation such as rocking or head banging may be observed. In addition, refusal to eat and physical complaints with a psychosomatic basis (headache, dizziness, abdominal pain) are frequent. These children may also display behavior appropriate of much younger children, such as prolonged muteness and bed-bound incontinence or clinging behavior. They frequently show repetitive traumatic play (Terr, 1979, 1985, 1991). The small child may show generalized fears for events that resemble the original traumatic event, or for specific objects that had to do with the event, or fear of being left alone in a room (Goodwin, 1988). Children may appear withdrawn or apathetic and lack normal curiosity. It is often difficult identifying what is bothering them. Yet they often turn out to be capable to reproduce more or less reliable details of traumatic events (Eth & Pynoos, 1985A; Goodwin, 1988; Pynoos & Nader, 1988). The emotions of loss and grief, however, are often frightening and may impede the freedom to talk. The child may be fearful of its own overwhelming emotions and be afraid to disturb the parents with its own anxiety. Posttraumatic stress syndromes (PTSS), depressive disorder, separation anxiety disorder, grief reactions and secondary adversities compose an interactive matrix that strongly influences the (post-)conflict or post-disaster recovery of children and adolescents. Persistent post-traumatic stress symptoms may have a direct role in the onset and severity of secondary depression (Pynoos et al., 1998). Many of the children become victims of a continuous strain trauma. Such trauma may result in personality disorders and even have knock-on effects on descendants, even though the phenomenon of transgenerational traumatization has not been shown to exist on a group level (de Jong, 2000).

Among *school-age children* cognitive restriction and difficulties in concentration—and consequently a decline in school performance—are often mentioned (Eth & Pynoos, 1985a; Pynoos & Nader, 1988). It is assumed to be caused by the introduction of a cognitive style of forgetting and suppressing spontaneous thoughts to avoid reminders of the traumatic events. In case of a taboo or secretive character of the experiences, this effect tends to be stronger (Goodwin, 1988). Other ways of dealing with traumatic memories are denial and dissociation. Associated depressed affect may play a role in declining school performances. School-age children often present medically unexplained pain, such as headaches, stomachaches, feeling dizzy or tired (Eth & Pynoos, 1985; Goodwin, 1988). Reminders of the event may trigger pain or other somatic memories, similar to somatoform dissociation among adults, rather than triggering verbally retrievable memory. School-age children may also show aggressive behaviour, loud or wild playing, irritation and incapability of cooperation with other children; or they are extremely quiet and well-mannered and never express feelings or wishes. In an extreme form children may show symptoms of silent withdrawal or hyperactivity accompanied by violent behavior or an alternation of these two types of behaviour. School-age children may become participants, in action or in fantasy. Issues of responsibility and guilt play a more important role in this age. Sometimes children cherish plans for revenge or worry about how they might have prevented the trauma from happening (Eth & Pynoos, 1985; Goodwin, 1988). Because of a growing ability to identify with others, the school-age child may also feel concern about others and stay worried about siblings or parents (Pynoos & Nader, 1988).

Adolescent behavior. The same patterns of behaviour may also be shown by adolescents. Acting out at this age may be more dangerous because adolescents can have access to weapons. It may also express itself in skipping school, promiscuity, substance abuse, antisocial or rebellious behaviour and delinquency. Re-enactment can be life-threatening, and adolescents may show self-destructive behaviour and accident-proneness (Eth & Pynoos, 1985; Pynoos & Nader, 1988; Goodwin, 1988). Adolescents may need acting out and substance abuse to distract their mind from feelings of guilt and anxiety and painful memories. Both re-enactment and acting out are phenomena often seen in child soldiers. Adolescents have a more developed sense of responsibility: they may be very preoccupied with their own share in the events. This may lead to detachment, shame and guilt (Pynoos & Nader, 1988) and be an obstacle for the shaping of their personality. The self-consciousness about feelings and the fear of being labelled abnormal may hinder emotional processing. Since the developmental task of the adolescent is to take decisions about later life, e.g. about schooling and occupation, difficulties often arise in these domains (Pynoos & Nader, 1988; Eth & Pynoos, 1985; Goodwin, 1988). The traumatic events and the inability of emotional processing may lead to a premature entrance into adulthood and closure of identity formation (e.g. to leave school or to marry). It may be difficult for the adolescent to determine and maintain aims and direction. He or she can lean too much on role models. But some youths may also identify with the helping profession and prepare themselves for future positions in a society without war or violence (Jensen & Shaw, 1993). Table 5 summarizes studies on children under extremely difficult circumstances.

Table 5. Summary of Results of Studies on Refugee Children in (Post-)conflict Situations (a) and in the West (b)

Author	Country	Summary of results of study of refugee children in
(a) *Post conflict situations*		
Abu-Nasr (1985)	Lebanon	A study of 3- to 9-year-olds in Lebanon indicated that war was the major topic of conversation in 96% of the children, of play in 80%, and of drawing in 80%.
Thabet and Vostanis (2000)	Gaza	In a longitudinal study a dose response with respect to PTSD was found. The presence of moderate to severe PTSD at follow-up is best predicated by the total number of traumas experienced by the child at the initial assessment. The study did not look at mediating factors. PTSD decresed from 41 to 10% between 6 and 10 months after the war in the months after the Oslo Agreement.

Table 5. *Continued*

Author	Country	Summary of results of study of refugee children in
Baker (1990)	Palestine	The study explored the effect of violence on a sample of 796 Palestinian children. A total of 80% started out fighting each other, 25% exhibited destructive behavior, one third suffered headaches, and one third difficulties sleeping, 12% bit their nails, and 43% felt depressed.
Boothby et al. (1991)	Mozambique	A study of child refugees in Mozambique showed that 77% of the children had witnessed murder, 37% had witnessed family members killed, and 51% had been physically abused or tortured. A total of 64% of the children were abducted, and of these 75% were forced to serve as porters and 28% were trained for combat. 63% witnessed rape or sexual abuse, 16% admitted being raped, and 9% admitted to having killed people.
Dawes et al. (1989, 1990)	South Africa	A study of women and children who were involved in riots in South Africa. Nine % of children suffered from PTSD, especially among children whose mothers suffered from PTSD.
Dyregrov and Raundalen (1993)	Iraq	A study on the effects of the Gulf war in Iraq, found that 90% of children had lost an average of four friends.
Harrel-Bond (1986)	Uganda	The drawings of Ugandan refugee children refer to experiences of violence, death, and starvation. Drawings depict soldiers shooting their mothers, infants bleeding to death, decapitations, dogs eating human corpses, and people crouching in the forests with jutting ribs and swollen bellies. In a follow-up after 1 year, these children were still producing such drawings.
Macksoud and Aber (1996)	Greater Beirut	A study of 224 children between the age of 10 and 16 years in Greater Beirut. A total of 94% had been exposed to shelling or combat, 70% experienced bereavement, 68% displacement, 45% violent acts, 17% separation from their parents, 12% deprivation of food, water or shelter, and 5% had been injured. Twenty-two % had experienced one to three stressors, 21% seven to nine stressors, and 15% 10 to 20 stressors.
Nader and Pynoos (1993)	Kuwait	Among 51 Kuwaiti children between the age of 8–21 years, 86% knew people who had been captured, 76% people who had been injured, 65% saw injured or dead people, 59% had known a deceased person. Of the 10 possible exposures, the average child experienced five. Thirty-one per cent had severe post-traumatic reactions, 40% moderate, 29% mild, and 4% of children reported no reaction. Total exposure correlated significantly with number of PTSD-symptoms and with each of the PTSD symptom categories re-experiencing, avoidance and arousal.

Table 5. *Continued*

Author	Country	Summary of results of study of refugee children in
Paardekoper et al. (1998)	Uganda	Sudanese refugee children in North Uganda suffered significantly more from the war than the Ugandan children in the same area: 94% of the families lost their property, 81% lost a family member, 92% suffered from a lack of food or water, 62% had no medical care when illness occurred, 28% of the children had been tortured, and 25% been lost or kidnapped. Compared to the Ugandan children, the Sudanese children reported significantly more PTSD complaints such as trouble sleeping, nervousness, traumatic memories, behavioral problems, depressive symptoms, and psychosomatic complaints.
Punamäki (1989, 1996)	Palestine	The study showed that 35% of a sample of Palestinian children had symptoms of fear, 22% showed withdrawal behavior, 27% difficulties sleeping, 92% nightmares, and 80% were afraid that the Israeli army would attack their homes. She later found that strong ideological commitment in children between the age of 10 and 16 had a moderating effect on anxiety, insecurity, and depression (Punamäki 1996). The more the mother is socially embedded, politically active, and ideologically (or religiously) committed, the better her mental health and that of her children (Punamäki 1989).
Punamäki (1987)	Israel Palestine	185 Israeli and 168 Palestinian children were interviewed during the first Intifadah. 45% of the Israeli children had seen or heard an explosion, an act of terror or shelling incident. 87% of the Palestinian children had been involved in violent confrontations with soldiers or 'border guards'. 29% of the Israeli and 37% of the Palestinian children had a relative wounded. 76% of the Israeli children's fathers and 40% of the Palestinian children's fathers took part in the war and 67% of the Palestinian children had a relative in prison.
Straker et al. (1995)	South Africa	A 3-year follow-up study of 60 young people in South Africa was carried out. They wanted to find out to what extent exposure to political violence, and violent conduct within that context can become generalized in behavior in other situations. Despite their adverse backgrounds, their militancy, and their endorsement of violence as a political tool, they did not see violence as an end in itself. Only a minority saw violence as a means to further personal gain and revenge.
Qouta (2000)	Palestine	Palestinian children aged 11–12 years showed that the more traumatic experiences they had and the more they participated in the Intifada, the more concentration, attention, and memory problems they had. 25 percent of Palestinian children in Gaza had psychogenic fits (Abu Hein et al., 1993).

Table 5. *Continued*

Author	Country	Summary of results of study of refugee children in
Rosenbaum and Ronen (1992)	Israel	A study of 277 Israeli children to explore the effects of violence. A high rate of anxiety was found, especially in the evening, which was very high in the first weeks after the trauma, but started to decrease in the fifth week. Females were more anxious than males, and there were similarities between the perception of the child and that of his or her parents concerning the danger.
Solomon (1994)	Israel	The study compared Israeli children in a high-exposure area with a low-exposure area. Children from the shelled area reported more coping activities than children in a non-shelled area. Children focusing on threat reported more psychological stress than children who focused on avoidance.
Ventura (1997)	Angola	Three groups of Angolan adolescents differing in their degree of war exposure, were studied 6 months after the 1993 war. The results show that the prevalence and symptoms of PTSD were greater in the refugee group (90%), followed by the non-refugees living in Lubango (82%), and the Angolans who at the time of the study had resided for more than 1 year in Portugal (22%). There was a relationship between increased war exposure and an increase in anxiety, depression, adjustment, and behavioral problems and a decrease in intellectual functioning and self-concept.
(b) The West		
Arroyo and Eth (1985)	USA	One third of 30 Central American refugee children (17 years or less) met criteria for PTSD.
Hubbard et al. (1995)	USA	In a 15-year follow-up of 59 Cambodian young adults, a prevalence of 24% for PTSD, and a lifetime prevalence of 59% for the same disorder were found.
Kinzie et al. (1986)	USA	Among 40 Cambodian adolescents in the USA, 90% had lived in age-segregated camps in Cambodia, 83% had been separated from their family, 98% endured forced heavy labor, 68% 'looked like skeletons', 43% had oedema, 43% saw people and 18% family members killed, 68% had members of their escaping group to Thailand killed and 50% felt that even in Thailand their life was in danger. A 50% prevalence rate of PTSD and a 53% prevalence rate for depression was found, four years after they left Cambodia.
Kinzie et al. (1989)	USA	During a follow-up of 27 students from the previous study, 47% still suffered from PTSD, and 41% from depression.
Mghir et al. (1995)	USA	34% of 38 adolescent and young adult Afghan refugees in the US met criteria for major depression, PTSD, or both.

Table 5. *Continued*

Author	Country	Summary of results of study of refugee children in
Sack et al. (1993)	USA	Studying the student from the two Kinzie et al. studies six years later, among the 31 subjects 38% still met criteria for PTSD, 6% for depression, and 6% for an anxiety disorder.
Sack et al. (1994)	USA	A study of 209 Khmer adolescents in the US aged 13 to 25. Point prevalence and lifetime prevalence for PTSD was 21%, for depressive disorders 11% and 35% respectively. Over 58% of the mothers qualified for a current diagnosis of PTSD or PTSD-NOS, as did 33% of the fathers. Mothers demonstrated almost twice the depression rates of the fathers: 23 vs 14%.
Zivcic (1993)	USA	Depressive symptoms were equally elevated among Croatian children during the war and among those living in refugee circumstances. Refugee children reported more sadness and fear than local children who had not moved from their home residence.

Several conclusions can be drawn from these studies:
- Traumatic stressors among children in war circumstances vary a great deal across countries and ethnic groups. Percentages of children who witnessed killings vary from 43% in Cambodia to 77% in Mozambique. The percentage of children who were physically abused or tortured varies from 28% in N-Uganda to 51% in Mozambique. The percentage of children who were abducted or separated from their parents ranges from 17% in Lebanon to 64% in Mozambique. Bereavement ranges from 29% among Israeli children to 70% of the Libanese children. And extreme deprivation of basic needs such as food, shelter and medical care ranges from 12% of the Lebanese children to 56% of the Cambodian children. Whereas these figure are shocking, research might better benefit refugee children by trying to reach agreement on a range of stressors that should be minimally assessed to define high risk groups of children in (post-) conflict situations. Consensus on minimal requirements of research would facilitate comparison of the impact of conflicts on children and hence on minimal requirements for psychosocial and mental health programs.
- Psychological consequences also vary widely across conflict situations. Levels of PTSD range from 9% among South African children to 90% among children in Angola. Several studies show that behavioral problems are quite common. Among children who emigrated to the West, PTSD levels range from 21% to 59% among Cambodian adolescents, and depression from 41% to 53% among the same group. These studies could gain strength if researchers would agree on a minimal set of symptoms and diagnoses to further this field of study, if they would focus less on PTSD, and if they would diversify the ethnic groups that are studied among refugee children and adolescents in the West.

- Whereas in Gaza PTSD symptoms decreased from 40% to 10% over a 6–10 *month* period, among Cambodian adolescents in the USA the diagnosis of PTSD decreased from 53% to 38% over six *years*. These studies should be replicated, preferably among children in the same age range staying in their country of origin and among children with the same socio-economic background going to the West. Studies should include moderating variables explaining which factors influence resiliency or vulnerability. These factors can be used to improve preventive and curative programs. In addition, this kind of studies could help to answer the important question whether children are better off in their regions of origin or in the West. If for example 'fortress Europe' continues to close its gates, it would seem logical that funding that is now spent on asylum seekers or refugees should be invested to relief the plight of children in their regions of origin.

WHY PUBLIC MENTAL HEALTH?

Rationale for a Public Mental Health Approach of Traumatic Stress

The psychosocial and mental health consequences of (post-) conflict and (post-) disaster situations require a specialized framework for interventions. They cannot be easily handled with psychological and psychiatric approaches common to high-income countries. These approaches are often not successfully implemented because of the following reasons: First, approaches from the west require their application by highly trained professionals. Within Africa, Asia and parts of Latin America, there are only a small number of mental health professionals. Even if countries had mental health professionals, violence may have caused an exodus of intellectuals like in Algeria, or they may have been murdered as part of the genocide as happened in Cambodia or Rwanda. Secondly, health professionals in low income countries have not been trained to deal with mass traumatic stress and they often only know models of intervention that are unlikely useful in situations of massive stress. Thirdly, refugees and IDPs often belong to a different ethnic group and reside in peripheral or rural areas, which are not the preferred sites for urban intellectuals to work. For example, in Sri Lanka it is unsafe for Singhalese psychiatrists from Colombo to go to the predominant Tamil areas. However, even in the best of times few urban psychiatrists are likely to volunteer to go to remote, rural areas. Fourthly, the state mental health care sector is often weak, offering little opportunity for professional employment. The few existing professionals work in private not public practice. Fifth, many middle class urban professionals have difficulties relating to rural or refugee populations who express their plight in a specific discourse and use different explanatory models. Six, professionals have often been trained in models that are not appropriate to deal with mass traumatic stress. Siegler and Osmond (1974) presented eight mental health models: the medical, moral, invalidity, psychoanalytic, social, psychedelic, conspiracy, and family interaction models. Models implemented in a specific country are often determined by social or colonial history and often need thorough transformation to be effective in post-war circumstances. For example, the former Yugoslavia, the Caucasian republics, Cambodia, or Vietnam follow the Soviet approach with its emphasis on medical authority, hospital-based care, and the conspiracy model. This is an obstacle for efforts to establish interdisciplinary community-based interventions. Similarly, the centralized custodial hospital-based care in Portugal's former colonies Mozambique, Angola and Guinea Bissau do not provide an infrastructure for establishing mental health care services in the rural areas afflicted by the war. The French psychoanalytic model, which is *en vogue* in Algeria does not equip its mental health care professionals to do rapid outreach work in the communities suffering from the sequelae of violence and human rights violations. So even though Algeria has a few thousand psychologists and a few hundred psychiatrists, the Algerian professional community was ineffective in assisting the rural population (see chapter on Algeria).

As a result of these considerations, we argue that mental health programs have to resort to primary care and community models within a public mental health approach. In this book *public mental health* is defined as *the discipline, the practice and the systematic social actions that protect, promote and restore mental health of a population*. Since *public mental health* is part of *public health*, most public mental health concepts are derived from or overlap with public health views and policies. The Alma Ata declaration (1978) propounded a broad and consistent philosophy and strategy for the attainment of Health For All, known as the Primary Health Care (PHC) approach. The principles of Alma Ata also inspire the field of public mental health. We have further developed these principles and distinguish between policy and service delivery principles.

Guiding Principles: Policy and Service Delivery Principles

Guiding Policy Principles. In terms of policy principles, we believe that public mental health programs are most effective when they:

- are based on a public health paradigm emphasizing horizontal planning
- are culture-informed and adapted to local circumstances
- are built on culture-specific expertise and coping strategies
- emphasize implementation on the basis of local need
- encompass the social, economic, political and cultural determinants of mental illness

- use a multisectoral or intersectoral approach, that is, they recognize the multifaceted nature of the cause of mental illness and, therefore, collaborate e.g. with education, rural development and women's affairs
- aim at empowerment and emancipation
- aim at human capital by stimulating social cohesion and solidarity, and involve collaboration with the community
- stimulate health promotion and awareness of the consequences of mental and psychological problems, including traumatic stress
- aim at protection of overall human rights and those of patients with the help of adequate mental health legislation
- promote social reconstruction and reconciliation
- stimulate South-North and South-South exchange
- avoid ethnocentrism
- stimulate debate about the antecedents and consequences of violence
- destigmatize mental illness and aim at enjoyment of full citizenship for the mentally ill.

Guiding Service Delivery Principles. In terms of services delivery principles, public mental health programs are best when they:

- use a contextual, systemic and interdisciplinary approach
- try to achieve equity as a component of mental health
- are decentralized, community based and integrated in primary care
- aim at sustainability of a local program ran by local people
- are easily accessible within a natural setting
- use innovative, culturally appropriate and flexible technology
- engage in health promotion and focus on people's strength and resiliency
- include natural support systems such as rituals and healers
- strengthen local, regional and international research capacity
- are implemented using available scientific/evidence-based knowledge
- guarantee permanent availability of essential psychotropic drugs
- monitor and evaluate service delivery as an integral strategic part of ongoing project cycles.

In the following section I will clarify the philosophy behind these principles.

A CONTEXTUAL AND TEMPORAL APPROACH AND ITS IMPLICATION FOR PROGRAM DEVELOPMENT

I have operationalized the above-mentioned guiding principles along two dimensions. The first signifies context, referring to a systemic or ecological contextual approach. The second dimension signifies time. Figure 1 shows the relation between context and time.

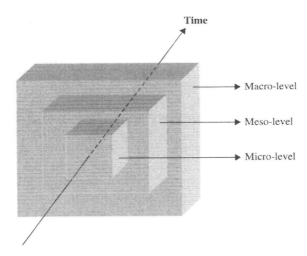

Figure 1. The dimensions of context and time. Macro-level: Society-at-large; Meso-level: Community; Micro-level: Family/Individual.

In this chapter I distinguish three levels of society (cf Bronfenbrenner, 1979). The *macro-level* is the society-at-large and the culture in which people live. The *meso-level* is the community. The *micro-level* is the level of the individual and the family.

The Interaction Between the Community-at-Large (macro-), the Community (meso-) and the Individual and Family (micro-level)

All human beings interact constantly with their environment. When violence such as war or ethnic cleansing is rampant on the level of the society-at-large, all families and individuals are afflicted. Similarly, violence even at the micro-level against or between individuals, for example in low intensity warfare, or in child abuse or domestic violence, is also or can be transposed to the meso-level of the community. Even in the case of violence on individuals, violence is rarely just a concern of individual victims. It too reaches families and communities, and occasionally almost everyone in society. In other words, the different levels of society are interwoven and linked to each other so that violence rarely, if ever, occupies only one niche. Before discussing each level, I want to point out the importance of the interconnections of all levels.

Interventions differ according to the level they try to influence although they may straddle two levels. Some interventions are appropriate on one level but unrealistic or adverse at another. This has led us to formulate the following guiding principle:

> Guiding principle 1: Public mental health programs should use a contextual approach, linking individuals, families, communities and society-at-large. Trauma needs to be conceptualized in terms of an interaction between these different levels, and not as an entity to be located and addressed within the individual or group psychology of those affected. Interventions that address one of these levels while taking account of its effect on other levels are optimal.

In the context of (post-) conflict, public mental health programs are determined by a range of political, social and cultural variables. To study these variables, it is important to employ a cross-level and cross-cultural methodology covering the range from the macro-level to micro-level.

Communities and societies have traditionally been studied by political scientists, economists, anthropologists, social psychologists, sociologists, historians or juridical experts. While individuals and families have been studied by psychologists, medical doctors, and epidemiologists. Since the distinction between the levels is abstract, and since the levels influence each other, it is imperative to address all levels at the same time. Thus the following principle:

> Guiding principle 2: For the implementation of mental health services and research into psychosocial and mental health programs it is essential to work across disciplines such as public mental health, psychology, psychiatry, anthropology, and epidemiology.

The Macro-Level or Society-at-Large

The macro-level or the level of society-at-large refers both to global political, economic and sociocultural processes as to the habitat of the people. Troubled political and economic processes create and maintain conflicts around the globe. These developments are often accompanied by ethnic and religious conflicts. Conflicts add to insecurity, oppression, dehumanization, ethnic cleansing and other human rights violations which can lead to "complex emergencies". Hence the following principle, which is in line with the *Global Action to Prevent War* (Institute for Defense and Disarmament Studies, 1999):

> Guiding principle 3: Prevention of trauma needs to aim at global action to prevent war. This entails a long-term complex set of measures, including (a) expanding global and regional security institutions, (b) strengthening non-violent means of preventing and ending armed conflict, and (c) clarifying the military's role of last resort for preventing and ending armed conflict.

The Meso-Level or the Community

At the community level, we find (1) the socio-political and economic context, and (2) cultural and biological adaptations *of the group* (Berry, Poortinga, Segall, & Dasen, 1992). Thus the community level includes religious and political institutions and movements; settlements of refugees and internally displaced people, settlements of local indigenous populations, and neighborhoods, slums, and ethnic subgroups. Relevant aspects within communities are the structure of family relationships; child-rearing practices; occupational training, education, and community health care. Hence the following principle:

> Guiding principle 4: Interventions should encompass the social, economic, political, biological and cultural determinants of mental illness.

Public health recognizes that individuals are embedded in their family, community and society (Green, 1992). This has important implications for the way interventions are planned at this level. One individual's lifestyle has repercussions on the community, whereas poverty, discrimination and threats to safety—all products of society—reduce the quality of life and the health of individuals and families.

Early public health efforts stimulated community development initiatives at the village level and tried to facilitate empowerment of communities and to provide means for their active participation in the process of development. The term *Health by the people* (Newell, 1975), reflected the idea that improvements in health required the involvement of communities as active partners rather than as passive recipients.

This line of thinking paralleled developments in community psychology, which also constructed its interventions in terms of empowerment (Rappaport, 1981; Hobfoll, 1998). Community psychology focused on simultaneously enhancing people's competencies and changing social systems to help people utilize these competencies in a productive fashion meaningful to their lives. This approach underscored the need to make necessary resources available and encouraged development along culturally appropriate lines.

To a large extent the thrust of mental health efforts in low-income countries has focused on the incorporation of a mental health component into Primary Health Care (WHO, 1990; de Jong, 1996b). Yet, the majority of people suffering from mental disorders do not seek care from health services. Only a small proportion reach primary services and even fewer find their way to secondary and tertiary levels of care (Goldberg & Huxley, 1992). More important in situations of massive stress is the virtual absence of mental health services. Therefore, intervening both at the community and at the primary care level is vital so that the majority of people with mental health problems can be targeted.

These considerations and TPO's field experience convinced us of the necessity to decentralize our interventions which was best accomplished by working at the meso-level to empower the community and family. As will be shown further on, the identification of problems is done in conjunction with communities and subsequent interventions are developed by mobilizing the community and its resources.

While in the initial stage we are typically asked for our professional expertise, we challenge expert-client models by promoting partnership, which in our view is the only way to achieve sustainability of our programs. Hence, the following principle:

> Guiding principle 5: Sustainability and equity can be realized by decentralizing mental health services to the community level. Empowerment involves the mobilization of local resources utilized in the natural setting of the community.

Much of people's cognitive and behavior repertoire is nurtured and mediated by community structures. Such behavior includes habits, skills, assumptions, and attitudes. For example, healing skills such as mourning, reconciliation or cleansing rituals are associated with community structures. This leads to the following principle:

> Guiding principle 6: Interventions benefit from including indigenous community structures such as the natural support systems of healers, and mourning, healing, cleansing and reconciliation rituals and ceremonies.

From a public mental health perspective both preventive and curative interventions have to focus on individuals and families nested in community structures. In our view individual psychosocial and mental health interventions need to be linked to initiatives on the community-level and the community-at-large. Two examples may illustrate this. Psychological issues must be balanced and linked to vital development priorities, such as water, food and shelter. Public mental health programs need to collaborate with rural development initiatives helping refugees and local populations to enhance their survival capacities and helping them increase their quality of life (see further on). A second example of linking up a psychosocial approach with other initiatives on the community-level is vocational training for adults and adolescents. For example, such training is important for demobilized soldiers, returning to the rural areas and lacking the expertise to function within the agricultural sector. Learning a way of living without a gun is essential to prevent an upsurge of war activities in countries such as Angola, Congo, Liberia, Sierra Leone, Sri Lanka or Uganda.

One can also argue that psychosocial programs *per se* influence the community positively by helping people to choose new ways of living including becoming economically active. The chapters on Cambodia and Uganda show that Cambodian widows and Ugandan ex-rebels found relief in (self-) help groups. When they felt that they had resolved enough of their psychological plight in their group, they set up economic activities.

What Fukuyama (1999) and other sociologists call social capital—the series of norms and values shared by all members of a group that enable people to cooperate, and to create order and security—is often disrupted or destroyed in post-conflict areas. One of the aims of our programs is to contribute to the restoration of social capital. It requires a multi-faceted approach to strengthen cohesion by aiming at various sectors of the community. Hence, the following principle:

> Guiding principle 7: To address vital priorities of affected populations and to restore social capital, several community structures have to be engaged in a multisectoral approach including the sectors of health, education, rural development, jurisdiction and gender-related organizations.

The Micro-level or Individuals and Families

The micro-level comprises the level of families and individuals. The micro-level is not only an important locus of suffering but also the focus of most psychosocial and mental health interventions. The following subsection describes TPO's theoretical model linking the micro-level to context and culture (Figure 2).

A Theoretical View of the Model

This theoretical model consists of a sequential and dynamic process that starts with the exposure to traumatic events and ends with the consequences that are directly and indirectly related to these events. The sequential mode of the model refers to the time perspective. The dynamic mode refers to the above-mentioned interaction between different contexts defined on the micro, meso and macro levels. In the following section I will walk through the different components of the model.

Stress and Traumatic Stress. In contrast to common stress models (Selye, 1956; Dunkel-Schetter & Bennett, 1990), Lazarus and Folkman (1984) argued that a definition of stress should not be restricted to objective environmental events because this approach would not explain why the same environmental event was stressful for one person but not for another. Characteristics of both the individual and the situation, in a dynamic interaction, were incorporated in the definition of stress. The problem is that in (post-) conflict and (post-) disaster conditions, however, Lazarus and Folkman are of little help. They were not interested in major stressors, because "extreme conditions result in stress for nearly everyone, and their use as a model produces inadequate theory and applications".

Hobfoll's theory (1998) on Conservation of Resources (COR) is based on the tenet that individuals strive to obtain, retain and protect the things they value. By emphasizing the resources that individuals retain COR theory has the advantage of highlighting observable events and circumstances, rather than perceptions of events. In situations of massive destruction the COR theory has the advantage of a model that helps to objectify the loss of resources.

The work of *traumatic stress* evolved quite independently from the above theories of stress and coping (Shalev, 1996). In fact there has been little interaction between the two fields of study. According to the stress literature, stress becomes

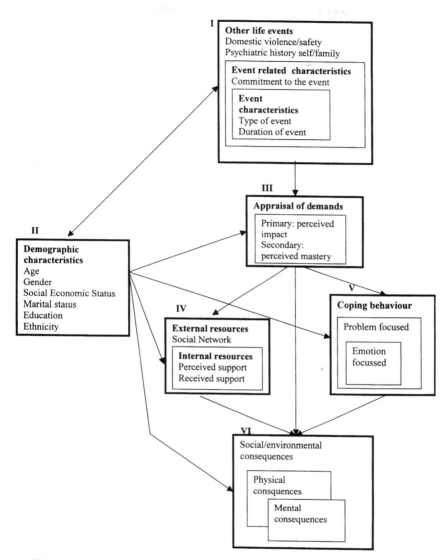

Figure 2. TPO's model for an interdisciplinary contextual approach to traumatic stress.

traumatic when psychological damage analogous to physical damage occurs. For example, damage to the histological structure of the nervous system leads to a breach in the shield against stimuli (Freud, 1920), or to the "self" (Laufer, 1988), or to one's cognitive assumptions (Krystal, 1978), to neuronal mechanisms governing habituation and learning (Kolb & Multipassi, 1982), or to one's memory network (Pitman, 1988), or finally to disrupting emotional learning pathways

(Ledoux, Romanski, & Xagoraris, 1989). In neurobiological terms traumatic stress may be explained as a hyper(re)activity of the amygdala which is not only the key structure involved in conditioning and responsiveness to fear but also in strengthening the level of arousal of emotional memory (Pitman, 2000). One problem with this is that the use of the term "stress" for both acute and chronic responses is problematic. Neuro-endocrinological studies show reduced cortisol levels in chronic reactions to stress like PTSD, while during acute stress there are elevated levels of cortisol. Thus supporting the distinction between acute stress and prolonged states of posttraumatic morbidity.

Stress research and the traumatic stress literature also differ in a number of methodological research dimensions. Most of the research on traumatic stress has focused on evaluating the relationship between trauma and subsequent disorders, thereby evaluating the traumatogenic nature of events rather than their stressfulness. The traumatic stress literature—in contrast to the stress literature—is mostly naturalistic, retrospective and observational.

Several authors conclude that PTSD can best be conceived as a chronic biopsychosocial disturbance (Van der Kolk, 1996), while Shalev (1996) argues that this biopsychosocial complex may not exist in stress-induced disorders. A biopsychosocial model explains:

- The permanent alteration of neurobiological processes, resulting in hyperarousal and excessive stimulus discrimination (Shalev, 1996).
- Psychological phenomena such as "freezing of affect" and subsequent loss of affective modulation (Krystal, 1978).
- Peritraumatic responses including (1) observable behaviors or symptoms (e.g. conversion, agitation, stupor); (2) emotional or cognitive experiences (e.g. anxiety, panic, numbing, confusion); or (3) mental processes or functions (e.g. defenses) (Marmar, Weiss, Schlenger, Fairbank, Jordan, Kulka, & Hough, 1994; Van der Kolk, McFarlane, & Weisaeth, 1996).
- The acquisition of fear responses to trauma-related stimuli.
- The change of cognitive schemata and the alteration of the three core assumptions of human beings that the world is a safe place, is meaningful and that the self is worthy (Janoff-Bulman, 1992).

PTSD symptoms can occur after a variety of stressors, so any *a priori* definition of specific characteristics of stressors that cause PTSD appears invalid (Breslau & Davis, 1987). This point of view is reflected in the DSM IV (APA 1994) definition of a traumatic event. It consists of two parts. Firstly, the situation is defined as one that involved actual or threat to death, serious injury, or a threat to he physical integrity of self or others; and secondly, the person's response involves intense fear, helplessness, or horror.

Another controversy concerns the impact of trauma of new life stressors that might activate stress reactions related to old trauma. Several studies (e.g. Solomon, Mikulincer, & Arad, 1991) mention a complicated pattern, in which symptoms of PTSD reinforce the coincidence of life stressors, especially in the social domain. This is relevant for our work, since after leaving a conflict zone, survivors are often exposed to a variety of daily hassles. This, for example, is typical in refugee camps.

We consider all the aspects of the situation, in addition to the characteristics and reactions of the individual useful in understanding traumatic events. The first block part of Figure 2—indicated with Roman cipher I—mentions the concepts of event characteristics, event related characteristics, and other traumatic life events. The aforementioned considerations have elicited the following guiding principle:

> Guiding principle 8: Public mental health programming needs to combine the traumatic stress approach—with its interest in epidemiology to describe the process of trauma and it's consequences—with a stress oriented approach to understand the relationships between trauma and its consequences.

Other Life Events. Examples are: (a) domestic violence (b) psychiatric status before the trauma, and (c) pre-trauma experiences. *Unrelated previous life events* influence an individuals' ability to cope with traumatic stressors. In some cases these provide the individual with tools to overcome previously experienced trauma and its consequences, and thus provide the individual with protective tools for future trauma. In other cases they may have harmed the individual and reduced or immobilized the person's basic potential to overcome trauma.

Traumatic Event-related Characteristics. Traumatic event related characteristics are factors that mediate and moderate the consequences of the experienced trauma. Two common examples include: (a) a person's commitment to activities or aspirations related to the event (e.g. political or religious commitment) and (b) migration.

Event Characteristics. Examples of event characteristics are (a) duration of event (e.g. one single traumatic event, multiple traumatic events, or chronic repetitive stress (cf Terr, 1991) (b) type of event. The magnitude and the intensity of the event, the dangerousness of the war or a rape incident, the intensity of a torture experience or the extent of physical injury contributes significantly to the development of PTSD (Van der Kolk et al., 1996).

Demographic Characteristics. The second block in the figure—indicated with Roman cipher II—refers to characteristics that define the uniqueness of the individual in his/her environment. These characteristics may play a role in the manifestation of symptoms after the traumatic event (Kessler et al., 1995). Examples are: (a) age (b) gender (c) social economic status (d) education (e) preparedness (f) religion and (g) ethnicity.

Appraisal. Appraisal—indicated with Roman cipher III—refers to the idea that the individual's experience of the traumatic stress can be perceived as positive, negative or overwhelming (cf Tedeschi et al., 1998).

The perceptual process can be broken down into two phases. The first is the primary appraisal which is defined as the individual's evaluation of the impact of the event in terms of harm and loss, threat or challenge. The secondary appraisal is defined as the individual's judgment whether or not the impact of the event can be mastered with the available individual resources (Lazarus & Launier, 1978; Folkman & Lazarus, 1980; Folkman, 1984).

Resources. One of the most important mediators for individuals and families faced with trauma—indicated with cipher IV in Figure 2—is social support (Dohrenwend, 1998). Social support is defined as an exchange of resources between at least two individuals that is intended to enhance the well-being or life circumstances of the recipient. To understand the effects of social support, it is important to distinguish between different modalities of support (i.e. perceived vs. received support; Cutrona & Russell, 1987); between different types of support (i.e., emotional support, esteem support, informational support and instrumental support (House, 1981); between different support sources (e.g., spouse, children, friends, (Tardy, 1985); and between different types of resources (Hobfoll, 1998). In our model we distinguish external resources (including social networks) and internal resources that consist of both perceived and received social support.

Coping Behavior. Coping behavior—indicated with cipher V—refers to the person's efforts to manage specific external and/or internal demands which are appraised as taxing or exceeding the available resources of the individual (Lazarus & Folkman, 1984). Coping can be problem-focused and emotion-focused (Thoits, 1986). Problem-focused coping refers to coping strategies to reduce the problem or change the situation. Emotion-focused coping are attempts to alter the impact of the event or emotions evoked by the event.

Consequences. We distinguish (a) social and environmental (b) physical and (c) mental health consequences, indicated with cipher VI. People not only suffer from stress, symptoms and disorders, but they are also confronted with disability.

Cultural Considerations Regarding the Model

The following section shows how the different components of the model are influenced by cultural aspects. Culture molds the relationship between events, moderators and outcomes. Obeyesekere (1985) wrote that "the work of culture is the process whereby painful motives and affects are transformed into publicly accepted sets of meaning and symbols". Each refugee, internally displaced person (IDP) or immigrant has to relate to and find an identity within the new environment. In the words of Tseng and Strelzer (1977): "as a result of enculturation, every individual learns a language, a religion, or other meaning system, specifying how the forces of nature operate in the world, as well as norms of behavior, and patterns of experiencing the environment". Examples of the importance of culture will be given by following the previous model with a cultural lense.

Events. We know little about the cultural influences on the measurement of traumatic events. We do not know if culture influences recall of traumatic events, and if so, in which way. Green (1993) has suggested eight generic dimensions of trauma: (1) threat to life and limb; (2) severe physical harm or injury; (3) receipt of intentional injury/harm; (4) exposure to the grotesque; (5) violent/sudden loss of a loved one; (6) witnessing or learning of violence to a loved one; (7) learning of exposure to a noxious agent; (8) causing death or severe harm to another. Some of these dimensions (e.g., 1–3) can be regarded as universal stressors in all cultures, but others are perceived differently in specific cultures.

In Uganda we found that group rape of abducted women can be dealt with by a collective purification ritual under the aegis of the elderly, whereas in Algeria, Cambodia, Nepal, or Namibia the shame caused by rape can lead to suicide or marginalization of the victim. Surprisingly, even in the latter cultures we found that most women were willing to talk about rape in an interview situation, and it appeared that the reluctance of the interviewers to discuss rape was sometimes greater than the reluctance of the survivors to discuss it.

Violence in the family is a possible consequence of continuous traumatic stress in many cultures. In some cultures—for example in Latin America and South East Asia—attitudes tend to be lenient toward wife battering, whereas in other cultures it is found to be unacceptable (cf Finkler, 1999).

In Buddhist and African cultures with a belief in reincarnation, the loss of a family member (dimension 5 and 6 according to Green) may have a different impact. The loss of an older loved person with children and some accumulated wealth can be acceptable in African animist cultures, since the person will travel to the reign of the ancestors and occupy an intermediary position between the living and the dead (de Jong & Van Schaik, 1994; Bagilishya, 2000). On the other hand, the death of a child in the same culture is a disaster (even though some Westerners think that parents suffer less in cultures with high exposure to child mortality). Similarly, political conviction may be an important factor in grief or mourning as has been described in Gaza (see chapter on Gaza; Qouta, 2000). Albanian Kosovar families who lost a family member in the war in 1999 regard their deceased family members as martyrs. This view may on the one hand alleviate their loss while on the other hand complicate the mourning process. The members of the international forensic exhumation and identification teams in Kosovo may be exposed to more corpses in a day than others would see in their whole life. Will their motivation to contribute to the just cause of bringing war criminals to the International Court outweigh their disgust of decayed bodies and the confrontation with cruelties? A child soldier who is a perpetrator (dimension 8) may be regarded as a hero in certain countries. Even exposure to the grotesque can be mediated by religious convictions such as the role of karma in Buddhism in Asia or divine persecution during the Holocaust (Abramson, 2000).

These culturally influenced subjective components are important in determining subsequent distress and psychopathology. Therefore, the assessment of the severity of traumatic exposure is a complex issue necessitating collaboration with cultural informants and social scientists.

Appraisal. We also know little about the ways people appraise property loss versus personal loss in different cultural settings. One can imagine that detachment, which is as an ultimate goal in Buddhism, decreases the impact of property loss. On the other hand, one may question whether detachment is the focus of concern of poor Tibetans or Cambodians struggling with survival? From our clinical experience it seems that relatively rich people who lose everything have more difficulty copying than those whose losses are smaller.

Resources. Cultural factors mediate the person's ability to utilize resources when trying to cope with a disaster. In the west, autonomy and individualization are important values which in other cultures may be perceived as selfish. The value of autonomy among many westerners is different from the dependency and interdependency in much of the developing world. But the interdependency and social support are challenged for example when a culture prescribes costly *rites de passage* that family members no longer can afford. Some cultures allow for creative solutions, but others require saving the meager resources until the ritual can be performed properly. People fear that the ghosts of the deceased may seek revenge if the mourning rituals have not been carried out in the proper way. This fear may lead to experiences of possession. If dowries cannot be paid, premarital sex, teenage pregnancies, and prostitution may become more common. Refugees often have to compete with local populations for resources like land and food, which were scarce even before the conflict started.

A social network may function as a protective factor when a family has an average size. But if many adults die due to war or AIDS, a large extended family may turn into a vulnerability factor. When I worked as a psychiatrist in West Africa, male clients were often struggling with the choice where to draw the boundaries of their responsibilities. If they chose to care for their nuclear family, the extended family would be angry and seek revenge through gossip, witchcraft or sorcery. If they chose to care for their extended family, their house would be inundated with family members requesting food or fees for education. As a result, their wives regarded themselves as the slaves of his extended family. Despite these controversies, families are often the main source of social capital and the main provider of mental health care for refugees and poor rural populations. Srinivasa Murthy (1998) mentions that the family is often been seen as a substitute for professional care, rather than as an essential component of mental support. Mental health programs in low-income countries would benefit from implementing ways that strengthen the positive aspects of rural life. Efforts have been made to understand the needs of families, to provide them with support and training skills, to help organize family groups, and to help families in networking. To prevent families from discarding their ill relatives, these needs must be addressed in a planned manner (Srinivasa Murthy, 1998). Hence, the following guiding principles:

> Guiding principle 9: In cultures where the extended family plays an important role, public mental health programs need to try to incorporate the extended family in its interventions and keep children within their family context. Interventions should preferably take place in the vicinity of the recipients' home.

Coping Behavior. In our model we distinguish problem-focused and emotion-focused coping. These too are influenced by culture. Cultures have developed coping strategies to deal with traumatic stress or mental illness. Once indigenous coping strategies and resources are identified and understood, they can be fostered and encouraged as a form of prevention or intervention. Our programs try to emphasize processes of salutogenesis, i.e. looking at resiliency and factors maintaining people's health. We try to strengthen these health promoting factors and useful coping styles. We also try to find a balance between a palliative and a curative approach, even though we realize the relativity of the concept of cure for people who have tremendously lost.

> Guiding principle 10: Interventions should be culturally appropriate and adapted to local circumstances. Interventions should be built on culture-specific expertise and coping strategies and focus on people's strength and resiliency.

Grief provides an example of the influence of culture on coping. Coping with grief is one of the essential tasks of survivors in (post-) disaster and (post-) conflict situations. There are several dimensions distinguishing cultures regarding grief and bereavement. In contrast to low-income countries, high-income countries use concepts such as counseling during the process of dying, grief, or terminal care. In low-income countries, people's attention is especially focused on various supernatural beliefs. These beliefs vary across cultures and include (a) that the dead communicate with the living, (b) that other people's supernatural abilities (e.g., witchcraft or sorcery) may cause death, (c) that the ghost of the deceased will take revenge if one does not complete proper rituals for the deceased, (d) that verbalizing the name of the deceased is dangerous, (e) that a newborn is a reincarnation of a deceased person, (f) that hearing or seeing the deceased person is normal, and (g) that tie breaking customs are useful to cope with loss (Rosenblatt, Walsh, & Jackson, 1976; Thomas, 1982; Goody, 1962; Irish, Lundquist, & Nelsen, 1993; de Jong & van Schaik, 1994; Parkes, Laungani, & Young, 1997). Thus in these cultures problems are expressed less in a psychological way and more as an interaction between the supernatural including the ancestors and the living.

Anger towards the deceased is another important difference in grief between African and Euro-American cultures. The common Christian habit is to encourage saying 'nothing but good about the dead' and this may hinder the expression of negative feelings towards the person who somehow left the living behind. As Wortmann and Silver (1989) have argued, in the West people often react in ways that are not comforting when people try to talk about feelings of loss. The bereaved person's social network frequently employs strategies to get the bereaved to inhibit displays of distress. These include discouraging of feelings ("tears won't bring him back"); minimizing the loss ("you had many good years together"); encouraging the bereaved person to recover more quickly ("you should get out and do more"); portraying their own past experiences as being similar to that the bereaved has experienced ("I know how you feel. I lost my second cousin"); and offering advice ("you should consider getting a dog. They're wonderful companions"). Very often the bereaved do not find any of these types of responses helpful.

In the African culture the expression of anger is often permitted in a ritual context. For example, on several occasions I witnessed funeral rites allowing the family to ridicule the dead in a kind of *comedia del arte* expressing avarice, laziness or stuttering. Another example is the wife of a deceased Afro-Caribbean head of a upper class family asking her children "to put four mud cunts in his coffin" so that he could enjoy adultery in afterlife as he sometimes did alive.

Unlike these cultures, in the West verbal expressions of distress are surrounded with ambivalence. According to several authors the disclosure of the 'conspiracy of silence' only took place in the seventies (Flanzbaum, 1999). Yet, western experts sometimes project a stereotypical opinion by stating that non-westerners do not want to discuss the past, and that the supposed willingness or 'working through' of westerners is a typical product of our western Judaic-Christian tradition of confession and catharsis (Tricket, 1995; Summerfield, 2000).

This stereotype is often supported by another stereotype, which is that non-westerners somatize rather then psychologize their distress, even though there is a substantial body of evidence supporting the view that somatizing is the rule rather than the exception around the globe (e.g. Üstün & Sartorius, 1995). In this case cultural consistency, rather than cultural differences, leads to misunderstanding.

The above two stereotypes may have added to a third one: the notion that it is impossible to do anything substantial or meaningful regarding massive traumatic stress. This erronous view had resulted in an avoidance of the issue of psychological suffering and of its economic consequences, which in turn has led to a 'conspiracy of silence'. So it seems that ideas such as 'it is good to forget the past' and 'time heals wounds' can be described as 'favorite' coping strategies in many areas around the world. On the one hand refugees may say that they never (want to) talk about their past and that their whole life is directed towards the future. On the other hand they often discuss their past with their fellow refugees. In our experience, people feel relieved after verbally expressing their distress of the past. Obviously, there are differences across cultures. For example, discussions with Africans from various socio-economic backgrounds show clearly that the issues of individual and collective grief and bereavement are perceived as much more important—both in terms of personal and economic consequences—in Africa than in the West. These differences are related to religion, the belief in ancestors—even after the advent of Christianity or Islam—and a variety of factors that are illustrated in several chapters of this book.

In addition to narration, the body mediates in perceiving and expressing grief and suffering. Time and again we realize the extent to which culture specific notions of anatomy and physiology interact with aetiologic factors causing misfortune or illness. For example, when the Cambodian team had to arrange a blood transfusion, it found out that nobody including the family was willing to give blood. It appeared that in Khmer culture everybody is gifted from birth onwards with a fixed amount of blood that is located in the upper part of the skull. Tapping blood means that the level of blood in the head decreases, but the blood that is given to another, cannot be substituted later in life. From a phenomenological perspective, Merlau Ponty describes the relation between body and culture as follows: "the body is the medium through which people experience their cultural world; bodily experience reflects the culture in which it occurs" (Becker, Beyene, & Ken, 2000). Kleinman (1988) adds an interactional component when he says that suffering is experienced within "the nested context of embodiment: collective, intersubjective, individual. Embodiment means that the body is seen as the threshold through which the subject's lived experience of the world is incorporated and realized." Translating these abstract words to the reality of psychosocial care implies that each aspect of our work is imbued with physical aspects. It ranges from diagnosing tropical and other disorders, synthesizing divergent explanatory models, clarifying the interaction between magic and supernatural causative factors and the body, and using the body as an important vehicle for healing, both for the people asking and providing support. When I ask our collaborators in Africa how they deal with the permanent flux of people and problems pressing on their shoulders, one important answer is invariably that dancing is their favorite way of keeping in balance.

To conclude, it seems that we are only at the initial stage of understanding differences and similarities across cultures. Apparently there exists a universal ambiguity in dealing with a traumatic past. Buddhist Asians may attribute their plight to kharma but simultaneously approach the ancestors and pre-Buddhist spirits to improve their fate (see the chapters on Cambodia, Sri Lanka and the Tibetans). People are also ambivalent about what they bring forward in their daily discourse and what they actually do or appreciate when it comes to coping with traumatic stress. The voices of the people in this book may say that they do not want to embarrass their fellow-survivors with their haunting past and yet find enormous relief when they can share their memories with others. Whether it happens in a self-help group, in an individual or family session, or during a ritual.

Getting beyond the surface will enable us to find out what are appropriate coping strategies satisfying universal human necessities while taking into account the specific sociocultural context. As mentioned before, building interventions on locally available coping strategies is an important guiding principle.

Consequences. The last part of the model explains the importance of culture in understanding the social, environmental, physical and mental health consequences to trauma. The lack of understanding the sociocultural context has been criticized both by clinicians and by culturally informed epidemiologists. Some aspects of this criticism can be summarized as follows.

1. Western psycho-diagnostic categories as defined in DSM-IV or ICD-10 often are not appropriate in non-western cultures. They may reify a western culturally constructed concept and use it in cross-cultural research procedures, a procedure called the "category fallacy" (Kleinman, 1977; Kleinman & Good, 1985). That is, one first defines the western category, then starts looking for that category in a non-western culture, and subsequently finds what was defined earlier leading to a *quod erat demonstrandum* ("that what had to be proven"). However, if one would carefully listen to people's phenomenological story, (also known as narrative, psychobiography or thick description), the reported complaints may not match the western category. For example, in most studies on PTSD—including one of our own (Shrestha et al., 1998)—investigators first define PTSD along DSM-criteria and then search for that 'disorder'. Even though most scholars find PTSD around the globe, the conclusion that PTSD is similar in all cultures is false, since the studies did not look for differences that might have yielded so far unknown (sub)types or variations of the disorder. For that reason, we cannot rule out the possibility that PTSD as an *a priori* culture-bound construct. I prefer the term (post-)traumatic stress syndromes [(P)TSS]. A similar reasoning may be applied to most psychiatric disorders.

2. Even if one agrees that most of the western categories do apply in low-income countries, there may still be considerable differences in the way people perceive or express their plight or illness. For example, stress and depression are often described as "thinking too much" in low-income countries. The expression of feelings of guilt and shame may vary from one culture to another. A person may have a number of physical sensations such as heat, cold, prickling sensations in some parts of the body, pulsating experiences, discomfort of the heart, creeping sensations under the skin, described in the literature (de Jong, 2001b). Or alternatively, the distress can be expressed in a variety of dissociative patterns, which even the local culture may find difficult to assess as normal or deviant (for example when people display a so-called 'hysterical state' or a possession trance).

These behaviors can be seen as typical templates that the culture gives to its members to express their plight.

3. The same holds for the way people express complaints or emotions in their language. The local language or *lingua franca* may use a number of expressions, metaphors, proverbs, or emotion words to express a complaint or an emotion that is quite different from western jargon. Therefore, one has to carefully make an inventory of the expression of distress in other cultures (the 'idioms of distress') before one can conclude that the way people perceive their problem is the same as the DSM/ICD categories. The chapter on Cambodia shows the arduous work to produce a culture-specific glossary of local expressions for stress as well as psychosocial and mental problems. If these challenges are not met, various diagnostic errors may occur. Either a clinician may miss the PTSD diagnosis because associated features are most prominent, or the associated features may be overlooked because of the presence of PTSD.

4. Blank (1994) has written a useful guide for the clinician evaluating post-traumatic responses, in which he repeatedly emphasizes the variety of reactions to trauma. He says that when assessing the plight of a refugee, one has to take into account that the reactions to trauma are often intertwined with the cultural transitions they are confronted with, along with acculturative stress, culture shock and cultural bereavement. This elicits questions regarding etiology and whether one is dealing with traumatic stress, the effects of daily hassles or a combination of coping style and acculturation. One may hypothesize that a comorbid disorder such as depression improves when life circumstances become stable and people are less confronted with adverse life events, but that the stronger neuro-biological component of PTSS may persist longer. This pattern of results was observed in our diagnostic studies among Bhutanese refugees in Nepal (Van Ommeren, 2000) and among Cambodian refugees in the United States (Sack et al., 1993).

5. A diagnostic or research instrument developed in one culture has to be tested before being applied in another culture. This helps to understand the concepts underlying the items of the instrument, testing them for their content, semantic, concept, and technical validity. This will show if a concept that may be relevant in one culture has significance in another culture. How to properly adapt instruments has been described elsewhere (de Jong, 1996; Van Ommeren et al., 1999).

6. Future epidemiological studies will probably not reveal that western diagnostic constructs are culture-bound. This might be because the algorithms, the exclusionary and the skip rules of the major diagnostic instruments such as the DIS and the CIDI, are such that dimensional analyses are impossible. In other words, western classificatory systems are limited because their decision rules to produce diagnoses are bound by the 'category fallacy'. In addition, current epidemiological techniques will not help us to solve the problem of

co-morbidity, which to a large extent is caused by the poor validity of Western diagnostic categories.

To conclude, one of the challenges of the next decades is a worldwide inventory of traumatic stress reactions. We expect that this will yield a neurobiological and universal core at the biological end of a continuum with a large variety of cultural induced phenomena at the sociological end of the continuum. These considerations lead to the following principle.

> Guiding principle 11: the best way to understand the expression of stress response syndromes is the use of a phenomenological approach employing a combination of qualitative and quantitative research methods within the sociocultural context.

Time in Relation to Traumatization and Healing

Figure 1 showed the relation between context and time. In the previous pages I explained the contextual, systemic and ecological dimensions of our work. This paragraph will discuss the dimension of time. Change over time is important both in relation to traumatization and healing as well as in the organization of services.

Time and traumatisation. The long-term sequelae of war traumas have been underestimated. Thirty to 45 years after a war, a large proportion of veterans were still suffering from PTSD and were at an increased mortality risk from tuberculosis, accidents, or coronary heart disease. Traumatized individuals have been found to be considerably more likely than others to have a high number of persistent physical problems and to account for a large consumption of health care services. Time per se does not necessarily heal wounds for a considerable amount of people.

We know little about the time aspects of other traumatic stress syndromes, both with regard to the latency time to manifestation of PTSS, and with regard to its course, both treated and untreated. However, in TPO's Multi-site Impact of Man-made disaster Study, we find the highest prevalence figures of depression and PTSD in Algeria, where the violence continues until today. We also see that in the course of time, traumatic stress manfestations are often overshadowed by a range of psychosocial issues and daily hassles as described in the different chapters. At the same time, we know little about the interaction of these hassles that are part of the daily plight of refugees with traumatic stress and with the host community. And whereas much research in the West is based on subjects who underwent one traumatic event, most survivors of armed conflicts went through an average of eight to fourteen horrific events. This process of sequential traumatisation confounds the previous questions about latency time and the course of (un)treated traumatic stress.

Another confounding time factor is the protracted course of conflicts with tides of warfare and peace that lead to complex emergencies. Although we hope that conflicts may fade out and refugees go home, the history of Afghanistan, the Middle East, or the Great Lakes Region in Africa teach us otherwise. Each civil war and human rights violation creates new waves of refugees who have to acculturalize across time. These are all time-related elements that are important for the organisation of services.

Time and the organisation of mental health services. International agencies, donors and organizations (including TPO) are seduced by the idea that there is a linear time-limited process leading from trauma to healing. Supposedly, the long-term outcome of a program can be determined by the original design. This approach often turns out to be unrealistic, especially with a view to the major changes that may occur among the target population. This attitude becomes manifest during different phases of programmes. For example, in the *preparatory phase* we at TPO have been requested to get involved in projects in some fifteen countries between 1999 and 2001. Only four projects were initiated because planning in the other sites was too difficult for a variety of reasons. In one of those country's, the refugees returned to their country of origin. In three other countries, civil war and an upsurge of hostilities prevented the formulation of a project in the complex emergency situation that characterizes these countries. Changes in priorities of the donors, who first showed interest, took place in several countries. And in others bureaucratic procedures slowed down the procedure to such an extent that projects were not initiated.

Similar problems with temporal planning may take place during the *implementation phase*. The following example shows a comprehensible lack of understanding of public health experts who were neither aware of the latency time nor of the course of traumatic stress syndromes, or the psychosocial aspects of refugee life. A few years ago a UN-agency asked our Nepali counterpart organisation CVICT to terminate their services in the camps of Bhutanese refugees in the Southeastern part of Nepal. The UN-agency's goal was to eliminate services in the camp in order to reduce the total amount of support for the refugees. The aim was to eventually close the camps. CVICT is a local NGO that began to provide physical health care right after the arrival of the refugees in the beginning of the nineties. Later CVICT asked TPO to add its expertise in the psychosocial field (Sharma & Van Ommeren, 1998). Everybody agreed that the quality of the work was excellent. Despite a request by the WHO's Head of the Mental Health Department to his UN-counterpart in Geneva and the promise of the latter to revert the situation, CVICT was forced to leave the camps. The whole project had to be handed over to the organisation responsible for general medical care. Yet, since this organization's primary care workers had no mental health experience, they had to be trained by CVICT-TPO (see chapter on Nepal).

A year before this incident we had a discussion with public health doctors of the UN-agency in their field office near the refugee camps. They asked us how many of the 90,000 refugees would suffer from psychiatric disorder and how long it would take to treat a patient. They then calculated that if x numbers of CVICT-staff would treat y number of patients a week, all the refugees including the torture survivors could be helped in z number of months and the project could be closed. This logical and straightforward linear approach might work for some somatic disorders, but in this case it is a reduction of a complex psychosocial reality into a over-simplified medical treatment model.

The chapter on the Tibetans illustrates the burden of different generations of refugees escaping Tibet in different time periods beginning with China's invasion in 1949. Each wave of refugees was confronted with typical acculturative stress upon its arrival in India as well as with problems of re-enculturalisation when they return to Tibet. Similarily, the chapter on Uganda mentions the different types of problems of Sudanese refugees over time after their arival in Uganda.

The above examples show that (post-)conflict situations require frequent adaptations of planning and intervention strategies. With this caveat in mind, our projects are implemented in project cycles that go from a pilot phase to an expansion and a maintenance phase. The key element of our strategy is highly similar to the DOTS strategy for tuberculosis control as promoted by WHO (Maher, Chaulet, Spinaci, & Harries, 1997; Maher, 1999). That is we first build commitment with our partner organization. We then select priorities for our interventions (ten of which will be mentioned shortly). We provide a range of preventive and curative interventions described at the end of this chapter. We set up monitoring and accountability systems to evaluate the outcome of our programs. These outcome data, in combination with epidemiological and cost-effectiveness data, are then fed back into the next project cycle of our intervention program to improve the quality of our services and to expand our program over the target population.

OBJECTIVES OF PUBLIC MENTAL HEALTH INTERVENTIONS

The afore-mentioned guiding principles resulted in the following objectives, which are reflected in the diverse descriptions of culture-specific intervention programs in the following chapters:

- The identification, management and prevention of psychosocial and mental-health problems caused by man-made or natural disasters
- The management of traumatic stress and the prevention of retraumatization
- The promotion of psychosocial well-being and the enhancement of quality of life

- The protection of human rights and the improvement of social conditions
- The initiation, consolidation and integration of culture-specific coping strategies to encourage human beings to help themselves in traumatic circumstances
- The development of culture specific intervention and training programs
- The support of local sustainable *community-based* organisations or programs including the institutional strengthening of the local organization
- The treatment of people with psychiatric problems which may or may not result from traumatic experiences
- The development, transfer and exchange of expertise and awareness of psychological and social consequences of violence, disasters and human rights violations on a local, regional and international level
- The development of a centre of expertise that (a) produces handbooks, training, and health promotion materials, (b) provides professional consulting services, and (c) provides advanced training
- The exchange of knowledge and expertise in the area of care for migrants and refugees between the West and TPO-projects elsewhere.

PUBLIC MENTAL HEALTH CRITERIA FOR THE SELECTION OF PRIORITIES FOR TRAINING AND MENTAL HEALTH INTERVENTIONS

A lesson learned from the large-scale psychosocial interventions in the last decade is that preplanning and selection of priorities is needed in order to cope with crises. TPO bases its psychosocial and mental health services for adults and children living in (post-) conflict or (post-) disaster situations on public mental health considerations mentioned in the previous part of this chapter. For the selection of interventions we handle criteria that are similar to the criteria for the selection of training priorities.

The next section will mention ten different criteria. It will explain the rationale for each one and mention some methods one can use to apply them in the field. It will conclude by stating that handling criteria is a subjective and judgmental process. Politics, policy considerations, professional discipline and expertise influence the weight one attributes to the different criteria.

The First Criterion: Prevalence and the Role of Epidemiology

The first criterion is the *prevalence* of the problem. In public health, prevalence is assessed to evaluate need. This assessment involves professional judgment about people's health status and their need for medical or psychosocial care.

The *prevalence* of the problem is determined with the help of a culture-informed epidemiological survey. This helps distinguish individuals who, once exposed to traumatic events, develop a disorder. Epidemiology helps explain the distribution and the determinants of disorders in populations. It is also an important tool in understanding the aetiology of post-traumatic stress syndromes (PTSS), because it provides a methodology for investigating the relative contribution of exposure, protective factors and individual vulnerability (cf De Girolamo & McFarlane in Marsella et al., 1996).

The role of the intensity of exposure is demonstrated by comparing prevalence rates to intensity of exposure (Mollica, McInnes, Poole, & Tor, 1998; De Jong et al., 2001a,b). The role of vulnerability and resiliency can be determined by the distinguishing characteristics of individuals who did and did not develop PTSS with similar levels of exposure.

Epidemiology is valuable in the design of treatment services after large-scale traumatic events because they provide the prevalence estimates that help define the size of the affected populations and help planning services.

> Prevalence and the assessment of DALYs (Disability Adjusted Life Years) help indicate how many people suffer from a disorder to develop services for them. Looking at mediating factors such as vulnerability and protective factors help designing preventive interventions.

In addition to prevalence, disability is an important indicator to develop services. Studies conducted after a significant period of time from the onset of the trauma provide essential information about the chronicity of symptoms and about the disability they produce. McFarlane and Yehuda (1996) wonder why disability has been so little investigated given the enormous costs of traumatic stress. They see disability as a critical issue for treatment because we should not assume that the interventions that improve patient's symptoms will automatically modify their ability to work or function within families. However, we know little about disability in chronic conflict situations in low-income countries.

The role that personality and attributes play in influencing adaptations to traumatic stress is important. Yet in view of the poor transcultural validity of personality constructs, studying personality in non-western cultures is hard even in peace-time, let alone in (post-) conflict areas. In general one may assume that a person living in a culture or a family promoting a stoical attitude is more likely to put symptomatic distress aside with a possible short-term benefit in terms of functioning. As I mentioned before, studies have shown that—at least in the west—such a coping style may have future adverse effects. Early intervention can prevent more serious long-term medical, psychological, and psychiatric consequences. Disclosing traumatic experiences is psychologically and physically beneficial. Inhibition of trauma-related thoughts or feelings appears to require a physiological and psychological effort that acts over time as a cumulative stressor. Subjects who failed to confide childhood or more recent traumatic experiences were more likely to have health problems such as cancer, hypertension, weight loss and skin rashes. Confiding or writing about traumatic memories and feelings exhibited improved immune system function, better school performance and decreased physician visits (Pennebaker & Susman, 1988; Pennebaker, 1993).

> One may conclude that chronicity of symptoms and the inability to work are important in arguing for service provision, and for secondary and tertiary prevention. Early intervention can prevent more serious long-term medical, psychological and psychiatric consequence. Disclosing traumatic experiences is psychologically and physically beneficial.

Epidemiological research contributes to understanding the relationship between PTSS and co-morbid disorders (cf Kessler et al., 1995; de Jong et al., 2001b). Although various disorders predispose individuals to PTSS, we found that the boundaries between DSM- or ICD-defined mood disorders and anxiety disorders are vague among non-western populations, in large part because they often overlap with somatization, dissociation and PTSS. This is an important issue for our projects.

> Studying the prevalence of co-morbidity and dimensional aspects in addition to categorical aspects of mental illness are other ways of identifying and focusing on high-risk groups.

Ideally, an epidemiological survey should include a study on help-seeking behavior. Help-seeking behavior is defined as 'the sequence of contacts with individuals, organizations and significant others, to seek help. It also refers to the help that is supplied in response to such efforts' (Rogler & Cortes, 1993). Help seeking behavior has *direction*, which is the sequential ordering of the individuals or organizations that are contacted during the effort of getting help. Help seeking behavior also has *duration*, which is the time lapse between the initiation of the help-seeking effort and the formation of contacts. Direction and duration are shaped by psychosocial and cultural factors. Cultural context not only affects the perception of potential problems, it also moulds the ways of dealing with the problem.

Studying help-seeking behavior provides information about the distribution of stress reactions and psychopathology in different health care sectors, e.g., whether people visit a healer or healing church, consult a family member or friend, or whether they prefer an allopathic health facility for their problems.

Figures about help-seeking seem to be somewhat contradictory. According to some colleagues only ten percent of a traumatized population may look for help. This ten percent is low in comparison with the results of epidemiological studies showing that PTSD rates among victims of wars and persecution vary between 15 and 50%, that rates of depressive disorder vary between 15 and 70%, and that a majority suffer from additional psychiatric disorders. On the other hand we know that trauma victims are disproportionate users of the health care system. Solomon (1997) reported more physician visits and higher hospitalization rates among former prisoners of war, rape victims, survivors of Nazi concentration camps, disaster victims, battered women, combat veterans, and crime victims than among the general population. Apparently, there seems to be a relation between under-utilization of services for psychological complaints and an over-utilization of health services for physical complaints.

The problem of service utilization is compounded in many war-affected areas where "treatment" in the Western sense is often absent. Therefore, studying help-seeking behavior contributes to the decision-making process of which services should be provided by e.g. health workers, teachers, local healers or relief workers.

> To develop curative and preventive interventions, we need information on the prevalence and distribution of disorders. Studying help-seeking behavior provides information on the indigenous, the allopathic or the lay services where people try to get support.

The Second Criterion: Community Concern

Community concern is the perceived need of people, communities, families and individuals to cope with their lives. Community concern is related to social structure, to mental health beliefs, and to the meaning given to the events. For example, it may make quite a difference whether a culture attributes its plight to deeds in a previous life, or to a heroic struggle for independence.

Addressing this need involves community involvement, community empowerment, and sustainability of services, which in turn help better understand help-seeking behavior and adherence or non-adherence to interventions (Andersen, 1995).

Measuring community concern belongs to the field of qualitative, operational and action research. Qualitative approaches are characterized by the description of social phenomena from the perspective of those being studied (i.e., an emic perspective). The research strategy is flexible and integrative (Bryman, 1992; Hudelson, 1994). Ager (2001) defends the scientific rigor of qualitative research by referring to concepts as triangulation, comprehensiveness, negative case analysis and transferability. In our programs we have used a combination of the following sampling and interviewing methods.

1. *Multiflex snowball sampling* is used to select key informants to utilise 'insider' knowledge and referral chains among people who possess common traits (Kaplan, Korf, & Sterk, 1987; Korf, 1997). Informants are selected on the basis of a particular trait, and are then asked to identify a number of people with the same trait. In this way a number of research participants are identified. From the set of those nominated, a random selection is made. The method is

especially useful with regard to identify people with 'hidden' or stigmatized problems. For example, rape survivors, perpetrators of violence such as boy-soldiers, people with stigmatising neuro-psychiatric disorders such as epilepsy, or people with HIV, or prostitutes.

2. *Key informant (KI) interviews* help us glean insight about a community. Key informants are selected on the following criteria:

- They are representative of the various ethnic groups and both genders.
- They hold a position of respect and trust.
- They have lived in the community for a considerable length of time.
- They have functions, which bring them into contact with many people within the community or with a particular section of it.

Examples of possible KIs include shopkeepers, teachers, religious leaders, local healers, traditional birth attendants (TBAs), members of political or women's organizations, or health workers. KIs can be interviewed either individually or in focus groups. The following information about KIs is recorded: demographic data, duration of stay in the community and their qualifications as a key-informant.

3. *Focus groups* consist of open group interviews with 5–10 persons to obtain qualitative information on priorities, needs, and attitudes (Krueger, 1994). Focus groups are used for a variety of reasons. They can be used, for example, as an orientation towards positive coping strategies, towards newly arisen problems in the area, for the evaluation of a program, for possible shifts in program priorities, or for the assessment of community dynamics. Focus groups to elicit community concern are organised on the macro, meso and micro-levels. It ranges from ministries, regional and district officials, to community leaders in the refugee settlements or family households. In some cultures there may be a formal or informal religious, political or traditional leader who gives the answers and the others may conform to his idea (i.e. group think) (de Jong, 1987). Group think may be caused by the strict hierarchy within a culture or family, or by mistrust which is often rampant in (post-) conflict and (post-) disaster situations. If group think is a problem, then it is better to organise individual KI-interviews.

4. *Sondeo method* is another approach to assess community concern. It differs from focus groups in that a multidisciplinary group of interviewers consisting of 3–5 members conduct the interview (e.g. a relief worker, an anthropologist, a psychologist or a rural development expert). Questions are asked from a variety of community members. The multidisciplinary approach widens the perspective, and lack of consensus may yield new program priorities, hypotheses, or problem solving strategies.

5. *Participant observation and phenomenological narratives or thick descriptions.* Participant observation is the preferred research technique of many anthropologists. A narrative is obtained in a sequence of steps that can be summarized as

follows. The first part consists of an autobiographically oriented story. The technique used resembles the personal interview taught to journalists, medical doctors and ethnographers. This part of the narrative or life history should be as broad as possible. The interviewer then asks more specific questions. Respondents are next asked to theorize about their lives and their 'problem'. Subsequently, the researcher must utilize guidelines to identify which data are worth further consideration, paying attention to primacy (what comes first in a story), uniqueness (what stands out in a story), omission (what seems to be missing from the story), distortion and isolation (what does not follow logically in the story), and incompletion (when the story fails to end in a satisfying way). In this stage, patterns of meaning and experience are sought and an analytic abstraction of the case is written.

6. *Community meetings*. Organizing a meeting with the community should be in accordance with local ways of gathering a community paying attention to representativeness of for example different age groups, gender and ethnicity.

Narratives and individual key-informant interviews can be used with individuals and families. On the community-level and the society-at-large-level one may make an inventory of priorities and responses of officials regarding the consequences of organized violence on each administrative level. This can be done with a focus group or with the sondeo method. More specific focus groups can be conducted if there are rumors or stories about certain problems. For example, groups with traditional birth attendants in cases of sexual violence or rape. Focus groups can be done with adolescents if they cannot express certain preoccupations in the presence of the elderly.

Community concern can be hard to assess in postwar circumstances because victims may have been so seriously deprived of basic human needs, such as shelter, water, or food for a considerable amount of time, that these issues form the whole gestalt of any interview. Or they may be so accustomed or conditioned to ask for material help from NGOs—the 'dependency syndrome'—that bringing forward any other issue does not come to their mind. They may also be so accustomed to the effects of traumatic stress that a distortion has taken place of the population norm with regard to normality and pathology. For example, during focus groups discussions in a war-ridden area in East Africa, the mothers stated that their children were not affected by the war. Since the results seemed hard to believe, we repeated the focus group discussions. It turned out that many children had night terrors and that children up to the age of 12 were wetting their bed in an area where being potty trained at the age of one year was not exceptional.

The assessment of community concern usually starts during the project preparation phase. It is an integral part of (rapid) appraisal methods and is reflected in a project proposal or policy document. Throughout the development of services, community concern is measured during the repetitive cycles that characterize multi-annual programs heading for sustainability.

In addition to the aforementioned techniques such as focus groups or key informant interviews, community concern can be assessed by looking at the type of problems that people present to community services or health services in the affected areas.

The presentation of specific problems provides insight into concerns that are complementary to the results of the aforementioned epidemiologic study or the research on help-seeking behavior. Assessing community concern is related to the psychosocial well being as perceived by people. The qualitative assessment techniques mainly belong to the domain of social science. In contrast, the aforementioned epidemiological studies pertain to the field of medicine and produce medically accepted disease categories. Before starting any service delivery, we like to do a survey to know details about prevalence and incidence of psychological and psychiatric disorder. However, current requirements for cross-cultural validity and translation of instruments is so time consuming, that a reliable epidemiological study takes about two to five years (de Jong, 1996a; Van Ommeren et al., 1999). Most programs in (post-)disaster-situations—but also in peace time—do not have that amount of time. TPO uses quick assessments assessing community concern as the major criterion used to set up a program. Over the years we add epidemiological research to obtain detailed information about the psychopathology we have to address. This information serves to fine-tune our intervention and training programs and to improve our training materials.

Community concern and epidemiology are complementary in several aspects as shown in Table 6. Another way of illustrating the complementarity between prevalence and community concern is by comparing figures of an

Table 6. Complementarity of Criteria One and Two: Prevalence and Community Concern

Prevalence	Community concern
Quantitative research: epidemiology	Qualitative research: participative social science
Assesses disorder and its distribution: e.g. depression, anxiety, alcohol, schizophrenia, PTSS	Assesses perceived concerns, idioms if distress, folk illnesses, culture-bound syndromes
Assesses morbidity, mortality, disability	Related to suffering
Related to health	Related to well being Related to community involvement
Technique: culture-informed psychiatric epidemiology	Technique: multi-method (focus groups, KI-interviews, in-depth interviews)
Cross-sectional, rarely longitudinal	Ongoing and cyclical
Survey plus reporting takes 2–5 years	Assessment plus reporting takes 2–8 weeks
Etic/emic	Emic

Table 7. Complementarity of Criteria One and Two: Psychiatric Morbidity and Presented Problems

Life-time prevalence of psychiatric morbidity according to MIM-study		Community concern according to presented problems, in rank order
Somatoform disorder	5%	1 Health (sleep, headache, body pain, epilepsy, neck/back/epigastric pain)
Anxiety disorder	25%	2 Mood (sadness, anxiety, aggression, nervousness)
Depressive disorder	12%	
		3 Family (domestic violence, child problems, disharmony)
		4 Mental illness (psychosis, falling)
		5 Abuse (alcohol, drugs)
		6 Social (lack of food, conflicts at work, poverty, unemployment)
		7 Cognitive (concentration and memory problems)
PTSD	29%	8 Trauma
Total amount psychopathology	39%*	9 Stress (stress, suicide, spirits)
Co-morbidity for 3 disorders	45%	
Co-morbidity for two disorders	37%	

*PTSD, Anxiety Disorder, Mood Disorder, Somatoform Disorder

epidemiological survey with the nature of the problems presented by people to a mental health and psychosocial program as shown in Table 7 (see also several chapters in the book).

The first column of the table shows the diagnoses identified in TPO's epidemiological survey, while the second column mentions the problems that people brought forward to our intervention programs in different countries.

Table 7 shows some overlap, but it also illustrates important differences when applying the two criteria. For example, whereas some professionals think that post-traumatic stress or PTSD should be the main focus of any program, it comes out as one of the last priorities as seen by the people themselves.

The Third Criterion: Seriousness

In immediate post-conflict situations, general distress and minor psychological disorders affect almost the whole population. After a certain amount of time a majority of the people generally cope with their problem without professional support. However, the management of psychosocial problems needs to be in balance with the seriousness of psychiatric disorders that are brought forward by the population. Because most programs struggle with a discrepancy between a need for services and a lack of funding, one has to weigh the seriousness of a disorder among a minority of the population against the enormous amount of distress among a majority that often dissipates in time. This choice is even more difficult because negligence of distress in an early stage may lead to serious mental and physical pathology in the future. Another complicating factor is that after a war or a disaster an increase in the incidence of major psychiatric disturbances may occur, partly caused by the absence of services during the war period (cf Cohen & Ahearn, 1991). A program may decide to focus on a specific problem that is considered important whereas the local cultural setting calls for another priority. For example, when we visited Honduras after hurricane Mitch it became clear that the effect of the natural disaster in rates of measured PTSD was leveled out by the much more traumatizing and omnipresent domestic violence that had also existed before the disaster.

Another source of confusion in considering the seriousness of a disorder is that subgroups among the population may show a different response when mental health services are offered. For example, when setting up mental health care services in Cambodia, we found that in areas with high concentrations of returnees from the Thai border camps, the consumption of mental health care services was many times higher than in areas that had never known any allopathic mental health care service. The reason for the difference was that, although both groups regarded mental disorders as a serious predicament, only the returnees from the border camps knew from their previous experience in Thailand that allopathic treatment for mental disorder exists (Somasundaram, Van de Put, Eisenbruch, & de Jong, 1999).

The Fourth Criterion: Treatability or Feasibility of Treatment

The criterion of susceptibility to treatment is important both with regard to the question of whether people with certain problems get support from their natural environment and whether there are sufficient resources in terms of personnel, time, and funds to treat specific problems. Prior to initiating interventions the likelihood of effective assistance, basic cost-effectiveness, and availability of resources must be evaluated. For example, in some areas of Africa and Asia, the prevalence of epilepsy is as high as 3.7–4.9% and it is often presented to psychiatric and primary health care services (de Jong, 1987; Adamolekum, 1995). In addition, especially in situations of massive stress, a large number of people show symptoms of dissociation varying from individual possession as an 'idiom of distress' to classical fugue states and epidemics of mass psychogenic illness with or without psychogenic fits (de Jong, 1987; Van Ommeren, Sharma, Komproe, Sharma, Cardeña, Thapa, Poudyal, & de Jong, 2001). In low-income countries one often still sees the classical dissociative phenomena described by Janet or Freud during their time in the Salpêtrière in Paris. While setting up services, one has to consider which health care sector is best equipped to deal with the high prevalence of all kinds of convulsions, whether neurologic or dissociative in origin (sometimes still referred to as 'conversion' or 'hysteria').

Offering treatment to those with epilepsy is a feasible option. A total of 95% of a sample of West African patients with generalized epileptic convulsions were correctly diagnosed and treated with phenobarbital by primary health care workers who received a couple of hours of training; the average seizure frequency decreased from 16 to 0.34 per month (de Jong, 1996b). Dealing with the equally highly prevalent dissociative states often requires sophisticated and psychotherapeutic skills, which are often not available. In many cultures, adequate management for both groups implies triage of the epileptic patients and referral of those with dissociative states to the local healers, healing churches or possession cults. Several authors in this book recommend closer collaboration between mental health systems and local healers. For example, incorporating the mutual development of treatment guidelines for disorders that are recognized in the local and the western nosological system, exchange of information, and referral of appropriate patients between the different health care sectors (Akerele, 1987; de Jong, 1987).

A similar problem exists with regard to the treatment of complex PTSD as a result of ongoing trauma in war-affected areas. In the West, the psychotherapy of complex PTSD requires a long-term commitment from both therapist and client. In most war-affected areas, psychotherapists are not or hardly available and long-term therapy is mostly alien to the local culture. This is one of the reasons why mental health care professionals often resort to short therapies, limiting themselves to the stabilization phase of the three- or five-phase model of Janet (Van der Kolk et al., 1996; Meichenbaum, 1997). The use of problem-solving short term treatment can usually be adequately done by a paraprofessional staff and seems to have the needed benefit.

It is obvious that on the previous criterion of seriousness, the neuropsychiatric consequences of HIV would receive high priority, but that on the criterion of feasible and effective treatment one can do little more than assist people in the process of dying. Those with strong spirit beliefs often do this with the help of the church. Although Obsessive Compulsive Disorder ranks high in terms of DALYs worldwide, in many service settings effective treatment is not available. One of the impediments to the treatment of various types of illnesses is that modern and often-complex types of psychotherapy such as cognitive-behavioral therapies are hard to apply among immigrants and refugees (de Jong, 1999).

The Fifth Criterion: Sustainability

The sustainability of a program depends primarily on the institutional capacity and the creation of enough human resources to continue the interventions. Sustainability has to be a top priority from the very beginning. This necessitates

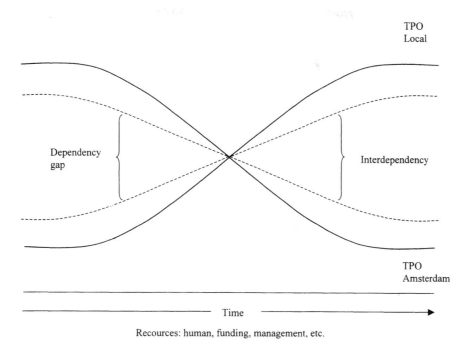

Figure 3. Interdependency relation between TPO Headquarters and its collaborative projects over time.

management, and on future means to guarantee funding for the interventions. In the context of an international NGO like TPO, it means that at the initial stage the field program depends on the central office and on expatriate support but that over time with proper training and preparation the project becomes more and more independent. Figure 3 shows this relation. The dotted lines indicate that when there are more means locally available, the dependency gap is smaller. Dependency changes into interdependency in the long-term. Figure 3 shows that in the beginning of projects, the input from TPO Amsterdam is large in terms of human resources, professional expertise, management, and funding. Over time this input decreases, while local resources increase by building up human resource capacity, management, a considerable coverage of the target group, logistic capacity and diversified funding sources. The chapters on Cambodia, Uganda and Nepal show that our programs are quite successful with regard to these functional aspects of sustainability when mutual commitment exists for a period of five till seven years.

With regard to the financial aspects of sustainability, the following is important:

1. Paradoxically, a large amount of external funding may hinder future sustainability. One should find a balance between external resources and

resources generated by the program itself. The larger the discrepancy between external and internal sources of income, the harder it is to build a sustainable program. Being poor may create an inverted relation between a large amount of initial external funding and long-term sustainability. That is indicated as the dependency gap in Figure 3, as mentioned previously. The dotted lines indicate that when there are more means available locally, the dependency gap is smaller. This may facilitate sustainability in the long term. Generating funds requires creativity and an unorthodox approach. For example, one may have to experiment with paying local staff in kind when donor-funding decreases over time. Another aspect of financial sustainability is that in general, mental health and human rights activities are hard to fund among marginalized people living in peripheral areas of host countries. In spite of the World Bank figures as expressed in DALYs, mental health still is the stepchild of health care among the donor community. In addition, there are only a few people in the world who dare to pose the question whether these activities are ever going to be financially sustainable.

2. 'Donor driveness' or 'demand driveness' may make a program vulnerable. Donors may emphasize certain target groups because they fall within their mandate. They may for example push a categorical program for (orphaned or street) children or ex-boy soldiers, which in the long run has little chance to restore the personal growth or the future prospects of these children within their society. Moreover, donors may be driven by media-hypes. For example, for a couple of years the West showed a voyeuristic interest in the plight and the 'wickedness' of child soldiers. A Mozambican NGO received large amounts of funds for an interesting rehabilitation project aimed at a small group of abducted children and some perpetrators. However, from a public mental health perspective, the project invested large amounts of funds in a relatively small target group. When the hype was over, it became extremely difficult to make the project sustainable. First, because funds followed the hype, and second because large amounts were spent on problems with small numbers of clients.

3. This example also illustrates the following important public mental health problem with regard to sustainability. There are tens of thousands of well-trained physical public health experts who know little of psychology and the treatment of traumatic stress. There are thousands of well-trained mental health professionals who are knowledgeable in the trauma-field but who virtually know nothing about public mental health. They often have little idea what it means to work beyond a western psychological model, let alone what it implies to set up a local sustainable organization in a low-income country. The Mozambican project was set up by professionals who just finished their training in the West and who with the best of intentions invested large amounts of money in a small group of children at the expense of hundreds of thousands other traumatized children and adults and at the expense of the sustainability of their own program.

4. Even though as a rule TPO works on a demand driven basis and reacts only to requests from afflicted areas, demand driveness also carries possible risks. For example, the Tibetan government in exile in Dharamsala depends almost entirely on donor funds and therefore has the wise policy to be cautious to create staff positions that it has to sustain. In such a situation even a long-term commitment from our side does not necessarily result in a local sustainable organization since the limited number of positions allowed by the government in exile can impede the sustainability of the program (see the chapter on the Tibetans). Another example is the rebel movement from South Sudan that requested us to set up a program. It is run by refugees who are trained by our program among the Sudanese in North Uganda. But the past human rights record of the rebel movements in South Sudan makes the program vulnerable if major political changes do occur among the competing rebel factions as happened so often in the past (Paardekoper, 2002).

5. Most donors increasingly require that programs should be demand driven and that the target groups should determine priorities. On the other hand, donors may have their own agenda imposed by political decision-makers requiring a shift in priorities that often endanger the continuation of a program. For example, after the last elections in the Netherlands the new minister of international cooperation—in line with some other European countries—sharply reduced the number of aid receiving countries. Wise or unwise, this new policy was a blow to the previous sermons on sustainability of the same ministry since many ongoing programs had to be ended. Therefore, receivers of funds may try to make themselves less vulnerable by looking for multiple donors and creating a buffer, which in turn may evoke distrust among donors. Even though one of our partners in Asia was always open about its multiple funding sources, one of the donors felt that 'something was going on' when it was informed about several donors and hence the project funding was stopped. Since projects depend on donors, they are extremely vulnerable when they want to protest. Donors and governments hardly ever admit their own failures while having considerably more civil servants than NGOs and at times retaliate after having to admit a mistake.

6. Work in (post-)conflict areas implies crisis interventions which must be rapidly implemented when violence flares up. This may happen at the expense of (a) rational project design, (b) adequate management, (c) developing preventive action, (d) interventions for a larger populations, (e) acculturation of services, or (f) adequate monitoring due to the volatility of the situation. Therefore, a program has to be flexible while also being insistent to become sustainable.

7. Becoming sustainable often requires working with local universities, a UN-agency or trying to transfer a program to local authorities or to the national government. This may imply adaptation of management and accountancy structures or require incorporation in government structures that may not be able to

pay salaries or that may change their health priorities. Public health-wise it may also imply being obliged to survive as a vertical mental health program because authorities do not see the advantages of horizontal integrated public health programs. Alternatively, the government may welcome a vertical program for development of the national mental health policy. In Cambodia, for example, we developed a community mental health program covering one fourth of the approximately twelve million inhabitants in a situation where no mental health services existed before. After six years the TPO-project became a local NGO and the government accepted our offer to hand over the mental health component to its new mental health department.

8. To guarantee continuation of the activities after repatriation of a refugee community or resettlement of IDPs, the program should train many (para-) professionals from the refugee community. This type of empowerment has a preventive effect on the community and decreases the 'dependency syndrome'. At first it is important to reflect on the career development of these trainees in order to work with the program and prevent a brain drain to other organizations, departments or countries. This can be accomplished by certification of the trainees or by training some psychiatrists or psychologists abroad.

9. Sustainability is also related to the provision of psychotropic drugs. As mentioned before, populations of refugees, displaced persons, or returnees will often contain individuals with serious psychiatric disorder or epilepsy. These patients need to continue their medication after resettlement or repatriation. This can be done by assuring that budgets reflect the need to continuous drug supply, and by assuring that psychotropic drugs figure on the List of Essential Drugs of the government of the new host country.

10. In our view, donors, governments and NGOs should abstain from engaging in mental health care services without a long-term commitment. Some donors customarily fund subsequent project phases on a 6-month basis. From an ethical point of view this is inappropriate. Donors cannot expect mental health care professionals to assist traumatized people if they have to disrupt their work every six months hoping for new funds to arrive.

11. Another aspect promoting the sustainability of a program is to take a politically neutral stance while implementing the program. This chapter clearly shows that this requires quite some flexibility and a need to be able to 'reculer pour mieux sauter' ("withdraw to jump better") from all the people involved. In Algeria, for example, during the period of civil war, the government was and is reticent to support NGOs because it fears that some NGOs might be used as a cover-up of fundamentalist Islamic groups. Our local counterpart organization, the SARP, gradually built up its program over two years while maintaining contacts with a range of government bodies. After the amnesty for fundamentalist groups, the program could come out and received coverage from local papers, radio and television (see chapter on Algeria).

The Sixth Criterion: Knowledge, Skills, and Availability of (Mental) Health Care Professionals

Before setting up a multisectoral intervention program, the number and types of mental health care professionals, general health workers, and other possible trainees from sectors such as education or social services should be assessed. The assessment can be done with the help of an instrument such as the Health Staff Interview, a 30-minute semi-structured interview developed by the WHO, which can be adapted to local circumstances (cf de Jong, 1987, p. 156). The interview can be used with existing (mental) health workers who will be trained and involved in the mental health care program. The assessment should answer questions regarding

- Ability to handle different types of psychosocial and mental health problems
- Normal duties and responsibilities
- Kind of problems they come across in their work
- Kind of training and supervision they need
- The extent to which the trainees themselves have been affected by the war

The training should address their own traumatic experiences so as to be able to support other people. After the training a second assessment should be carried out to find out whether the trainees are able to deal with the traumas of others.

Group and individual debriefing, supervision, and job rotation are useful measures to prevent burn-out expressing itself in emotional exhaustion, a tendency to develop cynical and negative attitudes towards others, and negative self-evaluation, especially regarding work. Debriefing provides support to mental health workers and maintains their availability for the program (WHO/UNHCR Refugee Mental Health; Friedman, Warfe, & Mwiti, 2000; Raphael & Wilson, 2000). For example, in Kosova TPO collected ante-mortem data on the 2500 people who were killed during the war. In addition, support is given to the forensic teams and to the affected Kosovar families. To prevent burn-out, the team organized a debriefing meeting once a week.

The Seventh Criterion: Political Acceptability

It is important to understand the sometimes hidden agenda of policy makers. For example, in epidemiological research and in stress research, it is necessary to measure traumatic stressors and life events before, during, and after the human-made disaster. Only by doing this can the effect of these independent variables on psychosocial well-being and psychopathology be measured. The results play a central role in designing culturally appropriate interventions. However, the results can also be used for other purposes, such as human rights work or advocacy against repressive governments or rebel groups, either at home or in a guest country. On several occasions, our collaborators were followed while collecting data on human rights abuse.

Governments may be ambivalent towards psychosocial and human rights research. On the one hand, the activities may stimulate democracy, respect for human rights, good governance and psychosocial support. On the other hand, governments may try to hinder a psychosocial program. Alternatively, a government may welcome human rights activists in case they themselves are imprisoned, thus needing the benefits of human rights protection, which their previous enemies tried to realize.

Governments are often reluctant towards mental health activities for a variety of reasons. Health Ministries often do not have a mental health department or a small division, and so mental health is not competitive with other health sectors, particularly within the sectoral approach. As a result a mental health division has to find ways to integrate its plans into a more comprehensive health plan, which then can be subsequently forwarded to donors. Also Health Ministries may not know the public health impact of mental health problems, and therefore do not regard mental health as a priority.

The Eighth Criterion: Ethical Acceptability

Programs must consider the possible harm that might be inflicted on others, e.g., by carrying out research that lacks cultural sensitivity or by carrying out research that does not result in provision or improvement of services. All too often scholars are eager to collect data to be published without questioning if the work will help in formulating preventive or curative interventions for the affected population.

Another ethical issue is the psychological impact of interviewing survivors of disaster or human rights abuse. We regard interviews, both during the preassessment of a program and as part of an epidemiological survey, as an intervention in itself. Clinicians who treat torture victims have described the emotional upset associated with recalling a torture experience (Allodi, 1991; Kolb & Multipassi, 1982). An open-ended interview using free recall may elicit the greatest emotional distress and poorest recall. Neutral retrieval cues, such as a list of possible events, produce more accurate responses and much less emotional distress. Our experience coincides with Mollica (1994) who considered that individuals who are interviewed feel relieved that they get an opportunity to talk about their trauma experience. Westermeyer (1989) also stated that asking about traumatic events does not create distress; rather it elicits distress already present. Nevertheless, one should take into account that an interview may cause such upset that counseling may be required immediately. Taking these precautions into account, why do we regard an interview as an intervention? As mentioned before, survivors tend to create their 'conspiracy of silence' because they do not want to embarrass others with their traumatic past, because everybody is occupied with surviving, or because the culture does not facilitate the disclosure of a traumatic past. Therefore, interviewees often perceive an interview as a unique event enabling them to share their problems, and feeling recognized in their suffering. It also gives them the possibility of giving testimony. The urge of being heard may create a dilemma for the interviewer. Knowing that neutral cues and a moderate amount of empathy create less distress for the interviewee may run counter to the need of the latter to disclose the past. Methodologically this dilemma also poses a problem. An interview format often imposes time limitations, and allowing time for specific events may create memory bias. To handle these ethical and methodological dilemmas requires careful navigating and careful preparation of interviewers, which can often be practiced in role-plays.

Another potential ethical problems is that Western-style informed consent with signatures on an elaborate consent form is expected in the West, but as Bromet (1995) argued after the Chernobyl accident, such forms may be perceived with distrust and suspicion. The procedure may evoke fear as we found out in countries such as Cambodia, Ethiopia or Gaza. One way of solving this problem is verbal informed consent, preferably in the presence of a family member or friend (cf ICH/CPMP, 1997).

Another ethical consideration relates to the above-mentioned sustainability of the project. Psychosocial and mental health assistance requires a long-term commitment. In low-income countries, it may take 5–7 years before a local training of trainers (TOT) group has been trained itself and before it has subsequently trained and supervised sufficient secondary- and tertiary-level staff to ensure continuity of the work. Without such long-term commitment it is not ethical to start a program.

The Ninth Criterion: Cultural Sensitivity

Culture defines reality for its members. It defines the purpose of life, sanctions proper behavior, and provides personal and social meaning. All this is learned through tradition and transmitted from generation to generation.

Culture serves two functions. It is *integrative*, i.e., it represents the beliefs and values that provide individuals with a sense of identity. It is also *functional*, i.e., it furnishes the rules for behavior that enable the group to survive and provide for its welfare, while supporting an individual's sense of self-worth and belonging. These two functions are analogous to the warp and woof of a tapestry (Kagawa-Singer & Chi-Ying Chung, 1994). The weaving technique is universal, but the patterns that emerge from each culture are particular.

Each aspect of a public mental health program has to be tested for its cultural assumptions and consequences. Local mental health care professionals—especially if they were trained abroad—should adapt their Western oriented knowledge and expertise to their countrymen who often have a different cultural background. In our opinion, Western mental health care professionals with the best of intentions have to be extremely cautious in offering their western culture-bound expertise in conflict-ridden areas elsewhere.

Another example of an issue influenced by culture is suicide. Suicide is taboo in many cultures. Yet, it may be highly prevalent among afflicted groups (and a relatively unexplored area of refugee care). Combat related guilt—in isolation or in combination with survivor guilt—has been shown to be a predictor of suicide attempts among perpetrators of violence in Vietnam (Hendin & Haas, 1991). In Thailand, medical personnel in the largest camp noted a dramatic increase in domestic violence and suicide attempts amongst camp residents (Mollica, 1994). In Namibia, an increase in suicide has been reported as well. High suicide rates in the northern part of Namibia motivated the Minister of Health to collaborate with our counterpart organization PEACE. The chapter on northern Uganda provides details on the size and the nature of the suicide problem among the Sudanese refugees.

The Composite International Diagnostic Interview (CIDI 2.1), used in our MIM-study, includes a suicide screening list that can help in detecting attitudes towards suicide, groups at risk, and risk factors operating on the group and individual level. Due to bias caused by social desirability we wonder, however, whether the answers to this CIDI-section are valid. Because of the taboo in a number of cultures we think that there is a serious problem of underreporting. Within a range of cultures, when a person commits suicide the soul may not reincarnate until the moment arrives that a natural death would have caused the death of that person. The soul may turn into a revengeful and capricious spirit attacking the living and causing misfortune, illness or death. This belief has a preventive effect caused by its stigma, because the person who wants to commit suicide knows that the act possibly has such a negative influence. Simultaneously, it may lead to underreporting of suicide attempts and suicidal ideation in epidemiological studies. The same may happen with the soul of a person who is killed by homicide or as the consequence of war. The anxiety-provoking whims of the wandering spirit may decrease if a proper burial ritual has taken place. But in a war it is often impossible to find the body, or part of it, that is required both in African local 'animist' cultures and in Islam to conduct a proper burial ceremony (de Jong & Van Schaik, 1994). Sometimes the culture finds a solution for this problem. For example, in Mozambique the healers' associations decided that when due to the war corpses were not available for ceremonies, a piece of cloth or another material possession of the dead would be acceptable and permit the soul of the deceased to take its place among the ancestors.

In fact we still know little on the influence of culture on guilt feelings or shame in relation to suicide. For example, when a culture handles an external attribution for the burden of war, such as when Cambodians say that "the war is the consequence of collective sins resulting in negative karma during a previous life", does this external attribution have a moderating effect on self-blame and suicidal ideation? What are the specific risk factors that lead some people to commit suicide in situations of massive poverty, violence, acculturative stress and marginalization in a host culture, whereas most of them hardly have any idea what the future may bring?

The Tenth Criterion: Cost-Effectiveness

There are at least five reasons to do research on the effectiveness of mental health programming in low-income countries affected by violence:

1. Thus far there is no empirical research establishing the effectiveness of care for traumatized people in (post-)conflict situations. (More general, there are no published results on effectiveness studies on mental health and psychosocial care in low-income countries). Given the current trend among international aid donors to fund mental health care of trauma survivors, it is pertinent to establish effectiveness information. If we do not develop information on what works and what does not work, it would be unethical to continue carrying out such programs. Without such information, program donors are likely to move their focus to other issues. On the other hand, if proven cost and time effective, the interventions could be of great importance in the large-scale mental health care of refugees and other victims of human-made disaster. The feasibility of different interventions is an important issue considering the realities of day-to-day running of community mental health services in troubled regions of the world.

2. Research is important because programs can be adapted to become more effective.

3. We need to develop information on effectiveness because it is theoretically possible that the current programs are doing harm. For example, by focusing on vulnerability of traumatized individuals, programs may cause unnecessary distress and helplessness (Summerfield, 2000). Mental health programs may create sick-roles among traumatized people, resulting in refugees and IDPs to undervalue their own capacities for survival

4. Almost all research on trauma has been conducted in the West. However, most trauma survivors live in low-income countries.

5. Western countries accept hundreds of thousands of refugees. It may be more cost-effective to help the refugees within the developing world. Western countries that restrict access for asylum seekers should spend their funds in the afflicted regions as a cost-effective measure to increase the quality of life.

Currently, TPO is implementing a cost-effectiveness study in six countries affected by massive violence trying to answer the following questions:

1. What is the outcome of the different treatment modalities employed in the different countries?
2. How is the effect of the treatment related to therapist/mental health worker/nurse/local healer variables, or interactively with such variables

as preliminary training, duration of the training and supervision of the treatment?
3. How is the effect related to the duration and the content of the specific interventions?
4. Will the outcomes of the interventions improve in the course of time? Are they related to improved and advanced training and supervision?
5. How can we provide the best cost-effective services?

Weighing the Ten Criteria

In the introduction of this section I mentioned that the application of the ten criteria depends on many factors. The following matrix lists priorities by attributing a figure on a Lickert scale from 1 (*not at all important*) to 4 (*very important*) to each of the ten criteria (Table 8). When varying the relative importance of certain criteria we found that the list of priorities changed substantially.

Based on Table 10, a mental health program can determine priorities by the rating and by multiplying them to obtain a total score. To illustrate the relative subjectivity if each criterion, the first row shows WHO's DALY figures (in italics) as compared to TPO's prevalence figures (in bold).

Table 8. Matrix to Determine Priorities Based on Ten Intervention Criteria

	Health Problem Rated 1–4				
DALYs[a]	*Major depression*	*Alcohol use*	*Bipolar Disorder*	*Schizophrenia*	*OCD*
	10,7	*3,3*	*3*	*2,6*	*2,2*
Prevalence[b]	**PTSD** **29%**	**Anxiety disorder 25%**	**Depressive disorder 12%**	**Somatoform disorder 5%**	
Community Concern x					
Seriousness x					
Feasibility x					
Sustainability x					
Knowledge x					
Political acceptability x					
Ethical acceptability x					
Cultural sensitivity x					
Cost-Effectiveness x					
Total score					

[a]*Italics* = Rank order of Standard DALYs (WHO—World Bank 1996): five of the ten leading causes of disability worldwide are psychiatric conditions.
[b]In bold: life-time prevalence based on MIM-study. One could develop a weighed score taking various epidemiological measures together, e.g. prevalence/incidence/DALYs.

It depends on policy, discipline or affinity which factor gets more weight. For example, an epidemiologist or a World Bank expert may decide that DALYs and prevalence figures are the real hard data and therefore should be emphasized. A field expert or gender specialist may feel that community concern and cultural sensitivity is all that counts because the only way of achieving a sustainable program is by empowering the people who will ultimately carry the program themselves. A mental health professional may want to focus on seriousness, feasibility or cost-effectiveness. A human rights activist may focus on political and ethical acceptability because these are considered as the roots of evil. In our view, a community oriented psychosocial and public mental health care program has to consider all the factors mentioned.

INTERVENTIONS: AN INTEGRATED MULTI-MODAL CONCEPTUAL MODEL

The last part of this chapter presents an outline of the conceptual model that we use to provide prevention and treatment services. Figure 4 shows an inverted pyramid with three levels of intervention. The three levels are in accordance with the contextual levels we described before. The first or macro-level is the society-at-large including (inter)national agencies and government. The second or meso-level is the community, and the third or micro-level the family and the individual.

The three levels overlap, are interconnected and presented in descending order of importance for the size of the coverage of the target group.

The interventions needed at the level of the *community-at-large* are meant for the majority of people. These include interventions aimed at primary prevention of conflict, wars or disasters. They often belong to the realm of international and UN-agencies, governments, politicians and policy makers. International laws, national laws and public policy can influence the outcome of exposure to traumatic events.

Interventions on the *second level or the community level* aim at the total population of refugees and IDPs. These include the provision of safety and shelter, empowerment of the community, and public education and capacity building. Interventions at the community level are often provided by NGOs, local governments or more specialized international agencies. Psychosocial interventions at this level try to cover most or all people and require less specific expertise in the field of mental health or trauma treatment.

On the *third level are the families and individuals*. This is the level of secondary prevention (or treatment) and tertiary prevention (maintenance treatment). Among refugees and IDPs these activities are mostly covered by NGOs. The goal of secondary prevention is to shorten the course of an illness by early identification and

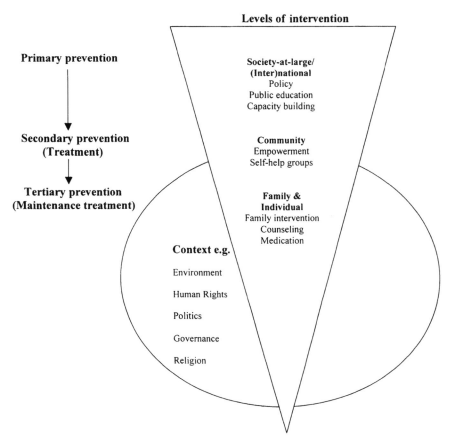

Figure 4. A conceptual model for psychosocial and mental health interventions from a public mental health perspective.

rapid intervention or crisis intervention (Kaplan & Sadock, 1985). For example, when primary prevention of a traumatic stress syndrome is impossible once a war has started, one can still prevent the problem of getting worse by providing crisis intervention or human rights protection to a family or a person.

The goal of tertiary prevention is to reduce chronicity through the prevention of complications and through active rehabilitation. In a public mental health context it often means maintenance treatment of serious mental illness with the goal of reducing relapse and of stimulating rehabilitation. The US Committee on Prevention of Mental Disorders in a volume called *Reducing risks for Mental Disorders: Frontiers for Preventive Intervention Research (1994)* relabeled secondary prevention as Treatment and tertiary prevention as Maintenance. Although their distinction may increase the goodness of fit of these terms for western-style mental health care systems, for low-income countries we regard this as an impoverishment of the original concepts.

On the individual level, a program requires the most trained and qualified staff for clinical interventions, secondary and tertiary prevention.

The left part of the circle in Figure 4 shows that many existing community and societal factors influence each of the interventions. These include those regarding human rights, governance, politics, environment, culture, traditions, socio-economic status and religion.

Universal, Selective and Indicated Preventive Interventions

Universal preventive interventions are targeted to the general public or a whole population group. This is critical, given that in many areas of the world there are insufficient resources to respond to large numbers of survivors. Universal interventions have advantages when their cost per individual is low, when the intervention is effective and accepted, and when there is low risk associated with the intervention.

Selective preventive interventions are targeted to subgroups of the population such as individuals whose risk of developing psychosocial or mental problems is higher than average. Some of these groups include child soldiers or groups of abducted people or rape victims.

Indicated preventive interventions are targeted to high-risk individuals who are identified as having minimal problems but show signs or symptoms foreshadowing neuropsychiatric problems. Examples are children with fits during a meningitis epidemic or a malaria attack, or torture survivors with head traumas.

Table 9 shows a theoretical matrix of the relation between primary, secondary and tertiary prevention, with the three types of preventive interventions. This matrix shows nine cells where different kinds of psycho-social or mental health activities can be located and can also be used to address the issue of complementarity between (post-)conflict emergency, rehabilitation and reconstruction efforts. For example, when UNHCR provides shelter and drinking water to a few hundred thousand refugees, it is a universal primary intervention at the community level. If in addition, UNICEF decides to set up a program for vaccination and psychosocial care for mothers and babies, it is a selective primary care intervention targeted at a whole subgroup. If the High Commissariat of Human Rights adds legal support to torture victims, it is an indicated primary preventive measure for individuals at high risk. And if WHO or an NGO decide to set up a project to prevent physically or mentally disturbed children to get worse or to prevent child soldiers to become criminals, it belongs to the realm of secondary prevention and it is a selective secondary preventive intervention.

Table 9. Matrix Showing the Relation Between Universal, Selective and Indicated Preventive Interventions, and Primary, Secondary and Tertiary Prevention

	Society-at-large/ (Inter)national	Community	Family and individual
Primary prevention	Universal interventions Selective interventions Indicated interventions	Universal interventions Selective interventions Indicated interventions	Universal interventions Selective interventions Indicated interventions
Secondary prevention (treatment)	Universal interventions Selective interventions Indicated interventions	Universal interventions Selective interventions Indicated interventions	Universal interventions Selective interventions Indicated interventions
Tertiary prevention (maintenance treatment)	Universal interventions Selective interventions Indicated interventions	Universal interventions Selective interventions Indicated interventions	Universal interventions Selective interventions Indicated interventions

Primary Prevention at the Level of the Society-at-Large, the Community, the Family and the Individual

The following paragraphs will show a range of preventive interventions that fit in the matrix presented in Table 9.

Table 10 shows a variety of primary preventive interventions that can be applied in an eclectic way in afflicted areas.

Primary Prevention in the Society-at-Large

Universal preventive interventions at the level of the society-at-large

(Inter)national laws. International and national laws, the criminal justice system and public policy can influence the occurrence or the outcome of traumatic events.

Defining and condemning traumatic events such as torture. Recognizing, defining and condemning the presence of traumatic events is a viable form of a societal intervention. For example, the United Nations' definition of governmental torture has brought considerable recognition to that form of traumatic event (cf Fairbank, Friedman, de Jong, & Green, 2001).

Research into the prevalence of events and their consequences. Efforts to define and measure traumatic events may result in an assessment of their prevalence and subsequently in a reduction of the frequency of these events. Our MIM-study provides data that helps us to improve and fine-tune our interventions. In addition, it verifies facts and helps to disclose the truth. This is in itself a form of non-monetary reparation that serves the moral and social welfare of the survivors.

Setting standards for intervention and training. Setting standards such as the WHO meeting in October 2000 on Mental Health of Refugees and Displaced Populations in Conflict and Post-conflict situations, the Guidelines for Progams

Table 10. Primary Prevention at the Level of the Society-at-Large, the Community, and the Family and Individual

	Society-at-large/(Inter)national	Community	Family and Individual
Primary prevention	**Universal preventive interventions**		
	(Inter)national laws		
	Public policy		
	Defining and condemning traumatic events such as torture		
	Research into the prevalence of events and their consequences		
	Setting standards for intervention and training		
	Free media and press		
	Expanding security institutions		
	Strengthening non-violent means of preventing and ending armed conflict		
	Voluntary repatriation		
	Define the military's role of last resort for preventing and ending armed conflict		
	Reinforcing peace initiatives & conflict resolution		
	Arms and landmine control		
	Economic pressure on nation states		
	Selective preventive interventions		
	War tribunals and the persecution of perpetrators Peace keeping forces		
	Indicated preventive interventions		
	Human rights advocacy (Co-occurring) Natural disasters: quality standards		
	Disaster preparedness training		

on Psychosocial and Mental Health Care Assistance in (Post-)Disaster and Conflict Areas (Aarts, 2000), the Guidelines on International Trauma Training (Weine, Danieli, de Jong, Fairbank, Saul, Shalev, Silove, Van Ommeren, & Ursano, 2000), the WHO-UNHCR Refugee Mental Health book (de Jong & Clarke, 1996), and hopefully this book as well, help to increase the quality of service provision to refugees and IDPs.

Free media and press. Support for free media and a free press is an important contribution to the recognition and the dissemination of information about events and to the exposure of human rights violations.

Expanding security institutions and strengthening non-violent means of preventing and ending armed conflict. Another set of universal preventive interventions is the prevention of conflicts that may lead to war, genocide or widespread violence. This entails a long-term action over a couple of decades. As mentioned before, it aims at a complex set of measures, including expanding global and regional security institutions, strengthening non-violent means of preventing and ending armed conflict, and *clarifying the military's role of last resort for preventing and ending armed conflict.*

Reinforcing peace initiatives and conflict resolution. Political leaders may be able to diminish hostility and can be stimulated by the international or regional community to build an atmosphere for social reconstruction or reconciliation (cf de Jong, 1995).

Voluntary repatriation. Another universal preventive activity is to work towards political solutions that allow for voluntary migration or repatriation to the place of origin as the chapter on Cambodia will discuss. When this is impossible and land is available, refugees can be allowed to settle in their new home country, as the example of Uganda will show.

Arms and landmine control. Arms control along with the banning of landmines is another universal preventive interventions. Despite the 1981 Land Mines Protocol, one out of every 236 Cambodians and one out of 1250 Vietnamese is handicapped as a result of the previous wars, and for every mine victim who makes it to the hospital, another died in the fields or on the way to the hospital (Asia Watch, 1991).

Economic pressure on nation states. Although economic pressure on states—including an economic boycott—often have an adverse effect on the marginalized people in a society, it is a way to undermine the credibility of populist politicians who prefer to increase the escalation of a conflict in their country. Economic pressure can only become an effective strategy when donor states do not compete with each other enabling the local politicians to thrive on this competition by divide and rule.

Selective preventive interventions at the level of the society-at-large

War tribunals and the persecution of perpetrators. In addition to the reinforcement of peace-increasing initiatives, the (inter)national community increasingly sees to it that perpetrators of gross violations of human rights or war criminals are brought to justice.

Peace keeping forces. Peace keeping and peace enforcing also play an important role in the prevention of re-escalation of armed conflicts.

Indicated preventive interventions at the level of the society-at-large
Human rights advocacy. Human rights advocacy can be regarded as a selective or indicated preventive measure. Every state has the responsibility to redress human rights violations and to enable victims to exercise their right to reparation. The UN and other intergovernmental organizations at the global and regional level can support and assist a proper consideration and management of reparation at national levels. Compensation to be paid in cash or in kind can also be viewed as a form of reparation. It includes health and mental health care, employment, housing, education and land (cf de Jong, 1995).

(Co-occurring) Natural disasters: quality standards. Sometimes natural disasters co-occur or are superimposed on previous traumatic events. The hurricanes in Middle America or the recent flooding in southern Africa or South East Asia are examples of these events. It is obvious that a number of (inter-)national initiatives can have a preventive effect. These can include setting quality standards for building in earthquake, landslide-prone areas or river bedding, or setting higher quality standards for the construction of nuclear power stations. Better accessibility of land in areas with land slides, better alarm systems for floods, cyclones or hurricanes, and sheltered areas of evacuation plans in areas that are hit by volcano eruptions or typhoons. Disaster preparedness training of the disaster-prone-segments of the population is an important preventive intervention.

Primary Prevention in the Community. Table 11 shows primary preventative universal and selective interventions *on the level of the community.*

Universal primary prevention at the community level
Rural development. In a previous paragraph I explained the relevance of rural development as a preventative and curative intervention. Rural development

Table 11. Primary Preventive Universal and Selective Interventions on the Level of the Community

	Society-at-large/ (Inter)national	Community	Family and Individual
Prevention (primary)	**Universal preventive interventions** Rural development Public education Empowerment Crisis intervention		

initiatives help refugees and local populations to enhance their survival capacities and increase their resiliency and quality of life. Rural development and vocational skills training instill hope and help survivors to acquire a sense of control and may thus help to prevent exacerbation of psychological disturbances. Since rural development is not part and parcel of the expertise of most mental health professionals, the following explains what we mean. Rural development refers to a process of change in rural areas leading to better living conditions and more secure livelihood for the population (Sterkenburg, 1987). This can be achieved through setting up small-scale income-generating projects such as palm oil presses, leather production, fishing, pottery, blacksmiths, cattle, rabit or poultry breeding. These income-generating projects may also compensate for a lack of land or space which is often inherent to the refugees' plight. Experience shows that IDPs and returnees are often unwilling to embark on long-term agriculture activities as they do not believe they will be able to stay long enough or be allowed to enjoy the benefits of these activities. Rural development may better fit their living situation as well as their aspirations to go back to their home country with a skill that they may apply later in life. These considerations have to be taken into account in the design and implementation of rehabilitation strategies for example by raising awareness of staff involved in relief and rehabilitation.

Because these activities also instill hope and help acquire a sense of control in precarious living conditions, they may help to prevent exacerbation of psychological disturbances and deterioration of social networks.

Public education is a community intervention with a potential to reach large numbers of people obtain information about aid, about legal rights, or any numbers of issues that will help them cope with their particular situation. Educational efforts can be used to educate those who have been through extremely stressful events, about what types of reactions are normal and common, as well as how to recognize unusual severe responses that require extra attention. In humanitarian crises, where normal modes of communication with the outside are damaged, public education can be used to quell rumors and help the community to have a more realistic view of the situation.

Public education can involve:

- Education of citizens on how to help those in the community who may be more vulnerable because they lost a family member or their possessions.
- Psycho-educational workshops on, for example, alcohol and drug use, child rearing, helpful styles of communication, mental disorders, and other mental health issues.
- Community campaigns through posters, leaflets, or group activities that promote positive mental health, for example, "Say NO to alcohol" or child rights campaigns.

- Media to heighten public awareness about types of behavior that are not well known or understood, such as abuse of physically or mentally disabled individuals. Public awareness can also be raised for the relation between specific physical disorders and mental disability (malaria, meningitis, AIDS) or between disabilities that are mistaken for retardation in school (bad vision or hearing).
- With regard to preventing violence of all types, toward children, spouses, the elderly and the disabled, young people can be trained in methods of conflict resolution as a way of settling disagreements.
- The use of educational material that promotes positive values, morals, and self-help can be presented in novel ways, like drama and story telling, that have the capacity to engage a larger or specialized audience. For example, the book of Baron (1994) to support children in conditions of massive trauma during their grief process, or the Kamla book that relates the tragic story of child prostitutes killed in the fire in Phuket in 1984 (Fairbank et al., 2002).

Community empowerment aims at revitalizing helping skills that are not utilized by the local people due to demoralization, collective apathy or a lack of appropriate knowledge. Empowerment activities involve community members to help themselves, their families, and their neighbors. These interventions lead to communal pride and a psychological sense of community (Sarason, 1974). They stimulate what Hobfoll calls "resource gain cycles" (Hobfoll, 1998).

These activities can be as simple as encouraging adults and children to get back to their normal routines, or as elaborate to develop activities that encourage interaction and promote self-esteem. Examples are:

- Activities that are conceptualized and implemented by the community itself, and contribute a sense of community efficacy. These may include religious activities, meetings, rallies, or the collaboration between healers and a psychosocial program. We work with collective healing and mourning rituals. Shraddhanjali is a mass grieving ceremony in Sri Lanka that promotes unity and collective action within the grief stricken community. Participation in such rituals may stimulate reflection on methods for rebuilding the community following a humanitarian crisis or dealing with a social concern.
- Strengthening coping skills among children. For example, among cattle-keepers from South Sudan, adolescent boys write poems for their initiation bull and poems about the traumatic events during the war. They tell each other dreams and analyze them in the group, because they consider that telling and analyzing dreams, like writing poems, is a way of healing the wounds of the past. For the same reason they weave problems from the past into the composition of songs (de Jong, 1995). These local coping styles were stimulated in our

program in Uganda and with Sudanese children in Ethiopia. In addition, we developed sport activities and children play groups to encourage constructive use of time. These activities also provide a venue for children to share their experiences with others (see the chapter on Uganda; Paardekooper, 2002). Some empowerment activities target the whole community. Other activities have a more selective character when they focus on vulnerable subgroups such as single and teen-aged parents, low socioeconomic or isolated families, the elderly or disabled, or children. For example, the TPO-Cambokids program in Cambodia created a save and stimulating context for children in Phnom Penh in the form of a guided playground. Both traumatized and non-traumatized children were seen there. They participated on a voluntary basis. Young children could create their own healing process under the guidance of an enthusiastic group of young adult volunteers. Traditional dance and music workshops as well as home-manufactured games offered room for the expression and structuring of emotions. Next to the therapeutic work with the children, the project served as a laboratory for the development of educational and healing games.

Other projects address children within the school setting, and involve teachers, school counselors, parent groups, and the media in protecting children's rights. The focus is on providing children with skills for self-articulation and increasing body awareness. The school uses various formats to support the children, such as puppet shows, street theatre, films/documentaries, discussion, and other creative exercises and games.

- Women centers for social and occupational activities and for baby care.
- After educating the community on how to help those who may be more vulnerable, social networks can be developed to promote solidarity and social support among peers within villages, neighborhoods, and housing units.

Capacity building is another preventive intervention, which according to the group being trained, can be a universal or a selective intervention. Most national health systems are not prepared for large-scale traumatic stress so there usually is a need for the training of local people to effectively engage in sustainable activities that fit to the culture, traditions and the language. Training activities should have immediate, mid- and long-term components, grounded in local educational and training structures, and prepare trainees for their future work.

To compensate for the lack of mental health professionals in low-income countries we construed a cascade of a 'TOTOT' (Training of Trainers of Trainers), followed by a 'TOT' (Training of Trainers) who then train subsequent levels within the local community. The TOTOT results in a group of qualified local and international trainers. From 2002 onwards TPO will organize—together with WHO and other partners—a Master's University Course to ensure that there will be more internationally qualified culturally sensitive trainers in the field of psychosocial and mental health care in low-income countries.

The TOTOT will share their expertise with the TOT (Training of Trainers). The TOT results in a Core Group of local (para-) professionals that depending on the size of the target group of refugees and IDPs may vary from six to twelve people per country. The Core Group builds on local experience and culture-specific coping styles and tries to achieve a synthesis between local and international approaches to deal with traumatic stress. On the one hand the participants of the TOT or the Core Group receive training and supervision of the TOTOT, whereas after some time they start to cascade down and train and supervise subsequent levels of trainees. During this whole training process we use a multisectoral approach. Thus our training programs cascade throughout the existing government structures for health, education, social and women's affairs, to the communities and the people.

Mechanisms of training are different in refugee and IDP situations. For IDPs living in their own countries the local government is responsible and often motivated for training. Refugees, however, live in a foreign country. Though the central host government may in theory accept responsibility for their care, local government structures often feel burdened by the refugees and are not interested in capacity building. As the chapter on Uganda shows, the inclusion of nationals in a program may increase the motivation of the local government to endorse a psychosocial and mental health program.

Training programs are different in developed and developing countries and countries in transition. In developed countries training includes the use of interpreters and developing knowledge and skills in intercultural communication, diagnosis and treatment so that local indigenous professionals can assist people from a wide variety of cultures. In most countries in transition, both professionals and service providers need to develop additional skills in the field of psychosocial and traumatic stress. In developing countries where qualified professionals are scarce, training programs need to work with lay people, paraprofessionals and community leaders to build up a core group of resource people leading to more systematic training and educational institutions (Baron, Jensen, & de Jong, 2002).

The curriculum includes discussion about the normal response to trauma, basic helping or counseling skills, overview of psycho-social and mental health problems, symptoms and treatment, methods of crisis response and how to make a referral to other available helpers (De Jong 2000). Staffs of NGOs are often interested to learn relevant listening skills, since children and adolescents often choose to unburden themselves to youth workers rather than teachers or parents.

The different chapters in this book provide examples of this model in the different countries where the reader can see that there are variations in the duration and content of the training, and the availability of ongoing supervision and refresher training.

Security measures. Survivors of wars (and sometimes natural disasters as well) are often re-traumatized by robbers or gangs of armed bandits. Shelling, ambushes or land mines may increase their plight. Whereas in refugee camps the relief workers and the internationals often live in designated areas, the refugees who live in general areas may have to protect themselves. A simple universal preventive intervention at the community level is to create as safe an environment as possible, especially in camps with a majority of women and children.

Decreasing dependency. Many relief agencies focus on materials and logistics and do not regard psychological problems as an issue. Both in developing countries and in the West, refugee camps or reception centers easily become 'total institutions' (Goffman, 1961). A dependency syndrome may develop that reinforces the learned helplessness that quickly emerges in the wake of war or natural disaster. This can happen especially in those camps that reproduce the authoritarian regimes from which the refugees escaped, possibly reproduced by the militarist approach of some relief agencies or peacekeepers.

To make matters worse, after imposing learned dependency, donor agencies tend to complain about the dependent and inert behavior of the refugees. In combination with previous traumatic stress and other risk factors such as marginalization, discrimination, poverty, poor physical health, collapse of networks and acculturative stress, this process easily leads to secondary traumatization.

Many refugees are resilient people from cultures that have developed ingenious coping strategies. In addition to the above-mentioned attempts to empower refugees, we try to decrease dependency by involving refugees in management and administrative issues. Refugees can assist in setting up community interventions, monitoring the program, helping with health education and public education, stimulate their contribution in distributing food, or assist in PHC-activities. Some people may provide interpreter services, teachers can be involved in education programs for adults and children, and traditional birth attendants in reproductive health. We encourage religious leaders and healers to continue their ceremonies and we stimulate musicians, dancers, and storytellers to organize leisure activities.

Primary and Selective Prevention at the Level of the Family and the Individual

Universal and Selective primary prevention at family level

Family reunion/family tracing. In our view a supportive network, mentioned in Table 12—preferably the family—is the main vehicle for healing (Qouta, 2000; Paardekoper, 2002). As mentioned before, we see western-style orphanages or children villages as a last resort, because these kinds of facilities may create additional problems such as being a breeding place for bandits or prostitution. In collaboration with other organizations we promote abandoned or orphaned children being accommodated within their extended family or within foster families. Simultaneously we try to assess whether one or both parents or other first or second grade family members are alive.

Table 12. Primary Universal and Selective Preventive Interventions at the Family and Individual Level

	Society-at-large/ (Inter)national	Community	Family and Individual
Prevention (primary)			**Universal and Selective Interventions** Family reunion/family tracing Improvement physical aspects

Improvement of physical aspects. For the psychosocial well-being of refugees it is important that they are involved in the development of their life world including the physical aspects of the camp. This includes discussing acceptable amounts of water, decreasing overcrowding in camps, allotting land to grow vegetables, varying diets, or drainage of the terrain. Sometimes relief agencies are not aware of the cultural taboos that surround for example the disposal of waste or excrements. In 1997 fear of possession pervaded a Bhutanese refugee camp in Nepal (see the chapter on Nepal). Clusters of adolescents experienced attacks of 'spirits' in the form of medically unexplained somatic symptoms, especially fainting and dizziness. In addition to the belief that the spirits of two lovers who had committed suicide were still on earth, it was believed that these spirits were now disturbed by the camp's filth, caused by human waste, violation of cultural sanitary beliefs, and thoughts of premarital sex (Van Ommeren, Sharma, Komproe, Sharma, Cardeña, Thapa, Poudyal, & de Jong, 2001).

Secondary Prevention at the Level of the Society-at-Large, the Community and the Family

The goal of secondary prevention is to shorten the course of an illness by early identification and rapid or crisis intervention. Table 13 shows several secondary preventative interventions.

Reparation and compensation. A universal secondary preventative measure is reparation and compensation. An international forum concluded that every state has the responsibility to redress human rights violations and to enable victims to exercise their right to reparation (Van Boven et al., 1992). The UN and other intergovernmental agencies at the global and regional level should support and assist a proper consideration and management of reparation at national levels. Compensation is a form of reparation that is to be paid in cash or to be provided

Table 13. Secondary Prevention at the Level of the Society-at-Large, the Community and the Family

	Society-at-large/(inter)national	Community	Family and Individual
Secondary Prevention	Universal, Selective and Indicated Interventions[a]	Universal, Selective and Indicated Interventions[a]	**Universal, Selective and Indicated Interventions**[a]
Treatment	Reparation and compensation	Self-help groups for ex-combatants and ex-child soldiers, widows, unaccompanied minors, survivors of rape and torture, elderly and others	Family/network building Counseling Individual, group and family therapy Pharmacotherapy

[a]To reduce the complexity of the matrix, the three types of preventive interventions (universal, selective and indicated) are taken together.

in kind. The latter includes health and mental health care, employment, housing, education and land (Van Boven et al., 1992; de Jong, 1995).

Self-help groups. Self-help groups can function to help people with similar problems help each other. They help to eliminate the need of a trained helping person. Several chapters of this book show examples of organizing these groups for ex-combatants, ex-child soldiers, widows, unaccompanied minors, survivors of rape and torture, mothers of the vulnerable such as mothers with handicapped children, the elderly, and Alcoholics Anonymous (AA) groups for alcoholics.

Family/network building. These interventions promote the family network or another type of network to help those who have psychosocial and mental health problems. It also promotes families with similar problems to help each other. It includes the following interventions:

- Working with groups of families who share similar traumatic experiences like families of the disappeared, murdered, or abducted.
- Local ceremonies and rituals that promote family cohesion and solve all kinds of social conflicts. For example, conflicts regarding mutual obligations such as paying a dowry, assisting the family of in-laws, producing means of production by bearing children, or the distribution of scarce resources such as land.
- Engaging victimized families in human rights organizations.

Counseling. Counseling is an inflated word covering an ill-defined range of activities without clear criteria for the qualifications of the counselor. The metaphor of the Anglo-Saxon counselor as a post-modern shaman carries a title which has no equivalent in the major European languages. (Para-)professionals and volunteers engaged in the field of psychosocial care, mental health care, or legal issues of repatriation may call themselves counselors. People trained for three days in basic helping skills and university educated people can also be called counselors. We prefer the term mental health worker and we try to use the term psychosocial counselor in those countries where our trainees adhere to the title of counselor. We are working on developing international criteria for certification as a psychosocial counselor in our programs. Our main psychosocial counseling activities include:

- Paraprofessional counselors are recruited among the target population with a set of selection criteria (see the chapter on Uganda). They provide problem solving and supportive counseling for psychosocial and mental health problems. In situations of acute stress they may provide crisis counseling or psychological debriefing. Relaxation—and sometimes self-dialogue through the repetition of a word or verse—is practiced in our programs, often in conjunction with local cultural and religious practices (as explained in the chapters on Cambodia and Sri Lanka). Counseling is either offered in the home of a client or in community based counseling centers. Counseling may be conducted in a family setting, a group setting or on an individual basis.

Individual and family therapy. Psychotherapy requires extensive training and supervision. At the lower end of the aforementioned intervention pyramid the amount of people requiring this form of treatment is small but present. In many developing countries this level of treatment is hardly available due to a lack of expertise. The approach can be individual, couple, family or group therapy. Examples are:

- Trauma therapy
- Testimony work
- Group therapy for traumatized children
- Group therapy for survivors of violence
- Systemic family therapy

In countries in transition and in some low-income countries with a considerable number of psychologists such as Algeria, South Africa and Namibia, professionals may want to use forms of psychotherapy that are commonly used in high-income countries. These would include cognitive-behavioral therapy including exposure therapy, cognitive therapy, cognitive processing therapy, stress inoculation training, systematic desensitization, assertiveness training and relaxation training. Exposure therapy is the most rigorously evaluated individual intervention. Exposure treatment methods involve confronting fearful memories within the context of a safe therapeutic relationship. The process involves intentionally experiencing and maintaining the distress associated with the traumatic event(s) until the distress diminishes. Other approaches are psychodynamic therapy or more recently developed techniques such as EMDR (Shapiro, 1995) or Thought Field Therapy (Callahan).

Pharmacotherapy. Because psychobiological abnormalities are involved in sequential traumatic stress and PTSD, medication can be used, alone or in combination with psychotherapy or counseling. Pharmacological treatments include tricyclic antidepressants or selective serotonin reuptake inhibitors (SRRIs), inhibitors of adrenergic activity and mood stabilizers.

Tertiary Prevention at the Level of the Society-at-Large, the Community and the Family

The goal of tertiary prevention is to reduce chronicity through the prevention of complications and through active rehabilitation. Usually, the concept of tertiary prevention in mental health care relates to the problem of institutionalization of patients. Institutionalization results in the disruption of social skills and rejection by family members and by others in the patient's usual social support network.

All TPO projects function in areas where mental health facilities are far away and hardly or not accessible, or where institutions are destroyed or disrupted. The interventions take place in collectivistic cultures where—as long as family members are around—rejection by the family is exceptional. These circumstances provide us with ample opportunities to provide after-care and involve the family to increase compliance with long-term treatment. It is remarkable that

Table 14. Tertiary Preventative Interventions

	Society-at-large/ (Inter)national	Community	Family and Individual
Tertiary Prevention (Maintenance Treatment)	Universal, Selective and Indicated Interventions[a]	Universal, Selective and Indicated Interventions[a] Public education	**Universal, Selective and Indicated Interventions**[a] Treatment of the chronic mentally ill and of people with epilsepsy Self-help (family) groups for children/adults with handicaps

[a]To reduce the complexity of the matrix, the three types of preventive interventions (universal, selective and indicated) are taken together.

most of our programs cover large populations with no or very limited possibilities to admit people in hospitals. Table 14 mentions several tertiary preventative interventions on a community level.

Psychotropic drugs are used for people with reactive or chronic psychoses, depression, anxiety disorders or epilepsy. Self-help groups including family members are set up for children who are mentally disabled, for people with epilepsy, and for those who suffer from a serious chronic mental disorder such as schizophrenia.

The principles of this first chapter will be illustrated in the following chapters of this book. Each program applies them in an eclectic way and moulds them to the requirements of the specific sociocultural context.

REFERENCES

Aarts, P. G. H. (2000). *Guidelines for programmes: Psychosocial and mental health care assistance in (post-)disaster and conflict areas.* Utrecht, the Netherlands: NIZW International Centre.

Abas, M., Broadhead, J. C., Mbape, P., & Khulamo-Sakatukwa, G. (1994). Defeating depression in the developing world: A Zimbabwean model. *British Journal of Psychiatry, 164,* 293–296.

Abramson, H. (2000). The esh kodesh of rabbi Kalonimus Kalmish Shapiro: A hasidic treatise on communal trauma from the Holocaust. *Transcultural Psychiatry, 37*(3), 321–335.

Abu Hein, F., Qouta, S., Thabet, A., & El Sarraj, A. (1993). Trauma and mental health of children in Gaza. *British Medical Journal, 306,* 1130–1131.

Abu Naser, J. (1985). *Effects of war on children in Lebanon.* Beirut, Lebanon: Institute for Women's Studies in the Arab World.

Adamolekum, B. (1995) The aetiologies of epilepsy in tropical Africa. *Tropical and Geographical Medicine, 47*(3), 115–117.

Ager, A. (2001). Psychosocial programmes: Principles and practice for research and evaluation. In F. Ahearn (Ed.), *Psychosocial wellness of refugees: issues in quantitative and qualitative research.* Oxford, England: Berghahn Books.

Akerele, O. (1987). Bringing traditional medicine up to date. *Social Science and Medicine, 24,* 177–181.

Allen, T. (1991). Understanding Alice: Uganda's holy spirit movement in context. *Africa, 61*(3), 370–400.

Allodi, F. (1991). Assessment and treatment of torture victims: A critical review. *Journal of Nervous and Mental Disease, 170* (1) 4–11.

American Psychiatric Association (1994). *Diagnostic and statistical manual of mental disorders* (4th ed.). Washington, DC.

Andersen, R. M. (1995). Revisiting the behavioral model and access to medical care: Does it matter? *Journal of Health and Social Behavior, 36,* 1–10.

Arroyo, W. & Eth, S. (1995) Children traumatized by Central American warfare. In R. S. Pynoos & S. Eth (Eds.), *Posttraumatic stress disorder in children* (pp. 103–120). Washington DC: American Psychiatric Association.

Asia Watch & Physicians for Human Rights (1991). *Land mines in Cambodia: The coward's war.* New York/Boston.

Baker, A. (1990). The psychological impact of the intifada on Palestinian children in the occupied West Bank and Gaza: An exploratory study. *The American Journal of Orthopsychiatry, 60,* 496–505.

Baron, N. (1994). *A little elephant finds its courage.* Colombo, Sri Lanka: Author.

Baron, N., Jensen, S. B., & de Jong, J. T. V. M. (2002). The mental health of refugees and internally displaced people. In B. Green, M. Friedman, J. de Jong, S. Solomon, J. Fairbank, T. Keane, B. Donelan, & E. Frey-Wouters (Eds.), *Trauma in war and peace: Prevention, practice and policy*. New York: Kluwer Academic/Plenum Publishers.

Bagilishya, D. (2000). Mourning and recovery from trauma: in Rwanda, tears flow within. *Transcultural Psychiatry, 37*(3), 337–353.

Becker, G., Beyene, Y., & Ken, P. (2000). Health, welfare reform, and narratives of uncertainty among Cambodian refugees. *Culture, Medicine and Psychiatry, 2*, 139–163.

Berry, J. W., Poortinga, Y. H., Segall, M. H., & Dasen, P. R. *Cross-cultural psychology: Research and applications*. Cambridge, England: Cambridge University Press.

Blank, A. S. (1994). Clinical detection, diagnosis and differential diagnosis of PTSD. *The Psychiatric Clinics of North America, 8*, 351–384.

Bromet, E. J. (1995). Methodological issues in designing research on community-wide disasters with special reference to Chernobyl. In S. E. Hobfoll & M. W. De Vries (Eds.), *Extreme stress and communities: impact and intervention* (pp. 267–283). Dordrecht, the Netherlands: Kluwer.

Blue, I. & Harpham, T. (1998). Investing in mental health research and development. *British Journal of Psychiatry, 172*, 294–295.

Boothby, N., Upton, P., & Sultan, A. (1991). *Children of Mozambique: The cost of survival*. Washington, DC: U.S. Committee for Refugees.

Breslau, N. & Davis, G. C. (1987). Posttraumatic stress disorder: The etiologic specificity of wartime stressors. *American Journal of Psychiatry, 144*(5), 578–583.

Brewin, C. R., Andrews, B., & Valentine, J. D. (2000). Meta-analysis of risk factors for posttraumatic stress disorder in trauma-exposed adults. *Journal of Consulting and Clinical Psychology, 68*(5), 748–766.

Bronfenbrener, U. (1979). *Ecology of the family as a context for human development: Research perspectives*. Cambridge, MA: Harvard University Press.

Bryman, A. (1992). *Quantity and quality in social research*. London: Routledge.

Cheng, A. T. A. & Chang, J. C. (1999). Mental health aspects of culture and migration. *Current opinion in psychiatry, 12*, 217–222.

Cohen, R. E. & Ahearn, F. L. (1991). *Handbook of mental health care for disaster victims*. London: John Hopkins University Press.

Cohen, R. E. & Deng, F. M. (1998). *Masses in flight: The global crisis of internal displacement*. Washington, DC: The Brookings Institution.

Cohon, J. D. (1981). Psychological adaptation and dysfunction among refugees. *International Migration Review, 15*, 255–275.

Corcoran, J. D. T. (1982). The concentration camp syndrome and USAF Vietnam prisoners of war. *American Journal of Psychiatry, 10*, 991–994.

Corradi, J. Weiss Fagen, P., & Garreton, M. (1992). *Fear at the edge: state terror and resistance in Latin America*. Berkeley, CA: University of California Press.

Craig, G. & Fowlie, A. (1997). *Emotional freedom techniques: The manual*. Novato, CA: Author.

Cutrona, C. E. & Russell, D. W. (1987). The provisions of social relationships and adaptations to stress. *Advances in personal relationships, 1*, 37–67.

Davidson, J. R. T. & Foa, E. B. (Eds.) (1993). *Posttraumatic stress disorder: DSM-IV and beyond*. Washington, DC: American Psychiatric Association Press.

Dawes, A. (1990). The effects of political violence on children: A consideration of South African and related studies. *International Journal of Psychology, 25*, 13–31.

Dawes, A., Tredoux, C., & Feinstein, A. (1989). Political violence in South Africa: some effect on children of the violent destruction of their community. *International Journal of Mental Health, 19*, 16–43.

De Girolamo, G. & McFarlane, A. C. (1996). The epidemiology of PTSD: A comprehensive overview of the international literature. In A. J. Marsella, M. J. Friedman, E. T. Gerrity, &

R. M. Scurfield (Eds.), *Ethnocultural aspects of posttraumatic stress disorder* (pp. 35–36). Washington, DC: American Psychological Association.

de Jong, J. T. V. M. (1987). *A descent into African psychiatry*. Amsterdam: Royal Tropical Institute.

de Jong, J. T. V. M. (1995). Prevention of the consequences of man-made or natural disaster at the (inter)national, the community, the family and the individual level. In S. E. Hobfoll & M. W. de Vries (Eds.), *Extreme stress and communities: Impact and intervention* (pp. 207–229) Boston: Kluwer.

de Jong, J. T. V. M. (1996a). A comprehensive public mental health programme in Guinea-Bissau: A useful model for African, Asian and Latin-American countries. *Psychological Medicine, 26,* 97–108.

de Jong, J. T. V. M. (1996b). *TPO program for the identification, management and prevention of psychosocial and mental health problems of refugees and victims of organized violence within primary care of adults and children* (7th version). Amsterdam: Transcultural Psychosocial Organization. Internal document.

de Jong, J. T. V. M. (1999). Psychotherapie met immigranten en vluchtelingen [Psychotherapy with immigrants and refugees]. In T. J. Heeren, R. C. van der Mast, P. Schnabel, R. W. Trijsburg, W. Vandereycken, K. van der Velden, & F. C. Verhulst (Eds.), *Jaarboek voor psychiatrie en psychotherapie* (pp. 220–238). Houten, the Netherlands: Bohn Stafleu Van Loghum.

de Jong, J. V. T. M. (2000). Psychiatric problems related to persecution and refugee status. In F. Henn, N. Sartorius, H. Helmchen, & H. Lauter (Eds.), *Contemporary psychiatry* (Vol. 2, pp. 279–298). Berlin, Germany: Springer.

de Jong, J. T. V. M. (2001). Remnants of the colonial past: The difference in outcome of mental disorders in high- and low-income countries. In R. Littlewood & D. Bhugra (Eds.), *Psychiatry and colonialism*. Delhi, India: Oxford University Press.

de Jong, J. T. V. M. & Clarke, L. (1996) (Eds.). *Mental health of refugees*. Geneva: World Health Organisation. (TPO has produced an Arabic, a Nepali, a Khmer, a Dutch, a Portuguese and a Tamil version of this book).

de Jong, J. T. V. M., Eisenbruch, M, Van de Put, W. A. M., Van Ommeren, M., Ketzer, E., Sharma, B., Somasundaram, D., Mandlhate, C., & Komproe, I. (manuscript submitted for publication). Bringing order out of chaos: The identification, management of prevention of psychosocial and mental health problems of refugees and victims of organized violence within primary care. *Journal of Traumatic Stress*.

de Jong, J. T. V. M., Komproe, I. H., Van Ommeren, M., El Masri, M., Mesfin, A., Khaled, N., Somasundaram, D., & Van de Put, W. A. M. (2001a). *Lifetime events and post-traumatic stress disorder in four post-conflict settings. Journal of the American Medical Association, 286*(5), 555–562.

de Jong, J. T. V. M., Komproe, I. H., Van Ommeren, M., El Masri, M., Mesfin A., Van de Put, W. A. M., & Somasundaram, D. (2001b). *Prevalence and co-morbidity of psychiatric disorders in traumatised communities from Algeria, Cambodia, Ethiopia, and Gaza*. Manuscript submitted for publication.

de Jong, J. T. V. M. & Van Schaik, M. M. (1994). Culturele en religieuze aspecten van traumaverwerking naar aanleiding van de Bijlmerramp [Cultural and religious aspects of coping with trauma after the Bijlmer disaster]. *Tijdschrift voor Psychiatrie, 36*(4), 291–304.

Desjarlais, R., Eisenberg, L., Good, B., & Kleinman, A. (1995). *World mental health: Problems and priorities in low-income countries*. New York: Oxford University Press.

Dohrenwend, B. P. (Ed.) (1998). *Adversity, stress and psychopathology*. New York: Oxford University Press.

Dunkel-Schetter, C. & Bennett, T. L. (1990). Differentiating the cognitive and behavioral aspects of social support. In B. Sarason, I. Sarason, & G. Pierce (Eds.), *Social support: An interactional view* (pp. 267–296). New York: Wiley.

Dyregrov, A. & Raundalen, M. (1993). *A longitudinal study of war-exposed children in Iraq*. Presentation at the International Conference on Mental Health and the Challenge of Peace, September 13–15, 1993, Gaza, Palestine.

Eisenbruch, M. (1984). Cross-cultural aspects of bereavement: I, A conceptual framework for comparative analysis. *Culture, Medicine and Psychiatry, 8*(3), 283–309.

Eisenbruch, M. (1984). Cross-cultural aspects of bereavement: II, Ethnic and cultural variations in the development of bereavement practices. *Culture, Medicine and Psychiatry, 8*(4), 315–347.
El Sarraj, E., Punamäki, R. L., Salmi, S., & Summerfield, D. (1996). Experiences of torture and ill-treatment and posttraumatic stress disorder symptoms among Palestinian political prisoners. *Journal of Traumatic Stress, 9,* 595–606.
Eth, S. & Pynoos, R. S. (1985). Developmental perspective on psychic trauma in childhood. In C. G. Figley (Ed.), *Trauma and its wake.* New York: Plenum Press.
Farias, P. (1994). Central and South American refugees: Some mental health challenges. In A. J. Marsella, T. Borneman, S. Ekblad, & J. Orley (Eds.), *Amidst peril and pain: The mental health and well-being of the world's refugees* (pp. 101–115). Washington, DC: American Psychological Association.
Fairbank, J., Friedman, M., de Jong, J. T. V. M., & Green, B. (2002). Integrated intervention strategies for traumatic stress. In B. Green, M. Friedman, J. T. V. M. de Jong, T. Keane, & S. Solomon (Eds.), *Trauma in war and peace: Prevention, practice, and policy.* New York: Kluwer Academic/Plenum Publishers.
Finkler, K. (1997). Gender, domestic violence and sickness in Mexico. *Social Science and Medicine, 45*(8), 1147–1160.
Flanzbaum, H. (Ed.). (1999). *The americanization of the Holocaust.* Baltimore: John Hopkins University Press.
Folkman, S. (1984). Personal control and stress and coping processes: A theoretical analysis. *Journal of personality and social psychology, 46,* 839–852.
Freud, S. (1920). Beyond the pleasure principle. In J. Strachey (Ed. and trans.), *The standard edition of the complete psychological works of Sigmund Freud* (Vol. 17). London: Hogarth Press.
Friedman, M. J. & Jaranson, J. (1994). The applicability of the post-traumatic stress disorder concept to refugees. In A. J. Marsella, T. Bornemann, S. Ekblad, & J. Orley (Eds.), *Amidst peril and pain: The mental health and well-being of the world's refugees.* Washington, DC: American Psychological Association.
Friedman, M. J. & Schnurr, P. P. (1995). The relationship between trauma, post-traumatic stress disorder and physical health. In M. J. Friedman, D. S. Charney, & A. Y. Deutch (Eds.), *Neurobiological and clinical consequences of stress: From normal adaptation to post-traumatic stress disorder* (pp. 507–524). Philadelphia: Lippincott-Raven Publishers.
Friedman, M. J., Warfe, P. G., Mwiti, G. K. (2002). Mission related stress and its consequences among UN peacekeeers and civilian field personnel. In B. Green, M. Friedman, J. de Jong, S. Solomon, J. Fairbank, T. Keane, B. Donelan, & E. Frey-Wouters, E. (Eds.), *Trauma in war and peace: Prevention, practice and policy.* New York: Kluwer Academic/Plenum Publishers.
Fukuyama, F. (1999). *The great disruption: Human nature and the reconstitution of social order.* New York: Free Press.
Geffray, C. (1990). *La cause des armes au Mozambique. Anthropologie d'une guerre civile* [The origins of armed struggle in Mozambique: The anthropology of a civil war]. Paris: Karthala.
Giel, R. (1998). Natural and human-made disasters. In B. P. Dohrenwend (Ed.), *Adversity, stress and psychopathology* (pp. 66–76). New York: Oxford University Press.
Goffman, E. (1961). *Asylums: Essays on the social situations of mental patients and other inmates.* Garden City, NY: Doubleday.
Goldberg, D. & Huxley, P. (1992). *Common mental disorders: A bio-social model.* London: Routledge.
Goody, J. (1962). *Death, property and the ancestors: A study of the mortuary customs of the Lodagaa of West Africa.* Stanford, CA: Stanford University Press.
Goodwin, J. (1988). Posttraumatic symptoms in abused children. *Journal of Traumatic Stress, 1,* 475–488.
Green, A. (1992). *Introduction to health planning in developing countries.* Oxford, England: Oxford University Press.

Green, B. L. (1993). Identifying survivors at risk: Trauma and stressors at cross events. In J. P. Wilson & B. Raphael (Eds.), *International handbook of traumatic stress syndromes* (pp. 135–144). New York, Plenum.

Green, B., Friedman, M., de Jong, J., Solomon, S., Fairbank, J., Keane, T., Donelan, B., & Frey-Wouters, E. (2002). *Trauma in war and peace: Prevention, practice and policy*. New York: Kluwer Academic/Plenum Publishers.

Halpern, E. (1982). Child help steps in a natural setting: Children's support systems in coping with orphanhood. In N. A. Milgram, C. D. Spielberger, & I. Sarason (Eds.), *Stress and anxiety* (pp. 261–266). New York: Hemisphere Publishers.

Harrell-Bond, B. (1986). *Imposing aid: Emergency assistance to refugees*. Oxford, England: Oxford University Press.

Helzer, J. E., Robbins, L. N., & McEvoy, L. (1987). Post-traumatic stress disorder in the general population: Findings of the Epidemiological Catchment Area Survey. *New England Journal of Medicine, 317*, 1630–1634.

Hendin, H. A. & Haas, P. (1991). Suicide and guilt as manifestations of PTSD in Vietnam combat verterans. *American Journal of Psychiatry, 148*(5), 586–591.

Hobfoll, S. E. (1998). *Stress, culture and community: The psychology and philosophy of stress*. New York: Plenum Press.

House, J. S. (1981). *Work, stress and social support*. Reading, MA: Addison Wesley.

Hubbard, J., Realmoto, G. M., Northood, A. K., & Masten, A. S. (1995). Comorbidity of psychiatric diagnoses with PTSD in survivors of childhood trauma. *Journal of the American Academy of Child and Adolescent Psychiatry, 34*(9), 1167–1173.

Hudelson, P. M. (1994). *Qualitative research for health programmes*. Geneva: World Health Organization.

ICH/CPMP. *Guideline for good clinical practice including the Declaration of Helsinki and the Belmont Report*. London: ICH (7 Westferry Circus, Canary Wharf, London E14 4HB).

Institute for Defense and Disarmament Studies. (1999). *Global action to prevent war: A coalition-building effort to stop war, genocide & internal armed conflict* (May 2000, rev. 14). Cambridge, Mass.: Author. Available http: www.globalactionpw.org/gapw-mainpages/rev14.shtml.

International Federation of the Red Cross and Red Crescent Societies. (1993). *World disasters report*. Dordrecht, the Netherlands: Martinus Nijhoff.

Irish, D. P., Lundquist, K. F., & Nelsen, V. J. (Eds.). (1993). *Ethnic variation in dying, death and grief: Diversity in universality*. Washington, DC: Taylor & Francis.

Janoff-Bulman, R. (1992). *Shattered assumptions: Towards a new psychology of trauma*. New York: Free Press.

Jensen, P. S. & Shaw, J. (1993). Children as victims of war: Current knowledge and future research needs. *Journal of the American Academy of Child and Adolescent Psychiatry, 32*, 697–708.

Jeyaraja Tambiah, S. (1992). *Buddhism betrayed?: Religion, politics, and violence in Sri Lanka*. Chicago: University of Chicago Press.

Kagawa-Singer, M. & Chi-Yung Chung, R. (1994). A paradigm for culturally based care in ethnic minority populations. *Journal of Community Psychology, 22*, 192–208.

Kaplan, C. D., Korf, D., & Sterk, C. (1987). Temporal and social contexts of heroin-using populations. *Journal of Nervous and Mental Disease, 175*(9), 566–574.

Kaplan, H. I. & Sadock, B. J. (1985). *Comprehensive textbook of psychiatry* (Vol. 4). Baltimore: Williams and Wilkins.

Keehn, R. J. (1980). Follow-up studies of World War II and Korean conflict prisoners. *American Journal of Epidemiology, 111*, 194–211.

Kessler, R. C., Sonnega, A., Bromet, E., Hughes, M., & Nelson, C. B. (1995). Posttraumatic stress disorder in the National Comorbidity Survey. *Archives of General Psychiatry, 52*(12), 1048–1060.

Kinzie, J. D. & Manson, S. (1983). Five years experience with Indochinese refugee psychiatric patients. *Journal of Operational Psychiatry, 14*, 105–111.

Kinzie J. D., Sack, W. H., Angell, R. H., Clarke, G., & Ben, R. (1989). A three-year follow-up of Cambodian young people traumatised as children. *Journal of the American Academy of Child and Adolescent Psychiatry, 28*, 501–504.

Kinzie, J. D., Sack, W. H., Angell, R. H., Manson, S., & Rath, B. (1986). The psychological effects of trauma on Cambodian children: I, The children. *Journal of the American Academy of Child and Adolescent Psychiatry, 25*(3), 370–376.

Kirmayer, L. J. (1996). Confusion of the senses: Implications of ethnocultural variations in somatoform and dissociative disorders for PTSD. In A. J. Marsella, M. J. Friedman, E. T. Gerrity, & R. M. Scurfield (Eds.), *Ethnocultural aspects of posttraumatic stress disorder: Issues, research, and clinical applications* (pp. 131–163). Washington, DC: American Psychological Association.

Kleinman, A. (1977). Depression, somatization and the new cross-cultural psychiatry. *Social Science and Medicine, 11*, 3–10.

Kleinman, A. (1988). *The illness narratives: Suffering, healing and the human condition.* New York: Basic Books.

Kleinman A. & Good, B. (Eds.). (1985). *Culture and depression.* Berkeley, CA: University of California Press.

Kolb, L. L. & Multipassi, L. R. (1982). The conditioned emotional response: A subclass of the chronic and delayed post-traumatic stress disorder. *Psychiatric Annals, 12*, 979–987.

Korf, D. J. (1997). The tip of the iceberg: Snowball sampling and nominating techniques, the experience of Dutch studies. In *Estimating the prevalence of problem drug use in Europe* (EMCODA scientific monograph series no. 1). Brussels: Council of Europe.

Krueger, R. A. (1994). *Focus groups: A practical guide for applied research* (2nd ed.). Thousand Oaks, CA: Sage.

Krystal, H. (1978). Trauma and affects. *Psychoanalytic Study of the Child, 33*, 81–116.

Laufer, R. S. (1988). The serial self: War trauma, identity and adult development. In J. P. Wilson, Z. Harel & B. Kahana (Eds.), *Human adaptation to extreme stress from the Holocaust to Vietnam* (pp. 33–45). New York: Plenum Press.

Lazarus, R. S. & Folkman, S. (1984). *Stress, appraisal and coping.* New York: Springer.

Lazarus, R. S. & Launier, R. (1978). Stress-related transactions between person and environment. In L. A. Pervin & M. Lewis (Eds.), *Perspectives in interactional psychology* (pp. 287–327). New York: Plenum.

Ledoux, J. E., Romanski, L. & Xagoraris, A. (1989). Indelibility of subcortical emotional networks. *Journal of Cognitive Neuroscience, 1*, 238–243.

Litz, B. T., Keane, T. M., Fisher, L., Marx, B., & Monaco, V. (1992). Physical health complaints in combat related posttraumatic stress disorder. *Journal of Traumatic Stress, 5*, 131–141.

Lobel, M. L. & Dunkel-Schetter, C. (1990). Conceptualizing stress to study effects on health: Environmental, perceptual, and emotional components. *Anxiety Research, 3*, 213–230.

Machel, G. (1996). *The impact of armed conflict on children.* New York: United Nations. Report submitted to General Assembly resolution 48/175.

Macksoud, M. S. & Aber, J. L. (1996). The war experiences and psychosocial development of children in Lebanon. *Child Development, 67*, 70–88.

Maher, D. (1999). The internationally recommended tuberculosis control strategy. *Tropical Doctor, 7*, 185–186.

Maher, D., Chaulet, P., Spinaci, S., & Harries, A. (1997). *Treatment of tuberculosis: guidelines for national programs.* Geneva: World Health Organization.

Mahjoub, A. (1995). *Approche psychosociale des traumatismes de guerre chez les enfants et adolescents palestiniens* [A psychosocial approach of war trauma among Palestinian children and adolescents]. Tunis, Tunisia: Editions de la Méditerranée.

Marmar C. R., Weiss, D. S., Schlenger, W. E., Fairbank, J. A., Jordan, K., Kulka, R. A. & Hough, R. L. (1994). Peritraumatic dissociation and posttraumatic stress in male Vietnam theater veterans. *American Journal of Psychiatry, 151*, 902–907.

Marsella, A. J., Bornemann, T., Ekblad, S., & Orley, J. (Eds.). (1994). *Amidst peril and pain: The mental health and well-being of the world's refugees.* Washington, DC: American Psychological Association.

Martin, S. F. (1994). A policy perspective on the mental health and psychosocial needs of refugees. In A. J. Marsella, T. Borneman, S. Ekblad, & J. Orley (Eds.), *Amidst peril and pain: The mental health and well-being of the world's refugees* (pp. 69–83). Washington, DC: American Psychological Association.

McFarlane, A. C., Atchison, M., Rafalowicz, E., & Papay, P. (1994). Physical symptoms in posttraumatic stress disorder. *Journal of Psychosomatic Research, 38,* 715–726.

McFarlane, A. C. & De Girolamo, G. (1996). The nature of traumatic stressors and the epidemiology of posttraumatic reactions. In B. Van der Kolk, A. C. McFarlane, & L. Weisaeth (Eds.), *Traumatic stress: The effects of overwhelming experience on mind, body and society* (pp. 129–154). New York: Guilford.

McFarlane, A. C. & Yehuda, R. (1996). Resilience, vulnerability, and the course of posttraumatic reactions. In B. Van der Kolk, A. C. McFarlane, & L. Weisaeth (Eds.), *Traumatic stress: The effects of overwhelming experience on mind, body and society* (pp. 155–181). New York: Guilford.

Médecins sans Frontières. (1997). *Refugee health. An approach to emergency situations.* London: Macmillan.

Meichenbaum, D. (1997). *Treating post-traumatic stress disorder. A handbook and practice manual for therapy.* New York: Wiley.

Mghir, R., Freed, W., Raskin, A., & Katon, W. (1995). Depression and posttraumatic stress disorder among a community sample of adolescent and young adult Afghan refugees. *Journal of Nervous and Mental Disease, 183,* 124–130.

Mollica, R. (1994). Southeast Asian refugees: Migration history and mental health issues. In A. J. Marsella, T. Borneman, S. Ekblad, & J. Orley (Eds.), *Amidst peril and pain: The mental health and well-being of the world's refugees* (pp. 83–100). Washington, DC: American Psychological Association.

Mollica, R., Donelan, K., Svang, T. O. R., Lavelle, J., Elias, C., Frankel, M., & Blendon, R. J. (1993). The effect of trauma and confinement on functional health and mental health status of Cambodians living in Thailand-Cambodia border camps. *JAMA, 270*(4), 581–586.

Mollica, R., McInnes, K., Poole, C., & Tor, S. (1998). Dose-effect relationships of trauma to symptoms of depression and post-traumatic stress disorder among Cambodian survivors of mass violence. *British Journal of Psychiatry, 173,* 482–488.

Mrazek, P. J. & Haggerty, B. J. (1994). *Reducing risks for mental disorders: Frontiers for preventive intervention research.* Washington, DC: National Academy Press.

Müller, M., de Jong, J. T. V. M., Komproe, I., & de Jong, B. (2002). *Traumatic stress and its consequences in Uganda.* Manuscript submitted for publication.

Murray, C. & Lopez, A. D. (1996). *The global burden of disease.* Geneva: World Health Organization.

Murthy, R. S. (1998). Rural psychiatry in developing counties. *Psychiatric Services, 49*(7), 967–969.

Nader, K. O., Pynoos, R. S., Fairbanks, L. A., Al-Ajeel, M., & Al-Asfour, A. (1993). A preliminary study of PTSD and grief among the children of Kuwait following the Gulf crisis. *British Journal of Clinical Psychology, 32,* 407–416.

Newell, K. (Ed.). (1975). *Health by the people.* Geneva: World Health Organization.

Novick, P. (1999). *The Holocaust in American life.* Boston: Houghton Mifflin.

Obeseyesekere, G. (1985). Depression, Bhuddism and the work of culture. In A. Kleinman & B. Good (Eds.), *Culture and depression* (pp. 134–152). Berkeley, CA: University of California Press.

Paardekoper, B. P. (2002). *Children of the forgotten war.* Doctoral dissertation, Vrije Universiteit, Amsterdam.

Paardekoper, B. P., de Jong, J. T. V. M., & Hermanns, J. M. A. (1999). The psychological impact of war and the refugee situation on South Sudanese children in refugee camps in northern Uganda: An exploratory study. *Journal of Child Psychology and Psychiatry, 40*(4), 529–536.

Parkes, C. M., Laungani, P., & Young, B. (Eds.). (1997). *Death and bereavement across cultures.* London: Routledge.

Pennebaker, J. W. (1993). Mechanisms of social constraint. In D. M. Wegner & J. W. Pennebaker (Eds.). *Handbook of mental control* (pp. 200–219). Englewood Cliffs, NJ: Prentice Hall.

Pennebaker, J. W. & Susman, J. R. (1988). Disclosure of traumas and psychosomatic processes. *Social Science and Medicine, 26*, 327–332.

Pitman, R. K. (1988). Post-traumatic stress disorder, conditioning and network theory. *Psychiatric Annals, 18*(3), 182–189.

Pitman, R. K. (2000). *Stress hormones and the amygdala in PTSD: Possible implications for secondary prevention.* Presentation at the 16th Annual Meeting of the International Society for Traumatic Stress Studies, San Antonio, Texas.

Punamäki, R. L. (1987). *Children under conflict.* Tampere, Finland: Tampere Peace Research Institute.

Punamäki, R. L. (1989). Political violence and mental health. *International Journal of Mental Health, 17*, 3–15.

Punamäki, R. L. (1996). Can ideological commitment protect children's psychosocial wellbeing in conditions of political violence? *Child Development, 67*, 55–69.

Punamäki, R. L. & Suleiman, R. (1990). Predictors and effectiveness of coping with political violence among Palestinian children. *British Journal of Social Psychology, 29*, 67–77.

Pynoos, R. S., Groenjian, A. K., & Steinberg, A. M. (1998). A public mental health approach to the postdisaster treatment of children and adolescents. *Child and Adolescent Psychiatric Clinics of North America, 7*(1), 195–210.

Pynoos, R. S. & Nader, K. (1988). Psychological first aid and treatment approach to children exposed to community violence: Research implications. *Journal of Traumatic Stress, 1*(4), 445–473.

Pynoos, R. S. & Nader, K. (1993). Issues in the treatment of posttraumatic stress in children and adolescents. In J. P. Wilson & B. Raphael (Eds.), *International handbook of traumatic stress syndromes* (pp. 535–549). New York: Plenum.

Qouta, S. (2000). *Trauma, violence and mental health: The Palestinian experience.* Unpublished doctoral dissertation, Vrije Universiteit, Amsterdam.

Raphael, B. & Wilson, J. (Eds.). (2000). *Psychological debriefing: Theory, practice and evidence.* Cambridge, England: Cambridge University Press.

Rappaport, J. (1981). In praise of a paradox: A social policy of empowerment over prevention. *American Journal of Community Psychology, 9*, 1–25.

Rogler, L. H. & Cortes, D. E. (1993). Help-seeking pathways: A unifying concept in mental health care. *American Journal of Psychiatry, 150*(4), 554–561.

Rosenbaum, M. & Ronen, T. (1992). *How did Israeli children and their parents cope with the threat of daily attacks by scud missiles during the Gulf war?.* Presentation at the ministry of Education Conference on the Stress Reaction of Children in the Gulf War, Rmat Gan, Israel.

Rosenblatt, P. C., Walsh, R. P., & Jackson, D. A. (1976). *Grief and mourning in cross-cultural perspective.* New Haven, CT: HRAF Press.

Sack, W. H., Clarke, G., Him, C., Dickason, D., Goff, B., Lanham, K., & Kinzie, D. (1993). A 6-year follow-up study of Cambodian refugee adolescents traumatized as children. *Journal of the American Academy of Child and Adolescent Psychiatry, 32*(2), 432–437.

Sack, W. H., McSharry, S., Clarke, G. N., Kinney, R., Seeley, J., & Lewinsohn, P. (1994). The Khmer adolescent project: I, Epidemiologic findings in two generations of Cambodian refugees. *Journal of Nervous and Mental Disease, 182*, 387–395.

Salimovich, S., Lira, E., & Weinstein, E. (1992). Victims of fear: The social psychology of repression. In J. Corradi, P. Weiss Fagen, & M. Garreton, *Fear at the edge: state terror and resistance in Latin America* (pp. 72–89). Berkeley, CA: University of California Press.

Sarason, S. B. (1974). *The psychological sense of community: Prospects for a community psychology.* Washington, DC: Jossey-Bass.

Selye, H. (1976). *The stress of life* (Rev. ed.). New York: McGraw-Hill.

Sen, A. (1997). *On economic inequality.* Oxford, England: Oxford University Press.

Shalev, A., Bleich, A., & Ursano, R. J. (1990). Posttraumatic stress disorder: Somatic comorbidity and effort tolerance. *Psychosomatics, 31*, 197–203.

Shalev, A. Y. (1996). Stress versus traumatic stress: From acute homeostatic reactions to chronic psychopathology. In B. Van der Kolk, A. C. McFarlane, & L. Weisaeth (Eds.), *Traumatic stress: The effects of overwhelming experience on mind, body and society* (pp. 77–101). New York: Guilford.

Shapiro, F. (1995). *Eye movement desensitization and reprocessing: Basic principles, protocols and procedures.* New York: Guilford.

Sharma, B. & Van Ommeren, M. (1998). Preventing torture and rehabilitating survivors in Nepal. *Transcultural Psychiatry, 35,* 85–97.

Shisana, O. & Celentano, D. D. (1987). Relationship of chronic stress, social support, and coping style to health among Namibian refugees. *Social Science and Medicine, 24*(2), 145–157.

Shrestha, N. M., Sharma, B., Van Ommeren, M., Regmi, S., Makaju, R., Komproe, I., Shrestha, C., & de Jong, J. T. V. M. (1998). Impact of torture on refugees displaced within the developing world: Symptomatology among Bhutanese refugees in Nepal. *JAMA, 280*(5), 1–6.

Sieswerda, S., Komproe, I., Hanewald, G., & de Jong, J. T. V. M. (2002). *Mental health and pychosocial problems of Sudanese refugees living in Ugandan camps.* Manuscript submitted for publication.

Siegler, M. & Osmond, H. (1974). *Models of madness, models of medicine.* New York: Harper & Row.

Solomon, S. D. (2002). Overview. In B. Green, M. Friedman, J. T. V. M. de Jong, T. Keane, & S. Solomon (Eds.), *Trauma in war and peace: Prevention, practice, and policy.* New York: Kluwer Academic/Plenum Publishers.

Solomon, S. D. & Davidson, J. R. T. (1997). Trauma: Prevalence, impairment, service use, and cost. *Journal of Clinical Psychiatry, 58*(suppl. 9), 5–11.

Solomon, Z. (1994). The pathogenic effects of war stress: The Israeli experience. In S. E. Hobfoll & M. W. de Vries (Eds.), *Extreme stress and communities: Impact and intervention* (pp. 229–247). Boston: Kluwer.

Solomon, Z., Mikulincer, M., & Arad, R. (1991). Monitoring and blunting: implications for combat-related posttraumatic stress disorder. *Journal of Traumatic Stress, 4,* 209–221.

Solomon, Z., Mikulincer, M., & Habershaim, N. (1990). Life-events, coping strategies, social resources, and combat complaints among combat stress reaction casualties. *British Journal of Medical Psychology, 63,* 137–148.

Somasundaram, D., Van de Put, W. A. M., Eisenbruch, M., & de Jong, J. T. V. M. (1999). Starting mental health services in Cambodia. *Social Science and Medicine, 48*(8), 1029–1046.

Sterkenburg, J. J. (1987). *Rural development and rural development policies: Cases from Africa and Asia.* Utrecht, the Netherlands: Rijksuniversiteit Utrecht, Geografisch Instituut.

Straker, G., Mendelsohn, M., Moosa, F., & Tudin, P. (1996). Violent political contexts and the emotional concern of township youth. *Child Development, 67,* 46–54.

Straus, A. (1987). *Qualitative analysis for social scientists.* Cambridge, England: Cambridge University Press.

Summerfield, D. (2000). Childhood, war, refugeedom and 'trauma': Three core questions for mental health professionals. *Transcultural Psychiatry, 37*(3), 417–435.

Tardy, C. H. (1985). Social support measurement. *American Journal of Community Psychology, 13,* 187–202.

Tedeschi, R. D., Parc, C. L., & Calhoun, L. G. (Eds.). (1998). *Post-traumatic growth: Positive changes in the aftermath of crisis.* London: Lawrence Erlbaum.

Terr, L. (1979). Children of Chowchilla: A study of psychic trauma. *Psychoanalytic Study of the Child, 34,* 547–623.

Terr, L. (1985). Psychic trauma in children and adolescents. *Psychiatric Clinics of North America, 8*(4), 815–835.

Terr, L. (1991). Childhood traumas: An outline and overview. *American Journal of Psychiatry, 148,* 10–20.

Thabet, A. & Vostanis, P. (2000). Post traumatic stress disorder reactions in children of war: A longitudinal study. *Child Abuse and Neglect, 24*(2), 291–298.

Thoits, P. A. (1986). Social support as coping assistance. *Journal of Consulting and Clinical Psychology, 54,* 416–423.

Thomas, L. (1982). *La mort Africaine: Idéologie funéraire en Afrique noire* [African death: Funeral ideology in black Africa]. Paris: Payot.
Toole, M. J. & Waldman, R. J. (1993). Refugees and displaced persons: war, hunger and public health. *JAMA, 270,* 600–605.
Tricket, E. J. (1995). The community context of disaster and traumatic stress: An ecological perspective from community psychology. In S. E. Hobfoll & M. W. De Vries (Eds.), *Extreme stress and communities: impact and intervention* (pp. 11–25). Boston: Kluwer.
Tseng, W.-S. & Strelzer, J. (Eds.). (1997). *Culture and psychopathology: A guide to clinical assessment.* New York: Brunner/Mazel.
Tylor, C. E. (1984). *The uses of health systems research: Public health papers.* Geneva: World Health Organization.
United Nations High Commissioner for Refugees (2000a). *Refugees and others of concern to UNHCR, 1999 Statistical overview: Table I.1, Indicative number of refugees and others of concern to UNHCR by region, 1998 and 1999.* Available http: www.unhcr.ch/statist/99/overview/tab101.pdf October 20, 2000.
United Nations High Commissioner for Refugees (2000b). *Refugees and others of concern to UNHCR, 1999 Statistical overview: Table II.2, Indicative refugee population and major changes by origin, 1999.* Available http: www.unhcr.ch/statist/99/overview/tab202.pdf October 20, 2000.
UNICEF. (1997). *The state of the world's children: 1997.* Oxford: Oxford University Press.
United States Committee on Prevention of Mental Disorders. (1994). *Reducing risks for mental disorders: frontiers for preventive intervention research.* Washington, DC: National Academy Press.
United States Committee for Refugees (1996). *World Refugee Survey 1996.* Washington, DC.
United States Committee for Refugees (1997). *World Refugee Survey 1997.* Washington, DC.
United States Committee for Refugees (1999). *World Refugee Survey 1999.* Washington, DC.
Üstün, T. B. & Sartorius, N. (Eds.) (1995). *Mental illness in general health care.* Chichester, England: Wiley.
Van Boven, T., Flinterman, C., Grünfeld, F., & Westendrop, I. (Eds.) (1992). *Seminar on the rights to restitution, compensation and rehabilitation for victims of gross violations of human rights and fundamental freedoms.* Maastricht, the Netherlands: University of Limburg.
Van de Goor, L., Rupesinghe, K., & Sciarone, P. (1996). *Between development and destruction: An enquiry into the causes of conflict in post-colonial states.* London: MacMillan.
Van der Kolk, B. (1996). The body keeps the score: Approaches to the psychobiology of PTSD. In B. Van der Kolk, A. C. McFarlane, & L. Weisaeth (Eds.), *Traumatic stress: The effects of overwhelming experience on mind, body and society* (pp. 214–242). New York: Guilford.
Van der Kolk, B., McFarlane, A., & Weisaeth, L. (Eds.). (1996). *Traumatic stress: The effects of overwhelming experience on mind, body and society.* New York: Guilford.
Van Ommeren, M. H. (2000). *Impact of torture: Psychiatric epidemiology among Bhutanese refugees in Nepal.* Doctoral dissertation, Vrije Universiteit, Amsterdam.
Van Ommeren, M., Sharma, B., Komproe, I. H., Sharma, G. K., Cardeña, E., Thapa, S., Poudyal, B., & de Jong, J. T. V. M. (2001). Trauma and loss as determinants of culture-bound epidemic illness in a Bhutanese refugee community. *Psychological Medicine, 31,* 7:1259–1267.
Van Ommeren, M., Sharma, B., Sharma, G. K., de Jong, J. T. V. M., & Cardeña, E. (2001). *The relationship between somatic and PTSD symptoms among Bhutanese refugee torture survivors.* Manuscript submitted for publication.
Van Ommeren, M., Sharma, B., Thapa, S., Makaju, R., Prasain, D., Bhattarai, R., & de Jong, J. T. V. M. (1999). Preparing instruments for transcultural research: Use of the translation monitoring form with Nepali-speaking Bhutanese refugees. *Transcultural Psychiatry, 36*(3), 285–301.
Ventura, M. M. F. (1997). *O stress postraumático e suas sequelas nos adolescentes do sul de Angola* [Posttraumatic stress and its consequences among adolescents in South Angola]. Unpublished doctoral dissertation, Minho University, Minho, Portugal.
Vines, A (1991). *Renamo terrorism in Mozambique.* Bloomington, IN: Indiana University Press.

Weine, S., Danieli, Y., de Jong, J. T. V. M., Fairbank, J., Saul, J., Shalev, A., Silove, D., Van Ommeren, M., & Ursano, R. (2000). *Draft guidelines for international trauma training*. Manuscript in preparation.

Westermeyer, J. (1985). *A clinical guide to alcohol and drug problems*. Philadelphia: Praeger.

Westermeyer, J. (1986). Planning mental health services for refugees. In C. Williams, & J. Westermeyer (Eds.), *Refugees' mental health issues in resettlement countries*. New York: Hemisphere.

Westermeyer, J. (1989). *Psychiatric care of migrants: A clinical guide*. Washington, DC: American Psychiatric Press.

Williams, H. A. (1990). Families in refugee camps. *Human Organization, 49*, 100–109.

Wilson, K. B. (1992). Cults of violence and counter-violence in Mozambique. *Journal of Southern African Studies, 18*, 531–582.

World Health Organization (1990). *The introduction of a mental health component into primary health care*. Geneva.

Wortmann, C. B., & Silver, R. C. (1989). The myths of coping with loss. *Journal of Consulting and Clinical Psychology, 57*, 349–357.

Yesavage, J. A. (1983). Dangerous behavior by Vietnam veterans with schizophrenia. *American Journal of Psychiatry, 140*, 1180–1183.

Yip, R. & Sharp, T. W. (1993). Acute malnutrition and childhood mortality related to diarrhea: Lessons from the 1991 Kurdish refugee crisis. *JAMA, 270*, 587–590.

Zivcic, I. (1993). Emotional reactions of children to war stress in Croatia. *Journal of the American Academy of Child and Adolescent Psychiatry, 32*, 709–713.

2

The Cambodian Experience

W. A. C. M. VAN DE PUT and MAURICE EISENBRUCH

CAMBODIA

Along a muddy road some twenty kilometers from the town of Pursat there is a signboard with information on psychosocial problems. We asked people about this, and were taken to the mee-phum, the village chief. He told us that this community had many problems. There were many people who felt hopeless about their lives, even so many years after the war and the Khmer Rouge regime. Some had simply given up, could not work any longer, and remained in their houses. People who were already poor became even poorer, and were even more hopeless. Other started drinking or gambling, and had violent fights at home or with others. Some were just feeling ill, could no longer care to look after their children.

As mee-phum and head of the village development committee, our informant was sincerely interested in how things could get better. He had therefore been interested when he was visited by two women who started talking to him about these kind of problems. They had proposed to discuss problems such as alcohol abuse, domestic violence, and feelings of hopelessness with the villagers. They had had several animated discussions, and found that the presentations of the women had helped them see their problems in a different perspective.

The women organized group meetings to further discuss specific problems. Some women from the village then started their own weekly 'meetings', and slowly people began to talk more about the gruesome events of the past and difficulties of more recent times. It turned out that this was not just causing old wounds to open, but actually could make people feel better. People began to realize that they might help each other improving these conditions. A man who had now joined the discussion told us he had actually tried to stop drinking. He had not stopped completely. At times grief would still overcome him and he could not help himself but by drinking. But things had become much better now that he felt he could at least control himself to a degree. He could work again, and was better able to look after his family.

The woman who then joined said she had learned a lot about emotional problems. After her husband died she started drinking heavily too. Now, she tried to help other families, and was enthusiastic about her weekly meetings with the women's group. She said the new information on causes of suffering and the relation with things that happened in the past had helped them to look again at problems and see that something could be done. Not everything would be solved—but at least life had become worth living at times.

INTRODUCTION

Cambodia had a history of violence and oppression when at the end of the 1960s the country was torn apart by civil war. In 1975 the 'Khmer Rouge' started their infamous nation-wide experiment in social engineering that has come to be known as 'the killing fields'. This affected every family, every community and all aspects of public life in Cambodia. Millions died, the country uprooted, religious life shattered and educational systems stopped. The Khmer Rouge regime of 'Democratic Kampuchea' was toppled by Vietnamese troops in 1979, but 'low-intensity-warfare' continued throughout the 1980s. In the 1990s the political situation slowly began to improve. After the second elections, in 1998, a process of normalization seems to have taken root in Cambodia, where the war has given way to enduring poverty, the legacy of landmines, and a disastrous AIDS epidemic.

Much has been written about mental health problems of the hundreds of thousands of Cambodians who fled to other countries (Eisenbruch, 1990a,b, 1991; Boehnlein, 1985; Kinzie, 1997; Mollica, 1994). Less is known about how the people in Cambodia cope with their experience. The authors of this chapter had independently worked in Cambodia and were struck by the obvious psychological suffering of the population. In 1992, through discussions with Cambodian representatives of the Ministry of Health, the Ministry of Women Affairs, and the University of Phnom Penh, the idea for a psychosocial intervention program was born.

A program to implement the community mental health approach of the Transcultural Psychosocial Organization (TPO) was started in 1995, with the aim of identification, prevention and management of psychosocial problems (de Jong, 1997). The program sought to develop interventions to enable people and communities overcome traumatic events. In this chapter we describe the context, the implementation and some of the results of this program. After a brief introduction of Cambodia's recent history we sketch the cultural and social context in which we worked. We then describe how we attempted to develop and implement appropriate interventions that could complement the already existing local systems of care.

TRAUMA IN CAMBODIA

Cambodia is one of the many low-income countries that provided the battlefields for the cold war. It was, and still is, a rather homogenous society.

'Pre-Revolutionary Cambodia was 80 percent peasant, 80 percent Khmer, and 80 percent Buddhist. First, it was an overwhelmingly rural economy. Its village society was decentralized, its economy unintegrated, dominated by subsistence rice cultivation. Compared to Vietnam, its villagers participated much less in village-organized activities. They were often described as individualistic; the nuclear family was the social core' (Kiernan, 1996).

Warfare and cruelty have always been part of Cambodian history, as the bas-reliefs on the monuments of the Angkor period testify. From the perspective of the present day generations of Cambodians, the last decades have been a succession of periods that each brought special difficulties.

Towards the end of the 1960s the whimsical Prince Sihanouk, who had ruled Cambodia as the 20th century version of the mythical-historical god-king, lost his grip on domestic developments and Cambodia was drawn into the war in Vietnam. The coup by Lon Nol in 1970 started a five-year civil war that killed at least 10% of the population. Many deaths were the effect of the American bombing campaigns that served little strategic purpose (Shawcross, 1979). The 'Khmer Rouge', the sobriquet Sihanouk gave to the communist resistance in the 1960s, recruited many young people from the destroyed villages. Social life was brought to a standstill, the eastern half of the country was destroyed and fronts kept shifting. Hundreds of thousands fled to Phnom Penh, and when the city fell to the Khmer Rouge in April 1975, the people welcomed them vaingloriously as saviours from this horrible war.

'Democratic Kampuchea', as the country was formally named, turned out to be an unprecedented experiment in social engineering while it marked the only period between 1970 and 1991 wherein the country was not at war. The complete, absolute rule of the anonymous party (*'Angkar') over ordinary people was mixed with intrigue, machination and 'cleansing' between factions of various revolutionary ideologies. It will always remain difficult to separate the mass graves made by Khmer Rouge cadres from the ditches used to bury the victims of American bombs, but a total of 1.5 million is seen by many as an acceptable estimation of those put to death. This amounts to 25% of the Cambodian population of 1975.

The fabric of social life suffered under the unprecedented violence of civil war in Cambodia, but the Khmer Rouge attempted to actively destroy it. Many people were killed for political reasons, but most deaths were the result of policies aimed at transforming a traditional, family centered Asian society overnight into a state-centered, self-supporting communist model (Vickery, 1984; Kiernan, 1996). Urban groups exposed to hard labor in the rural areas were the first victims. When communal eating was forced upon all families it was clear for all Cambodians alike that the *Angkar was out for some new shape of society that nobody could imagine or understand. Pagodas were destroyed. Monks were defrocked and forced to marry. Traditional healers were used simply for their knowledge of herbs—but as servants, breaking the respect they had in villages. Mass marriages were arranged between men and women selected by the party. Families were torn apart. Many of the young Khmer Rouge cadres were given positions of authority over much older people, with a 'license to kill'. Traditional rituals were debunked by new party rituals. Traditional Cambodian life as people knew it was almost snuffed out.

On 7 January 1979, after 3 years, 8 months and 20 days, the state of Democratic Kampuchea was thrown over by Vietnamese troops. The horrors of the Khmer Rouge regime came to the attention of the world as refugees started arriving in Thailand. Although clear signals about what was happening in Cambodia had been given before (e.g. Ponchaud, 1978), there was now a worldwide outcry about the massive scale of terror and the enormous number of victims. The scope of events seemed unique, autogenocide was coined as a term, and the 'killing fields' became famous.

Cold war logic made the Khmer Rouge, the enemy of the Vietnamese, an acceptable ally for Western powers for another eleven years. Aid was organized for refugees in camps at the border between Cambodia and Thailand. The 'border camps' housed up to 350,000 refugees until the repatriation of 1993. A huge variety of programs were set up by many international organizations in these camps, while Cambodia itself remained unaided by the West, supported instead by Warsaw Pact countries (Myslewic, 1988).

The world fabricated an explanation of what had happened, and this 'Standard Total View' (Vickery, 1984) reduced the complex Cambodian reality to a story of a harmonious, innocent, self-supporting society, made up of smiling people, that was suddenly disrupted by the terror of a group of barbarous communists. It allowed all those for whom it was politically convenient to see the rule of the Khmer Rouge as a breach in timeless Khmer history. The context of a long existence of cruelty in Khmer history and the more recent effect of the massive bombing campaign of the United Sates in 1972–3 escaped attention. The relief and rehabilitation programs in the border camps, and later on in Cambodia, unconsciously adopted such a view. The representation of the suffering of the Cambodian people in books, films and aid-programs was filtered through this two-dimensional version of reality. Thus a picture was built of Cambodians being victims of one of these extreme yet incomprehensible cases of 'Asian cruelty'.

Meanwhile, in Cambodia, the Vietnamese control of the country caused intense fear amongst the population. Cambodian masters over decades had labelled the Vietnamese as the archenemy of the Cambodian people. Many expected no less than total eradication. Khmer Rouge guerillas penetrated deep into the countryside and had bases everywhere. In the infamous K5 projects many Cambodians were dragooned by Vietnamese to build a fanciful bamboo wall to keep out the Khmer Rouge in deforestation projects in highly malaria-endemic and mined areas—many did not survive.

Low intensity warfare continued to harass the population even after a peace agreement was brokered between the parties in Paris in 1991. A massive peacekeeping, elections-enforcing and disarmament intervention by the United Nations in 1992–4 did not succeed in disarming the parties, but brought back the refugees from the Thai border and organised elections in 1993. The coalition patchwork government blew up in July 1997.

The Khmer Rouge was holding out along the Northern and Eastern borders. Within months of exposure and show trial in a jungle makeshift court room by his former generals, Pol Pot expired in April 1998. Weeks later, twenty-three years after they had taken control of Cambodia, the Khmer Rouge ceased to exist as a military force. Elections were held in 1998, and at the time of writing Cambodia has a government that seems to be the most stable since the time of Sihanouk in the 1960s.

The Need for a Cambodian Perspective

Cambodian history is complex and tragic. In order to find out whether Cambodian people could be helped to help themselves, one has to understand the country, the culture, and its people at various levels. The orchestrated way the Vietnamese authorities organized 'days of hate' and fabricated political explanations strengthened the tendency of individual people to refer to 'standard histories'. This safe representation of what had happened to Cambodia as a whole served to avoid political risk, while there was little interest among families in details of what had happened to others. In understanding problems of people we had to discover 'local histories'. Some people considered the civil war and the massive bombarding a more difficult period than the Khmer Rouge years. Others suffered more after the fall of Pol Pot, when they were caught between warring factions at the Thai border or were forced to join the 'K5' projects.

What are the coping mechanisms of all those that still function—how do people cope with loss, and what do they believe to be causes of illness and misfortune? When people try to explain how they have coped with the loss of a child, cultural concepts such as the 'former mother'—the mother of the baby in its previous life who may reclaim the baby—are essential to know what people mean. And when people talk about hope, desperation, suicide, guilt, anger and acceptance, one needs to know what is meant.

Foetal and Neonatal Death

People in rural areas have few options to avoid the loss of children and must believe in some cosmic and physical reality to make sense of the spectre of high infant mortality. Healers offer hope and a system of response for parents who would otherwise remain totally helpless in facing the prospect of such loss.

> Whether a fetus dies in utero or the infant dies in early life, the general term used is 'diseased child' (*?aarih koon). Usually, the postpartum 'diseased child' refers to one of two main subtypes. In the first, the child suffers from 'child not harmonious' (*koon min kaap). In the second subtype, in which the child died at the hands of ancestral spirits or its preceding mother, the condition includes 'disease of the preceding mother' (*?aarih mdaay daem) or as *'skan of the disease of the preceding mother'. For the most part the healers attribute the child's illness to defects in its mother.

Traditional beliefs and traditional healers of many kinds are essential in offering people at least a thread of continuous identity in the massive turmoil that threatened their existence and their culture. Any intervention aimed at alleviation of psychological suffering needs to be complementary to—and at an absolute minimum, informed about, the work of these healers.

Coming to a full understanding of Cambodian tradition and culture is not the objective of the project in Cambodia. The idea was to build a shared understanding between the Cambodian and international members of the team. Based on literature, but much more on everyday conversations and working experience with villagers, we have tried to use these insights in the design of interventions. We will attempt to describe aspects of psychological and social suffering in Cambodia before we turn to these interventions.

PSYCHOSOCIAL AND MENTAL HEALTH PROBLEMS

In discussions with families throughout Cambodia everyday problems are easily related to the events of the past. People who have given up hope and stopped functioning in the sense of being able to do their daily tasks are known to all. Those that started drinking too much after the loss of a beloved one are to be found in any village. Domestic violence is widespread. Sleeping disorders, recurrent nightmares—it is all so common that it is not seen to be any special problem that might be helped. Families with more severe problems in coping with traumatic events of the past have, in many cases, lost all their possessions in their search for help. These families are easily identified by anyone in any village. Roughly 20% of families in villages assessed were considered to be dysfunctional by their fellow villagers, and this included anything from alcoholism to extreme poverty, from not being able to take care of children in the household to recurrent violence, abuse or chronic disease.

These problems do not always seem directly related to gruesome events in the past. To the outsider it even seems that many families blame past events for present-day problems that are found in any developing society: poverty, growing pressure on available land, a bad harvest or the impact of modern media on traditional values. The link between historical and social events and present day individual problems is easier understood when the effect of decades of civil war and social upheaval are taken into account, in a society that as such has been the focus of destruction. Whatever the material destruction wrought by bombs and artillery, the Khmer Rouge's aimed target was destruction of traditional social, family and religious life—resulting in a much deeper crater in the Cambodian psyche.[1]

In Cambodia the whole population, and not merely selected groups, lived through the years of horror. Only age might be used to distinguish between groups with different levels of exposure to traumatic experiences. But while some people are still haunted by memories of events that date back to the 1940s, others have experienced traumatic events recently, as the case of Vanna shows.

Case: Older Woman in Kandaal Province

...After discussing the aim of our work with a teacher in (the village) the team was directed to an older lady named Vanna who was living opposite his house. According to the teacher Vanna had problems, because she went bankrupt. The team found her in the space under her traditional Khmer house. She had never left her house since she went bankrupt, some months ago. Her business, transporting goods from the village to the market by oxcart, went bankrupt after one of the oxen she bought with borrowed money died. There was no more income, so Vanna had to sell the other ox and the cart in order to pay her debts, and than still she owed more money. She felt ashamed about that, and told us that she did not want to walk through the village anymore. Vanna belonged to a well-known family, her father had been the governor of the district when she was a young girl, and she felt awful about having lost everything.

When the team asked how she started the business she told that she needed an extra source of income after her son had married and went living with the family of his wife. She had two other sons and a teenager daughter. Two years ago her elder son's life ended upon standing of a landmine in the forest close to the village. Her younger son, still living with her, was severely mutilated in the same explosion, and his handicap rendered him almost unmarriageable. So she felt she could not refuse when a family in the village offered to marry their daughter to him without asking a dowry—even though she felt the marriage might not be right. Her mind remained preoccupied with the landmine-accident that had changed so much. What still hurts her is how

---

[1]The destruction of religious, ritual and family life challenged people's basic values and worldviews. In trauma-theory, this should lead to a compensatory search for meaning, which, when frustrated, leads to psychological and physical distress. Various theoretical approaches to explain the occurrence of stress disorders include the use of a behavioral conditioning framework, or a focus on a psychodynamic perspective, or an information and emotional processing model, or a constructivist perspective, while others explore the social dimensions of people's responses to traumatic events in terms of the loss of resources (Meichenbaum, 1995). In all these theories 'meaning' is an essential concept: people need to rebuild their worldview in order to overcome trauma. The search for meaning has been made virtually impossible by the continuity of dramatic episodes in Cambodian history.

she was not able to be with her son when he died. When the news of the accident came to the village, some neighbors took Vanna to the pagoda, to be with the monks who would know 'how to keep her calm'. Her sons were brought to the hospital. When she heard about the accident she ran to the hospital, although the monks had warned her not to go. She saw her sons, and when she came out of the hospital, she was so confused that she did not pay attention and was hit by a car. After some days in the hospital recovering from her wounds she was brought back to the pagoda. The villagers had brought her there in the first place because they remembered her strong emotional reaction in 1977, months after her second husband had been arrested by Khmer Rouge cadre (her first husband was killed by bombs in 1973). He had been too critical and was accused of being a spy. After some months Vanna saw him pass by as a prisoner on an oxcart. She was upset and angry with the militia, and villagers had trouble controlling her— which they needed to do for her own safety. After Vanna's husband came back from prison he was a broken man and died a few months after the Vietnamese invasion. Faced with the burden of bringing up the children on her own, her work kept her from thinking too much about the losses suffered. She had to 'keep going'. But when Vanna's sons were blown up by the landmine, everything fell apart for her. Now, being bankrupt, she could not avoid thinking about all that had happened to her, from the time her father was killed before her eyes by the 'Khmer Serei' faction when she was only a small child in the late 1940's. Vanna's father was an important man, a chief of the district. The family had barely survived that loss. She could have never guessed, at that time, that it was only the beginning.

Assessing Psychosocial Problems by Participatory Action Research

The assessment of real problems for real people in villages was part of the training of the project team (see below). In assessing families and individuals short versions of a more extensive battery of instruments were used, and this enabled the construction of a culture-specific questionnaire used in a survey. The final instrument included sections on demographics and social position, the illness and health seeking history of the individual and the family, a narrative report on personal history, traumatic events and coping styles. Sections of the WHO Composite International Diagnostic Interview (CIDI) were included.[2] A specially developed instrument was used to gather data on how the Cambodian people themselves would describe, explain and classify their problems.[3] In recording symptoms and signs, vernacular descriptions of the patient, the family, and traditional healers were used, in an attempt to avoid imposing western categories and which would be extrapolated to unreliable and invalid English-Khmer translations of constructs of emotional experience and behavior.

Beyond the familiar categories of events as they are often listed in trauma questionnaires, we asked for events that are typical for the situation in Cambodia. This includes dead, sick or missing relatives, marital and family related problems,

---

[2] The probe flowchart was adapted to the Cambodian setting.
[3] The Mental Distress Explanatory Model Interview was developed earlier, and adapted for this survey, by Dr. I. M. Eisenbruch.

gambling and domestic violence, social problems with neighbors or in-laws, and the presence of landmines and having land-mine victims in the family. These are 'new' events, in the sense that they did not belong to the range of life-events to be included in a normal life pattern before the civil war started in 1970. The complex structures of many families in Cambodia, for example, is a reflection of past traumas (forced Khmer Rouge marriages, lost relatives who returned later, widowhood) and more recent traumas (abandonment of wife and small children by breadwinner). Poverty is a constant stressor, especially in the rural areas.

Qualitative information was gathered through group discussions and in the narratives of the people met in the village where the teams set out to work. Group interviews were done in about a hundred *phum (villages) throughout the country. Topics included the history of these specific communities during different episodes, composition of the population, changes in daily life, and problems that were important for the villagers. Coping styles, idioms of distress, healing rituals and explanations for suffering were discussed in focus groups and in-depth interviews with key informants such as healers, monks, village leaders, teachers, youth and elderly villagers. Next to the narrative section in the survey, patients (about 1,400 at the time of doing the survey) seen in the five clinics supported by the program throughout the country added information about the personal experience of people who stayed in Cambodia, or had come back.

The survey was undertaken in three different districts throughout Cambodia. A team of especially trained interviewers accessed and conducted interviews in more than 650 families. The age range in the survey was from 16 to 65. About half the total population of Cambodia is younger. A study into Cambodian perceptions of illness in children shows that many problems (Figure 1) in this field are not easily recognized (Eisenbruch, 1994a). The overall majority of the population has been through events that are considered to be traumatic on any scale so far developed, and those born after civil war and social terror are growing up in a society where practically everyone has to cope with terrifying events.

This whole process of preparing the instruments and doing the survey helped to identify and understand personal and community problems, and to select the human resources with which to work (as referral potential, or as trainees). The research outcomes also provided basic knowledge needed for the development of monitoring instruments, and was instrumental in selecting specific areas of attention and specific target sub-populations in the villages. The documented group discussions, individual interviews, and observations of healing sessions recorded on videotape, were used for training sessions with the core group.

In documenting the personal narrative of the cases, we took care not to pre-configure the trauma or to assume it to be a punctuation of their life history during the Pol Pot years. The villagers defined their problems themselves. We did not find any respondent who did not experience at least several traumatic events as listed in the CIDI-PTSD module. We found that experiencing extreme events led to various reactions. Some showed symptoms, such as recurrent nightmares, consistent with the PTSD criteria. Many more, however, showed crippling complaints such as 'heat in the head', 'stabbing in the abdomen', 'thinking too much', and other complaints which do not fit neatly into any of the ICD or DSM criteria. Cases could be divided into three categories: people with clear physical illnesses, such as TB, consequences from road traffic accidents, epilepsy, or blindness; people with mental health problems including psychoses; and people with problems of depression, alcoholism, domestic violence, marital problems, sadness and anxiety. Roughly 20% had a physical illness, 35% had a psychiatric problem, and 45% can be described as having psychosocial problems.

Most were suffering quietly, not knowing where to go with their grief. In this state, they could not participate in daily living, stopped taking care of themselves and their families, and some in this state were regarded as *'ckuet'*—mentally ill. The total toll of these problems for village life is enormous.[4] Fifteen to 20% of families could not cope with the demands of daily life. Many are caught in a downward spiral of depression, hopelessness and poverty, where trouble takes many appearances.

Lovesickness—Malevolent Power Over the Heart

Despite the apparently trivial label, lovesickness is a common and potentially serious mental condition. It shows the ways in which sense is made of community stress such as poverty, and social disharmony such as conflict in marriage. The Khmer word for love is *snae*, and 'madness of lovesickness' is *ckuət snae*. There is the side of lovesickness in which the ritual specialist, in this case acting as sorcerer, *induces* lovesickness. This action is known as *dak snae* or 'putting love'. The other side is the healer who acts to treat someone under the influence of a love-charm. This action is known as *dah snae*, or literally 'dispelling the lovesickness'.

In Cambodia many men abandon wives and children for another woman, 'marry her' and have children in another family, returning from time to time to Wife Number One, only to impregnate her once more before wandering off again. These unfortunate women, known euphemistically as 'widows' and functionally female head-of-household, make up a big proportion of Cambodian villages.

At first, the victim daydreamed harmlessly about someone. In the second stage, the person fell hopelessly in love. At this stage the suitor simply craved love (or sex). Should she spurn his ardour, in vexation he hires a sorcerer to make her mad; if he can't have her, nor will anyone else.

If lovesickness might seem a trivial issue, in which family members come to terms with temporary lapses by a spouse, it can also be shorthand for potentially catastrophic family disruption.

---

[4] By way of comparison: In the 1993 World Development Report it was estimated that mental health problems the world over produce 8.1% of the Global Burden of Disease (GBD) measured in Disability Adjusted Life Years (DALY's), a toll greater than that exacted by tubercolosis, cancer, or heart disease (see Desjarlais, p. 34). In Cambodia the relative importance of psychosocial and mental health problems seem much bigger—which is to be shown by epidemiological survey methods now developed in the TPO programme.

> If a woman's husband finds a 'second wife', the matter seldom rests there. In the course of our work we observed commonly a pattern of a woman with young children and no husband to support them cascade into poverty (see below).
>
> The abandoned wife, visited from time to time by her husband, is made pregnant once more, which only escalates her poverty when her husband next abandons her. All this compounds her depression and she may be driven to suicide. The combination of lack of economic means and social support, along with her depression and a poor level of domestic hygiene and a lack of environmental stimulation for the children, can lead to malnutrition, chronic illness and poor psychosocial development among the children. Her husband during his visits may also bring with him the threat of syphilis and HIV/AIDS. Cambodia has an extraordinarily high rate of women as head-of-household, not simply because of a shortage of men, but because of the pattern we have sketched in this example. Lovesickness can help to frame this in local cultural terms, and shows how the traditional healers can possibly help to remoralise people who are otherwise deprived of power to influence their circumstances.

Ninety-six percent of the respondents reported exposure to at least one traumatic event in their lives, and on average respondents had experienced 4 of these events. More than two thirds of respondents were exposed to several traumatic events under Khmer Rouge rule. These events ranged from lack of food and shelter (40%) to separation from the family (34%), to suffering from severe illness with no access to medical care (22%).

Males and females were exposed to the same extent, but age groups above 22 reported significantly higher exposure. People in rural and border areas reported more events than people living in Phnom Penh. Thirty-six percent reported loss of a family member during the war and genocide, while 18% witnessed the torture or murder of a family member. These numbers seem low, taking into account that many people reported torture as common practice during the Khmer Rouge time. Usually, severe torture and mass killing took place in remote areas away from potential witnesses (the 'killing fields'). Next to that it was highly unlikely that the person taken to torture would survive, while the KR used to kill all family members, including children, when people were listed as traitors.

Similarly, fifteen percent reported imprisonment or serious injury. Although this figure seems high, it may not reflect the extent of imprisonment and torture during the KR time. The worst single example is the history of Toul Sleng prison in Phnom Penh, where only seven survivors are known out of more than 14,000 people imprisoned and killed (Chandler, 1999).

Exposure to war-related events declined after 1979. A temporal increase was noted around 1985, which might be attributable to the 'K5' projects mentioned above. Exposure to torture, injuries from landmines, imprisonment and witnessing violence in the community still exist until the time of the study. At the beginning of the 1980s Cambodia had a grossly imbalanced demographic structure with areas where up to 65% of the population was female. In the study

29% of women were widows, or separated from their husbands, or divorced—and all these women are called 'widows' in Cambodia.

Mental Disorders in Cambodia

The survey questionnaire included especially adapted cross-cultural instruments to measure prevalence of psychiatric disorders. The prevalence of anxiety disorder, posttraumatic stress disorder (PTSD) and major depression are of specific interest.

In a sample of 610 randomly selected Cambodians between fifteen and sixty-five years old, we found that lifetime prevalence of PTSD is 28%, and 11.5% suffered major depression.[5] In 9% of the respondents, PTSD and major depression were present together. Disorders were more common in people who were exposed to war events in the past or family and community violence today. Also, they are more common in older age groups than younger age groups. The effects of stress, grief and cognitive impairment caused by trauma were an important risk factor for disorders. The prevalence was higher in geographic areas that witnessed more social-upheaval due to war events, as well as current social structural change.

A quarter of all respondents reported at least one period of two weeks in which they felt sad or lost interest in their daily activities, and 11.5% met the criteria for at least one depressive episode (DSMIV-Major Depressive Episode). The prevalence in females was more than males (15.6% to 9.5%, chi = 4.86, $p < .05$), and older age groups reported more depression than young. Suicide is the most serious consequence of depression and is estimated to happen in 15% of all depressed people. It is noteworthy that from all respondents in Cambodia—not only the ones that scored on depression, 49.7% reported to have been 'thinking about death', 20.3% reported suicidal thoughts, 14.4% had planned for suicide and 13.7% had actually attempted suicide.

The highest prevalence of PTSD (40%) is found in the middle-aged group (36–55). This is the group of which the youngest people were about ten years old in 1970. One out of five of people born between 1972 and 1981 score on PTSD. The way people judge the quality of their life is not significantly related to their scores on mental disorders.[6]

---

[5]Compared to an overview given by de Girolamo and McFarlane (de Girolamo and McFarlane, 1996) these are high scores: Former political prisoners, Basoglu, 33% lifetime, 18% point; Laotian refugees attending an Indochinese Psychiatric program (Moore & Boehnlein, 1991) 88%; Vietnam veterans formerly wounded in action (Pitman, Altman & Macklin) 32% point, 40% lifetime.

[6]Based on the Cambodian adaptation of the short version of the WHO Quality of Life instrument (WHOQOL).

In the mental health clinics that were set up by the projects, it is significant that posttraumatic stress disorder (PTSD) accounted for only 1.1% of the diagnosis, as compared with the 28.4% found in the random sample of the population (20.6% for men, 34.2% for women). The reasons for the difference include that people do not see signs and symptoms of PTSD as a reason to look for help (in the public health sector). As PTSD usually does not produce severe, incapacitating dysfunction in quite the same way as does a psychotic illness, a mental health clinic would not be seen as an appropriate place to seek help. It could be expected that many with PTSD manifesting through somatic complaints (Kirmayer, 1996) would seek help in the traditional sector. They will be diagnosed differently in the public health services, where health staff might easily overlook PTSD, due to the level of training and experience and the role of transference as an obstruction in asking about trauma.

Forty percent of the sample showed anxiety disorder (14.4% for men, 49.1% for women), and more than half of all people interviewed (53.4%) have either anxiety disorder, PTSD, mood disorder or somatoform disorder. More than one third of these people were not exposed to violence related traumatic events. Do these high scores on concepts from western nosology point at a 'pathologic society'?

The constructs of PTSD and major depression are foreign to Cambodia. The popular Cambodian views of people suffering after the Khmer Rouge can be summarized as 'thinking too much' or 'headache' or 'Cambodian sickness' (Eisenbruch, 1991).

Madness of the Damaged Mind—A Khmer Rouge Creation?

Of all the types of mental disorders, the illness known as 'madness of *the sa?te? ?aaram*' seems to have a lot to do with stress, loss, bereavement, social and economic deprivation and family disruption—all of which lead to 'thinking too much' and to slow destruction of the mind. 'Madness of thinking too much' was the final stage of a cascade, for which there were terms for each stage. The person started with demoralization, literally 'small heart' (*tooc cət*). This progressed to worries, the thoughts literally 'broken'—the term *khooc cət* means literally 'broken down heart-mind'. This state progressed to *lap*, a term implying distractibility and doubled as *lap lap* to imply a progression of it. The epithet *'aa* is added, *aa-lap*, to jeer at such a person. Further deterioration led to muddling and 'lost and confused intellect or cognition' (*vɔəŋveeŋ smaardəy*). Anyone could have this mental state, not yet mentally ill.

A Cambodian traditional healer pays no less attention to how a person expresses thoughts than to what is thought. The indigenous terms for disorders of thinking have mainly to do with the person's speech. The healers also emphasized social context—did the speech upset people, and could they understand the person. Often, the abnormal content had to do with the Buddhist moral code. A person's talk was regarded as crazy if it put him outside the social fold. Patients with thought disorders talked to themselves in rambling unrelated sentences, known as 'no cadence or beat that bound them'. The term *rɔvəə-rɔviey* refers to a scrambled series of

> thoughts and, as a result, he can't get started on anything. This thought disorder can progress to the more severe form, *vɔəŋveeŋ-vɔəŋvoan. The word *vɔəŋveeŋ on its own simply means to have lost one's way, perhaps along the road. One difficulty for westerners in coming to grips with this concept is that the notion of *rɔvəə-rɔviey mixes disorders of thinking, perception, memory and concentration. The central feature is the social isolation and personal neglect, along with the gradual and chronic withdrawal and isolation. The healers are guarded in their optimism. They know the inexorable slide of such patients, few of whom have access to effective Western antipsychotic medication, and they tend to avoid false claims (Eisenbruch, 1996). They can offer some calming medication, but it is not a cure. They offer some family support and counseling.
>
> 'Madness of the senses' is often colored by memories of accumulating massive traumas and losses that envelop the patient's thinking—as indeed, of most 'healthy' Cambodians. A case could be made that Cambodian 'thinking too much' is as much a local idiom of PTSD as of schizophrenia, a proposition difficult to test in any war-torn society like Cambodia, which has endured successive waves of trauma and loss over more than two decades. There is no one-to-one 'discrete' trauma followed by a posttraumatic reaction (Eisenbruch, 1991, 1992b, 1994a). Further work is needed to sort out the contributions, not only of PTSD, but of ongoing social-economic privation and lack of safety and security.

The important question may not be whether PTSD is cross-culturally valid in Cambodia, but that a much deeper collective traumatization may not be expressed as an individual complaint. Trauma tends to be pervasive, massive, chronic, complex and multilayered as the case examples show. Given the widespread nature of the traumatization due to war, the reactions would have come to be accepted as a normal part of life (Somasundaram & Sivayokan, 1994). The prevailing cultural idioms of distress including tiredness (*ohkumlang), thinking too much (*kit chraen), and flashbacks of past traumas in the form of dreams and imagery which spill over into waking life (*sr amay), were so common as to be considered normal. Similarly the common occurrence of nightmares (71%), and what was termed depression or *pibak cet in 83% of Cambodian refugees in a Thai border camp (Mollica & Jalbert, 1989) in apparently functioning adults cannot be considered pathological.

Summarised one could state that in Cambodia every household bears the consequences of warfare, violence and repression. Individuals are often physically and mentally scarred and have to cope with loss on many levels. Many find themselves far away from what they consider to be their 'home land'. In a country where attachment to ancestors and their land is combined with a strong believe in reincarnation, it is striking to hear people say that the only hope they have left is not to be born as a Cambodian in the next life. Even more worrying is the significant number of people who have contemplated, and actually attempted, suicide, in a country where general belief holds that the very negative consequences of suicide have to be carried for the next five hundred lives. People see no use in talking to each other about the bad things in the past: everyone had similar experiences and it is 'better not to think about it'. 'Good' behavior is composed behavior, and when tears come, or anger, or outrage, it does not help and isolates a person even more. People feel tired (*ah kamlang*), they 'think too much' (*ki't craen*) or feel hopeless (*ah samkhum*). On the other hand one finds extreme violence, lack of control mechanisms, sexual and domestic aggression and crimes aimed at the most vulnerable people in society. In this atmosphere, sleeping disorders, nightmares, not being able to concentrate, a certain gloominess covering everything, have become symptoms of normal life.

COPING IN CAMBODIA: SOCIO-CULTURAL CHARACTERISTICS

Cambodia has a wealth of indigenous ways of dealing with illness, misfortune, stress, poverty and conflict. Various types of healers offer help to people in distress. Traditional social mechanisms could help solve conflicts. Pagodas are resources for advice, help, and consolation. Public health and social care is another potential resource for help. Currently systems of health care and social work are being developed and installed in Cambodia.

In order to develop sustainable and appropriate interventions, the project aimed at strengthening the systems already in place, and made an effort to introduce complementary skills at the right levels, through the right people. Active participation of the population is essential in installing sustainable care systems, and can only be achieved when new systems are complementary and acceptable to existing mutual support schemes.

In this section we will describe the existing resources for help used by the population, and present them in the context of special characteristics of Cambodian society. We will start with a helicopter view on society, and descent to have a closer look at the structure of communities and the world view of people in these communities. In the next section we shall then explain how we modeled interventions in accordance with the existing resources.

Understanding 'Communities' in Cambodia

To understand psychosocial problems in Cambodia it is necessary to consider long time characteristics of this society as well as present circumstances. Any separation between causes and effects where causes are defined in historical, and effects in psychological terms, is superficial. The notion that historic events caused the breakdown of the fabric of social life and traumatized the society as a whole is only one part of reality. The equally bitter other part is that some elements of the original structure of society gave room for catastrophic developments. In thinking about community work one needs to be aware of this.

Most social scientists who have worked to any extent in Cambodia agree that the level of social integration in Cambodia is unique (Chandler, 1993; Delvert, 1961; Ebihara, 1968; Martel, 1975; Ovesen, J., Trankell, I. & Ojendal, J., 1995; Porée-Maspero, 1962; Thion, 1993; Van de Put, 1992).[7] For centuries, Cambodia was made up of families who lived scattered over the country. Nowadays people are found in villages (*phum), and these are often seen as the basic unit for social change by rehabilitation or development programs. Yet the memory of living in smaller, scattered units is vivid in Cambodia: the *phum is not necessarily a natural habitat.

In Cambodia, Thailand and Vietnam alike, as in any peasant society, access to land is essential. Whereas pressure on the land by growing numbers of people forced the Thais and Vietnamese to keep up a strict system of social behavior, the Cambodians numbered far less and did not have to deal with large landownership until late in the 20th century. There was not the same need for communal organization as a collective defense mechanism as in the neighbouring countries. The Khmers lived in scattered compounds, containing less than ten houses. Relatives would be living together in an uxorilocal system—where husbands would join the families of their wives. These units of extended families were separated by dense forest.

Beginning under the French administration, people were forced to rebuild their houses following orders for relocation given by subsequent regimes, while Democratic Kampuchea reorganized public space completely. This process

---

[7]Some quotes:

'Que les phums soient miniscules ou qu'ils groupent plusieurs centaines de maisons, un fait apparait certain: l'absence d'une communaute rurale. Pas de maison commune. Pas de terrain commune' (Delvert, 1961).

The majority of families that live in that phum will be found scattered over the rural area, usually in groups of 8 to 12 houses. These are the '*kroms*' (= group) that are inhabited by members of the same family in matrilineal line. These kroms can be considered the core of social life in Cambodia, where 85% of the population lives in rural areas. Within these kroms, every nuclear family runs it's own household. (Van de Put, 1992)

The weakness, or the outright lack of institutional links among individuals may lead someone in authority, facing any form of challenge, to resort to immediate and violent retaliation. This is probably a result of the traditional basic education, handed down from the ancient times when a majority of the people were slaves of the rulers, which insists that authority should never, and cannot be, challenged—for any reason whatsoever. (Thion, 1993, p. 166)

Cambodian proverbs and didactic literature are filled with references to the helplessness of the individual and to the importance of accepting power relationships as they are. (Chandler, 1993–1, p. 105).

The Cambodian communal institution was far from having the same strong internal cohesion that was so noticeable in neighboring Vietnam. The real nucleus of the Khmer village is the pagoda. The difference in political organization is obvious at first sight even today. (Thion, 1993, p. 25)

(Greve, 1993; Davenport, 1995) led to the clusters of houses one sees nowadays all over the countryside, the *phums, and these cannot simply be taken as the natural focus of community interventions.

To come to a better understanding of what constitutes a community in Cambodia we assessed more than a hundred *phums. We looked for people and families with common interests, and potential mutual benefit in relationships with each other. The assessments led us to distinguish between vertical and horizontal structures in a groups living in the same area. Vertical relationships were to be found in any *phum between different income groups. Relative wealth was linked to ones position in this system that was loosely structured on the basis of kinship and links to the spiritual world in the area of birth. Horizontal relations, between people in the same income group, were less developed and less clear.

In order to identify individual people willing to work with us, compose groups willing to collaborate, organize effective self-help groups and to assess the presence of vulnerable families, we found it was useful to distinguish between three different types of *phums. There are 'old' *phums where a number of families have managed to stay together over time, without 'newcomers'. Having experienced hardships as a group, mostly related, there is a sense of continuity and solidarity. Here people would have their social networks mainly intact, and traditional healers could be accessed by all. Nevertheless, in these phums people have not found ways of helping each other cope with extreme emotions. In these phums interventions such as psycho-education sparked initiative and group discussions had considerable impact on the coping strategies used, as we will discuss below under 'community interventions'.

Another type is the *mixed phum, where 'new' people joined the old core of related families.[8] In these *phums it was effective to create bonds between the older and newer groups by 're-installing' traditional links between people in need and traditional resources.

A third type is the 'new' *phum. Created often for returnees, or, in the 1980's, for families in need of new land to work on, or, in the 1970's, for reasons of security and control, psychosocial problems are often serious in these *phums. Yet there is limited access to traditional resources, because healers, leaders and teachers do not belong to the same group. In these phums it was important to bring together people with shared interests, who would not necessarily have previous contact between them. Interventions such as psycho-education, group work and individual counseling were then productive per income group.

To understand the context of psychological suffering and some natural coping styles in Cambodia, we will narrow our focus and 'zoom in' to have a more detailed look at life within these *phums.

---

[8]New people were the people who had been ordered to leave the cities by the Khmer Rouge, versus the 'old people' who were supposed to be the original, real Khmer peasants in the rural areas.

Order and Hierarchy. Amidst all confusion and chaos in Cambodia since the end of the 1960s it is essential to realize that Cambodian cosmology is based on strict order. This order is normative, and translates in a hierarchical society. Order is preserved by proper behavior, by acting and behaving according to ones role in social life. Order is contrasted with wilderness. The well arranged order (*robab rap roy*) and the wilderness (*prey*) marks the difference between the untamed forest, the wild, and the cultivated, civilized, the predictable, the arranged (Chandler, 1996). The word for 'normal' is the same word for 'to be' (*chea*), and is the same word for healing. One gas to strive for order, and keep the dangerous wilderness at bay.

This importance of order, of respect for hierarchy, of the careful balance in man-occupied and cultivated land and wilderness, helps to explain the impact of forced relocation from cities and villages to 'the fields' or 'the forest' that happened all over Cambodia in the Khmer Rouge time. It also clarifies the literal meaning of being 'marginalised' when the poorest are always to be found in the outskirts of any community—far away from the ordered center, close to the evil and danger of the unordered wilderness. And it stresses the importance of the 'right behavior' and the position of the 'self' in Cambodian cosmology.

Violations of Codes of Conduct

There are disorders which are caused by violations of conduct: by people against their ancestors, by healers against former masters (*koh kruu*), or by misconduct, or by marital or community dysfunction (*ckuət cue cambuə*). Acute psychotic reactions can be involved.

The person's own ancestral spirits, the *cue cəmbuə* may induce madness of the ancestral spirits when they invade a person or withdraw their protection against spirits from the lower world. It is often brought on by relapse in conduct and the patient may know it. If, for a example, a young single woman commits a sexual indiscretion, she is violated but so is her family, including her ancestors. In retribution, her ancestral spirits makes her or her father mad. The *kruu* will diagnose it as caused by the ancestral spirits (remember how an individual problem will also affect the family, and eventually the community).

Ancestor madness seems to be grouped in three types. It can be based on genetic inheritance, or on violations of expected codes of conduct and respect towards parents and ancestors, or on punishment inflicted by spirits for similar violations.

Fixed Roles and Choice in Relationships. The core of Cambodian values delineates proper conduct, proper for one's position in society. There is a complex set of rules and regulations for the right behavior. One needs to know how to play the role of the mother, the father, the son, the cousin, client, or patron. Hierarchy is a condition for order, and prevails in interpersonal relations. An example came in a conversation with a high ranking official in the ministry of justice, who had been beaten and abused when he was in prison just a year before. When asked about any feelings of revenge to his abusers who were now his subordinates, he was surprised and said he would take action against them only when they stopped their abusive behavior towards prisoners—for that was how they were supposed to act. The role prescribes and justifies behavior. Tortures need not be revenged, as long as they were part of an overall imposed system. But immediate revenge is in place when ones role is mocked, when one is insulted in public, made ridiculous by people who have no right to do so.

This is not a unique Cambodian characteristic—one finds it in any Asian society. The special Cambodian characteristic is related to the above-mentioned level of social integration. Not being forced by socio-economic circumstances to develop and maintain relationships based on mutual dependency, there has always been a choice in engaging in certain relationships. Within any existing relation the rules are strict, but one can choose not to engage in that relationship—without the consequences that would lead to social exclusion in Thailand or Vietnam.

Magical Action Illness—Malevolent Power to Harm the Body

At the level of the village and community, individuals and groups inevitably come into conflict, reflected in the category of illness called 'magical action' or 'magical human intervention'. Modernisation, bringing in its wake complications in work, marriage and sexual relations, induces its own forms of social strain, and 'referrals' to traditional healers because of sorcery show no signs of decreasing. With the loss of the predictable social structure imposed by communism, and the advent of UNTAC and a market economy, the social strain went up and so did the level of accusation. One might say, ironically, that where sorcery is replaced as a means to blow off social strain, it is replaced by a tendency towards indiscriminate or disproportionate violence—two friends playing cards, or a married couple, suddenly in disagreement, and one blowing the other to bits at point blank range with a B-40 rocket launcher.

The common Cambodian disorder known as 'magical human interference' relates to what is usually described as sorcery. It is a key marker of social and domestic disharmony and, at the same time that its ritual treatment acts to restore social harmony. Beyond that, what psychiatrists might term as psychosomatic or somatoform disorders could be interpreted by the patient and family as a sign of a community disorder and, if not promptly treated, can turn into a chronic disability, misunderstood and misdiagnosed by western health services.

Magical sorcery is common in Southeast Asian societies. In Cambodia, magical human intervention leads to the acute onset of bizarre and socially disruptive behavior that, it would seem, can be ameliorated by the healer. The common signal that alerts the patient is a dream, which notifies him that something magical is in the process of invading his house, or his body—and the full-blown physical and mental symptoms follow the next day. The hallmarks of people suffering from magical human interference are swelling of the abdomen and, too, migratory stabbing pains.

One can blame magical action initiated by *people*—as opposed to spirits—if community relationships break down. The terms make sense according to the *agent* (non-human or human); the *mechanism* (invading spirits, a spell, or projected foreign bodies); the *physical effect* (disrupted body elements, causing swelling; pain, caused by the effects of foreign objects).

The healers are unconcerned with localizing the culprit. The resolution of community problems does not call for that and, more important than showing the victim who had done him in, the *community* has to see the sick person reintegrated in the course of the healing ritual.

A dramatic condition calls for a dramatic solution. This illness is the leitmotif of community rivalries and jealousies—and healers, as part of the community, cannot escape professional rivalries. The protagonists avoid the local healer, preferring to travel to a healer further away where they can reveal their problems with less chance of local gossip getting back to family and neighbors. For their part, patients who have been troubled by multiple episodes of 'magical human intervention' say that they have visited many healers in different localities, and no one, patient or healer, seems perturbed.

'Illness of magical human interference' is one of the most common disorders identified by healers. Whereas 'ancestral spirit disorders' can give rise to a variety of secondary illnesses, 'magical human interference' seems to be a *result* of trouble between the victim and someone in their community. The use of magic to induce illness reflects a need by people to control their social and personal environment.

Shifting Social Values, Growing Individual Confusion. The age-old notion of order, and the certainty that comes with obeying the order, is shifting. As long as roles where clear, there would be certainty on when they were played rightly or wrongly. The change in the last decades brought the need for new roles and new definitions to Cambodia.

Correct behavior was and still is important in social life. People adjust behavior, language, and appearance, to the status and role they have in relation to people in their company. Codes of conduct are important, and we have seen many clients for whom breaking the code of conduct was the origin of their illness ('incompatibility of sleeping' or *toah damneek*—see below). The traditional healers can only be powerful (that is, effective) only if they follow their codes of conduct. At the same time, such adherence has to be maintained in a society which seems to be 'on the loose' as a whole.

Whereas patronage, kinship, and the religious obligations used to organize social life in the past, short-term mutual interest between individual families is nowadays acting as an organizing principle for community life.[9] The relative isolation in which extended families lived made avoidance a rational alternative to complex systems of 'conflict management', and while heads of families used to try to limit the consequences of smoldering conflict, nowadays these mechanisms for social control have disappeared in many villages.

---

[9] See Thion, 1993, p. 152: kinship relations seem to be modeled on patron–client relationships, and used to promote individual ambitions.

> **Domestic Violence**
>
> As an example of change in response to problems one may look at the problem of domestic violence. Little is known about the prevalence of domestic violence before 1975, but informants told us that in the past, excessive brutal behavior within the family would not be tolerated. People who were able to put a stop to it were the elderly, provided that the original infrastructure of the village would be intact. People like the *aacaa, the Buddhist ritual assistant and functionary in the pagoda, had real authority in the village, and could use their influence with heads of the families (of which they themselves would often be one) to end unacceptable breaches of conduct.
>
> In the turmoil between 1970 and 1979 traditional uxorilocality was disrupted. Nowadays economic factors are decisive in deciding whether a newly married couple will live close to her or his parents—if there are parents (Nepote, 1992). This has consequences for the resources available to the women that end up in the village of their husbands—especially so if the marriage breaks down or the husband dies. Going 'home', back to their village of origin, is not a real option, since the woman is not seen as the responsibility of her kin once she found a husband and another place to live. As one village leader commented about his frustration at seeing how his son-in-law used physical violence against his own daughter, who lived with her husband's parents: 'there is nothing I can do. They were married, with my consent. The husband is her master. I cannot interfere'.
>
> Thus a rather 'natural' protective mechanism in favor of women has disappeared, and is not replaced by an alternative. Where there used to be the safety-net of well known and often related resources for help for the woman, such as the traditional healer and the *aacaa, nowadays many widowed or abandoned women find themselves living in an environment where they 'do not belong'.

Once we understood these mechanisms, we were able to find solutions for these problems. Women in distress could be linked to resources in their villages (see case study below). Repairing these traditional links was at once one of the more appreciated and successful interventions of the Cambodian project team, as an illustration of the usefulness of a 'new approach' to well known problems in traditional settings.

Much confusion results from the loss of role models and the balance which needs to be found by each individual between playing his role in traditional, strictly hierarchical Cambodian society and the present day chaos. Assessing Cambodian community from this angle helps in interpreting the use—or the lack—of social networks in coping, while at the same time providing the necessary background information to develop community level interventions.

Why would all this be important? First, it sheds light on the complex knot of cause-and-effect in recent Cambodian history. This 'looseness' in relationships was strengthened through the upsetting civil war in the early 1970s, while the Khmer Rouge went further and actually forced people to see themselves as individuals without any social responsibility but to the 'Angka'—the 'organization'. Assuming responsibility for even family members or friends was enough for instant execution. There is an uncomfortable continuity in the loose structure of traditional society (Evers, 1969, 1980), the age-long absolute rule by a distant monarch, the lack of models for conflict resolution and lack of societal capacity for organized resistance to totalitarian control. It could be argued that the success of the Khmer Rouge, a movement that numbered probably no more than about 60,000, mostly adolescent members, in mastering a society of 6 million for almost four years, has much to do with this fragmented character of society. Traditional bonds of trust between people were fragile, which in itself allowed the Khmer Rouge to destroy these fragile bonds even further.

Second, this forced erosion of bonds between people in Cambodia seems related to the difficulty in making sense of what has happened and creating new coping mechanisms. The traditional ways of living together have changed so often and so quickly, that there has been no time to find new rules. In many cases people found that as soon as warfare would cease to be the common threat, insecurity would come from within the community.

The political order imposed by the Khmer Rouge regime did not replace the old cosmological order—here continuity reached its limits. In traditional society order and hierarchy was balanced by a minimum of social responsibility and cohesion. People who had fled the last stronghold of the Khmer Rouge in 1997 had secretly continued performing the rituals explicitly forbidden by their new leaders for almost thirty years.

The Cambodian Self. The Western concept of the self is described as '... a bounded, unique, more or less integrated motivational and cognitive universe, a dynamic centre of awareness, emotion, judgement, and action organized into a distinctive whole and set contrastively both against other such wholes and against its social and cultural background.... is a peculiar idea within the context of world cultures' (Geertz, 1983). Cambodian culture constitutes another perception of the self.

The point here is not that Cambodia would be a 'collectivist' society as contrasted to an individualistic society (Kirn, Triandis, Kagitcibasi, Choi & Yoon, 1994). Cambodian individuals do not see themselves as 'set contrastively' against their social and cultural background, but rather think of themselves in terms of the sum of their relationships and ambitions. Relationships include family, friends, colleagues, authorities as well as relationships with the spiritual world. As shown above, the individual strives to lead a life following the roles that have been provided by birth. But at the same time it is personal ambition that defines each individuals choice in which relationships to engage in—and which not.

Karma and Reincarnation. The worldview of individuals people is shaped by the classical Theravada Buddhist doctrine as much as the beliefs in the supernatural world (Choulean, 1986). These beliefs are seamlessly woven together, and influence people's ambivalent responses to misfortune, poverty, psychosocial misery and mental disorders. An illustration of this effective mixture of religious doctrine and animistic beliefs is the fact that the *neak tha*, the spirit that is a symbol of man's domestication of the wilderness, is often presented and honored in the (Buddhist) pagoda.[10]

The boxes on mental illness in Cambodia throughout this chapter show that illness is contextualised by the patient's network of family, kin, neighbors, and the general community. What stands out is the large number of polymorphous spirits; the poor classification which straddles the world of the living and the dead; their immaturity and childishness; their ill-defined and unpredictable role as gatekeepers of moral behavior; and their capricious tendency to cause harm. The guardian spirits define not only where people may go in their environment, but also how they should behave. In spite of the recent modernization, the Cambodian beliefs in the guardian spirits appear to be firmly entrenched and are perhaps the last to be relinquished as an explanation for illness.

The spiritual world is therefore very much 'real'. Everyday decisions can often not be taken without consulting a medium, e.g. about the right time and route for a funeral. Karma and reincarnation are important aspects in daily life, too. People know that there will be more lives, in which they will bear the consequences of their behavior in this life. The theoretical texts of the Theravada tradition offer a basis to assess the self as an active and morally responsible agent, notwithstanding the explanation of the person, the I, as only conventional truth. Ultimate truth is in impersonal elements of existence (*dhamma*) (Collins, 1982). Fascinating as they are, these theoretical considerations are beyond the interest of most people in daily life. What counts is the effect of the belief in *kamma* (bad karma) and *b'aap bon* (good karma) in reincarnation in Cambodia.

The continuation of life and moral consequence may be illustrated by the example of the survivor of the civil war and the Khmer Rouge who managed to become a successful businessman. This man, who does not feel the need to share his wealth with his parents, or other relatives apart from wife and children, sees his survival and material success as proof of his good deeds in the past, in previous lives. He managed to gather enough *b'aap bon* to achieve what he has achieved today—and in his eyes, other people must have failed to do so.

So while karma and predestiny shape the present life, actions towards capricious deities may push one across the knife edge, with retaliatory action possibly resulting in misery and mental affliction. One has to be careful, and one needs traditional healers of many kinds to deal with the spiritual world—be it to know how to prevent misery or to deal with the effects of spiritual actions. And at the same time, many older people devote time to 'make merit', to build up *b'aap bon* for the next life. Some people go live at the pagoda, temporarily or for good.

---

[10]Lecture Ang Choulean, July 2000, Phnom Penh.

The *doon chhi* (buddhist nuns) are women who have chosen the spiritual life. Their quest for enlightening is an individual path, as fits exactly in Theravada Buddhism, where the role of Boddhishatva who returns on the threshold of the Nirvana to help others reach the same level of insight does not exist. Therefore it needs to be understood that the pagoda is always there for people who choose the religious path—but one should not assume that the monks or the *doon chhi* could be turned into 'community activists'.

Example of The Use Some Women Make of a Pagoda: The *Doon Chhi* (Nuns)

In the north west of the country there is a fertile province, Battambang, that for many years was the landmine-pocked battleground for the civil war with the Khmer Rouge. Ek Phnom is a district of that province. In Wat Ek Phnom, a well-known pagoda, there is a group of Buddhist nuns. The teacher of the *doon chhi* (nuns) living here is Pun Sim, 75 years old. She was trained at Wat Toul Tong, in Phnom Penh, in the 1960s and 70s. She originally came from Ek Phnom, and was sent back there by the KR in 1975. Wat Ek Phnom was destroyed, and in 1980 she was among the four women who started the rehabilitation of the *Wat*. A *doon chhi* center was started, and at some time the number of women present rose to more than 70. Women come from all over Cambodia to Wat Ek Phnom. Most of the women follow the *sel pram*, (five Buddhist precepts), some follow the eight Buddhist precepts, and some *sel dap* (ten precepts). A monk in theory strives to adhere to the full 227 Buddhist precepts; laymen strive to observe five basic precepts, and some lay people at certain stages of their lives, like these *doon chhi*, undertake to follow eight or ten.

There are women who stay in the *Wat* for a certain period of time, and there are women who stay for the rest of their lives. They have all come to the Wat to make merit. Wrong deeds have to be made good by making merit at the end of life. Younger women may feel that they have to make merit at some point in their lives too. Many women come for three months, the Lenten season. Then they go back home again, and some of them will come back for another three months the next year. At *Cool Wosa* (Lenten) there are more *doon chhi* than during the rest of the year, usually about 50 or 60 in Wat Ek Phnom.

Pinn Simm is the teacher. Her supreme master is Sah Matak Virihea Pok Soi, who resides in *Wat Andouk. As in *Wat Andouk, Ek Phnom also receives women who have mental health or psycho-social problems. They can be helped if they want to learn about the Buddhist way of life, the rules, the codes of conduct, the explanations of suffering (*toah*). Women who want to come to the *Wat are welcome, even if they have nothing, if they are in debt. Pinn Simm said, after we discussed our work with her, that TPO is trying to help 'from the outside', while the *doon chhi* approach the problem from the inside. But, she said, at *Wat Ek Phnom they also have to begin at the outside. A woman who is depressed needs to be dressed and fed, before they can start working on the 'inside'.

These notions of individuality and continuity had to be acknowledged in understanding the suffering and coping mechanisms of individual people. The importance of relations with the ancestors helps to explain the suffering of people who were never able to organize for the necessary rituals at the death of family members. The notions of 'making merit' and the effect it may have on the next life, as well as the certainty that no deeds will remain without consequences, are important notions in understanding psychological problems as well as potential solutions. In the interventions we used these notions, as we will show below.

The Community Resources

The Traditional Healing System. Healers and monks practice traditional healing methods all over Cambodia. Most communes have a Buddhist pagoda and most villages have at least one healer. The label 'traditional sector' in itself does not mean very much when the vast difference between various types of healers is taken into consideration. There are the Buddhist monks (*preah sang), their ritual assistants and much-respected heads of families, (*aacaa), and sometimes nuns (*doon cii) in the pagoda. There are male, and sometimes female, traditional healers (*kruu boran or *kruu khmer). There are female, and sometimes male, mediums (*kruu chool ruub). There are lay healers, fortunetellers, and traditional birth attendants (*cmap). Monks and traditional healers have often had many years of training and developed skills in some specialized aspect of healing. Some are renowned, for example, for treating children's diseases or illnesses brought on by human interference such as sorcery; many are experts in pharmacological treatment, gathering plants outside their houses, which they sometimes prepare in elaborate pharmacies. Each sort of traditional healer offers a particular target intervention: the monks, for example, tend to focus on advice and calming people's anxieties; the *kruu, the trained healers, provided medication and magical rituals to help rid people of invading spells and spirits and, through the public ritual, to reintegrate the person into the local community; the mediums, mostly women, offered an intercession with the ancestors and in this way acted as remoralizing counselors for women who cannot face their future; the traditional birth attendants help families through difficulties around childbirth and the puerperium. All healers have to follow strict rules of moral conduct.

Sick Healers

Violations of moral codes can be committed by ordinary people and by monks and *kruu who are entrusted with the transmission of cultural knowledge. There are particular forms of madness associated with violation of moral codes. The *kruu's former *guru can take his errant disciple out of the intergenerational chain, and in the process cultural transmission is vouchsafed. These mental disorders of moral turpitude serve cultural survival by ensuring that those entrusted with cultural knowledge—monks and *kruu—are kept in line.

Wrong kruu, *or Brahmanic Malpractice*

The most popular term for this condition was simply 'wrong *kruu' or sometimes as 'madness of wrong *kruu'—if the healer fell ill with 'wrong *kruu' inevitably he went mad. The illness being caused by the former master stationing on the head of the *kruu, it was not surprising that the symptoms began in the head. Generally the sick healer became disinhibited, shouting while walking all around the house. If no one knew how to prepare the offering, the disabled *kruu, lucid or not, would remain insane.

Nearly every healer had the same 'emergency response' when they felt the premonitory signs of 'wrong *kruu'. He or she rushed to prepare the offering and think of the good deeds of the former master. One had to get the angry former master on side as quickly as possible. The offering was called literally the 'equipment'(*rɔəndap) for the former master, a different construction than more common ways to express offerings made by people to deities.

Sickness of the Monk Who Deviated to the Left, or Buddhist Malpractice

If 'wrong *kruu' is the hallmar of illness striking down the *kruu for Brahmanic malpractice, 'madness of the dhamma' is the equivalent for the monks for committing Buddhist malpractice.

The most popular term was 'madness of the dhamma' (*ckuət thoa). The root cause was that the practitioner tried too hard, with the wrong reasons, using the wrong techniques, or with the wrong instruction, to transcend consciousness. The culprit in practicing Buddhist dhamma may unwittingly have 'deviated to the left', the expression denoting a violation from the rule, set up by their meditation teacher.

'Madness of the dhamma' affected those within the orbit of the Buddhist pagoda—elderly 'nuns', ritual assistants, those who observed the 10 Precepts, as well as the ordained monks—while living under the influence of the pagoda where the dhamma was so concentrated.

In some provinces there are exceptionally successful healers, some based in Buddhist pagodas, whose fame extends throughout Cambodia. Some of these monks, and *kruu, manage up to ten or fifteen inpatients, and some healers see more than one hundred patients per day. These healers do not claim that they can cure all serious psychiatric illnesses, but they believe they can ameliorate symptoms in a majority of cases. For the most part, patients do not pay more than they have to pay to visit the local hospital.

The more experienced traditional healers know their limitations and avoid treating cases of what would be called chronic psychoses in western nosology (Eisenbruch, 1994b). They help the family to understand why a person may have developed *çhkuet (literally 'mad') and in this way, open the door for reintegration of the patient into the community.

A female *kruu may also work as a TBA, combining the technical skill of midwifery with the cosmic power of the healer, especially when it involves women's illnesses. The traditional birth attendants are nearly always women. They reinforce the cultural prescriptions for pregnancy and childbirth which, when violated, are believed to lead to puerperal forms of insanity.

Mediums (*kruu chool ruub) have their clients mainly coming from considerable distances. In their own villages, the magic of their performance may be hindered by their personal ties to the community, while the personal character of many of the relational problems people take to the medium may cause them to cover some 'safe' distance from their homes. Mediums are usually women, sometimes men. Not only do the mediums act as general psychosocial supports, but they may also help to ameliorate the problems of patients afflicted by serious and acute psychiatric derangement such as 'magical human intervention' and spirit possession.

The medium focuses on the management of nagging and intractable psychosocial problems. In serious situations, such as a woman abandoned by her husband for another, with no livelihood or means to raise her four small children, shunned by her local village, at the bottom of a cycle of poverty, profoundly demoralised and depressed, the *kruu is a resource for help. The mediums, often women who experienced severe problems themselves and where then called by a spirit (*yee) to serve as their medium for healing, help people to find the cause their problem. They relate their clients to a cosmological setting shared by client and medium. The *yee can speak freely, through the medium, and is not tied to social rules or etiquette. The often strict hierarchy in social positions does not apply to the spirit. This may lead to a 'break-through' in communication when a family situation seems hopelessly blocked. Relational problems can be more openly discussed and sometimes solved with the help of the spirit through the medium. This discussion in itself is a special characteristic of the medium. People can talk to her or him. It is an opportunity to talk about the problems at hand, which one does not find easily in Cambodian society. The traditional healer or the monks know what needs to be done: their social status limits verbal contact with the client.

There is at least one *kruu in nearly every village. The *kruu, like the monks, are an integral part of the community, highly respected among most villagers. If monks and *kruu carry out similar healing rituals, the monks are seen to be spiritual healers, the *kruu the medical ones. Within the project we tried to avoid the 'category fallacy' (Kleinman, 1977) by working as much as possible within the cultural belief system, offering medical treatment only for the more severe symptoms or illnesses that did not find help elsewhere.

Other Resources in the Traditional Community. Traditionally, public life centred around the market and the pagoda, which was the original venue of the schools. Traditional resources for help included, next to the monks and the traditional healers, the teachers in a village, the people involved in village associations, official authorities, or people with a special position in the *phum. The most respected villagers are members of the 'pagoda committee', and together with the *achaa, the ritual assistant of the monks who is also in the pagoda committee, these men are family leaders and the locus of social control. These men are also important in 'associations', which can be seen as models for organizing mutual support. Examples of associations and ways of working together are: the 'pots and pans group' (*samakum chaan chhnang); the funeral association; construction associations; rice bank groups, and parents associations. The presence and functioning of these associations is closely related to the type of *phum (see above): the closer the relationships between the people who make up a community (the 'old' *phum) the higher the level of functioning associations.

Another avenue for social support is given with the habit of reciprocal work, usually called '*provas dai*' (giving a 'helping hand').

There are official authorities, such as the village chief (*mee-phum*) and members of the various committees. There are also informal leaders, people who are respected, and who act as patrons for others (e.g. the *mee-kchal*). Families need to relate to the village authorities inorder to begin finding solutions for very practical problems such as access to land. In case of domestic problems, some people may also need the assistance of authorities, e.g. in cases of domestic violence. All these local resources have roles in Cambodian society, and they can be effective in alleviating psychosocial distress.

The Public Health System. The Cambodian context includes resources beyond those traditionally provided in the community. In assessing the potential solutions people might use modern systems need to be included. State provided systems of care were weak in all respects. Ministries of women's affairs, social welfare and veterans, culture and religion, and rural development existed since the United Nations Transitional Authorities in Cambodia were installed in 1992. It would be beyond the focus of this chapter to give a detailed overview of the efforts made in all these ministries to set up systems of care for the most vulnerable groups in society. What all these have in common is a fundamental lack of means to effectively cater for the large target groups. In view of the efforts made by the project to contribute to sustainable solutions for psychosocial problems, we need to make one exception here for allophatic health services. There is overlap of course in psychosocial problems and rural and urban poverty, social exclusion and education. The illness metaphors and somatization used by individuals to understand their psychological suffering and find effective coping styles to alleviate it point at the health sector as a avenue for developing effective interventions. We will therefore briefly sketch the health system and its problems in Cambodia here, which should provide the contextual background for the interventions in the health sector as they are described below.

When the Khmer Rouge took over in 1975, the one mental hospital, *Takmou*, providing mainly custodial care, was closed, as were most other medical services. Few traditional healers and monks who had provided some care for the mentally ill (Eisenbruch, 1994a), were allowed to continue. After the fall of the Khmer Rouge regime in 1979 public health care was modelled on the experience in Vietnam. This effort to introduce a nation-wide system resulted in a situation where too many staff had had too little training, and were ill placed throughout the country lacking financial means and supervision. Although the traditional healing sector was affected by the years of war and terror, it was able to take a central place in the options for health care after 1979. In 1995, at the time the project started, psychiatric care was simply non-existing.

In general the health status of the Cambodian population is still among the poorest in the world. Average life expectancy is 54.4 years, much lower than in neighboring countries such as Vietnam (61.3 years), and Thailand (66 years). Maternal mortality rate is estimated at 900 per 100,000 live births, the highest in the region. Acute respiratory infections, malaria, and, increasingly, HIV related illnesses are the main causes of mortality. HIV prevalence in adults reached an alarming 4% by the end of 1999, the highest in Asia, and comparable to countries such as Ghana and Nigeria (UNAIDS, 2000). Fertility rate with 5.2 children is, after Laos PDR, the highest in Asia (Demographic Survey of Cambodia, 1996).

There is thus a very high burden of disease in Cambodia, and still a very weak infrastructure to address it. Seeking care in government health facilities is unattractive for most patients, because of its time-consuming and unpredictable character. Staff is often absent, the waiting time is long, and when people are seen by health staff they face an often disrespectful attitude and unpredictable costs (Van de Put, 1992).

Cambodians privately spend a lot of money to seek health care. This out-of-pocket contribution amounts to 82% of total health care expenditure, or US $33.3 per capita per year (World Bank, 1999), and constitutes with 13.2% of GDP far more than many households can afford. One illness episode can ruin a family, especially when they desperately need treatment with immediate effect to restore the working capacity of one of the family members. The population can hardly judge the real effect of the huge variety of health services offered in the traditional, private and public sectors.

Utilisation of public health facilities is on average throughout Cambodia 0.35 contacts per capita per year, which is dramatically below the WHO international standard of 0.60 for rural areas, and well below the contact rates as observed in the region (World Bank, 1999). Also the number of patients admitted in government health facilities is low, due to the absence of staff, poor hygienic conditions, lack of drugs, etc. In 1997, no more than one third of the necessary structures were in place, the health sector was seriously under-funded, and health staff received extremely low salaries (on average 15 USD/month—whereas average monthly household expenditure is 262 USD in Phnom Penh and 80 USD in the rural areas).

Low salaries not only makes it difficult for health workers to concentrate on their public duties, but also severely limits the effect of training efforts on behavior change in health workers. Experience in other projects since 1997 shows that training only yields results when combined with an incentive system that directly relates financial benefits with quality outcome of work. (Soeters & Griffiths, 2000).

The efforts of the project to help install basic mental health skills in integrated primary and secondary care (Somasundaram, Van de Put, Eisenbruch & De Jong, 1998) are described below. For now it is important to stress that people suffering from the psychological consequences of stress as well as the mentally ill could only find relief within the traditional sector as described above. There were no alternative choices, and there was no system in place capable to deliver social or medical services.

Coping in Cambodia and the Need for Interventions

We have presented some of the existing resources in the community within the context of characteristics of Cambodian culture and society. Given this variety of traditional resources, one might question the need for new interventions. We will conclude the first half of this chapter by showing this need as related to the characteristics of Cambodian coping styles. We will use the remaining part of the chapter to show how we have tried to overcome these barriers or even use some of them in developing appropriate interventions.

Cambodian Culture. The worldview of Cambodians stresses the continuous cycle of lives, the importance of *b'aap bon (good karma) in reincarnation, and the reality of the impact of spirits and ancestors on the environment. The importance of conducting the right rituals for the dead and the need to restore disturbed relations with the spiritual world are essential elements of coping. These essential elements need to be the point of departure for any effective approach to help people help themselves—it is not sufficient just to be aware of these beliefs. In our community approach we have stressed these elements as will be shown below under 'community interventions'.

Spirit Madness—Messing with the Non-human World

One has to propitiate one's guardian spirits by making the expected offerings. But one can also become ill if one interfered with the guardian spirits of a neighbor, even if this was done indirectly. In this way, madness of guardian spirits shares with madness of magical action the function of stabilizing community relations. Trouble in the community starts at home and the house spirit is the detonator in the guardian spirit bomb.

Madness caused by spirits was remarkable in that the patient spoke in the strange, sometimes high-pitched voice of the spirit. The most marked disturbances were in mood. They were capable of outbursts of murderous destruction. Madness of spirits, like madness of magical action, tended to be an acute illness.

Before attacking the spirits, the healer had first to 'put the patient's mind back together'—to assemble the brain's four body elements and to refresh the patient's perceptions and memory (*dah sa?te?*). After that, he could worry about the spirits, using a sequence of Pali stanzas to tie them up with one; expel them with one; chase them away with one; made them break up and disperse into little pieces (*bambaek) with one; dissipate them with one (*kamcat); stab them with one; and melt and liquefy (*rumliey) with another.

People quarrel and love, fall ill and recover, and all these human experiences, centred naturally on pathogenic processes in the patient's body, invariably take place along with the involvement of spirits and the supernatural. To oversimplify the formula, hurt or offended ancestors cause ancestral madness; offended people cause magical human interference illness or sorcery; and hurt or offended spirits cause spirit madness.

As said, for most Cambodians traditional health beliefs still prevail. Although it was clear from the outset that the construct 'psychosocial' was foreign to Cambodians, people had no difficulty in discussing the variety of problems they had to deal with—in which they did not distinguish easily between physical, mental or spiritual problems. Behaviour and health are embedded in beliefs about natural and supernatural forces in the environment of the village and the surrounding fields and forests. While traditional views on the world and the according life perspective are severely shaken, the health beliefs as they are illustrated in the textboxes throughout this chapter remain the main framework of meaning.

This means that these health beliefs need to be taken into consideration when looking for additional interventions. This requires careful translation and comparison of indigenous health beliefs and international concepts of psychiatry and psychology. A major effort was made in initial training and subsequent development of training materials to be used by others in Cambodia, as is shown below under 'training'.

The traditional sector is strong in Cambodia. People in the traditional sector make ideal resources for any community health programme because of the respect and familiarity given to the traditional healers in Khmer society, the relevance of explanatory belief systems and cosmology of the traditional sector, the acceptance by the general population, their wide availability in even the remotest village and the common use made of their services by those seeking help.

It would seem that the healers might act as 'trauma therapists' in many countries recovering from war. Traditional healers provide a means for people to resolve their personal sadness and their problems in the community more acceptable than the methods brought by the West. And more than that, the traditional methods are themselves a way of combating feelings of cultural loss caused by ongoing modernization and development projects. As new health services take off in Cambodia, we had hoped that the healers could work alongside them, with no detriment to either.

Social Setting and Social Change. There are also limits to what can be achieved by the healers within a changing society. There can be a social mismatch, an inability of the healer to deal with what was also part of her/his personal experience, and a mismatch in meaning and interpretation in traditional versus international taxonomies of illness.

On the level of a social mismatch it is important that the difference in social structure between villages leads to various levels of access for Cambodians to traditional healers. Many people have been displaced because they have either returned from refugee camps, were forcibly removed from their own land and had no chance to go back there, or went to live in the village of a husband who later left them. These people do not live in what should be their own, natural environment. Their attachment within their communities is different, and they often have less access to local helpers.

More important is that all healers, whether medium, *kruu, or monk, have shared the Cambodian history with their clients. For some of the healers the events of the past decades have even been especially difficult, because they were targets of prosecution (monks and traditional healers). Mediums (*kruu chool ruub) usually become mediators between the spiritual and human world at the request of a spirit who came to their assistance when they experienced severe personal problems, often the same emotional problems as their clients have.[11] While this may actually help some of the healers to help these clients, many healers said clearly that they felt powerless when faced by problems related to extreme violence, repression and warfare.

This emotional difficulty is related to the fact that the traditional taxonomy of problems applied by the different healers is often ill fitted for dealing with the results of modern warfare and extreme violence. There are examples of how healers adapt their explanations and tools, but health beliefs are shifting in general, patterns of health seeking behavior are changing, and healers are now in competition with other sectors that offer help. Next to a confrontation between explanatory models this includes a more vulgar aspect: healers have to maintain their families as small independent entrepreneurs within a rapidly changing society.

The competitors from other sectors have their share of problems too. As was said in the discussion of the public health care system, there are many reasons why institutional weakness prevents successful introduction of new skills. There is a clear need for integrated basic psychiatry in primary care, but at the time the necessary conditions of a motivated, salaried and skilled staff were simply non-existent. Yet a beginning had to be made, and below we will briefly describe the efforts made.

We found that there was no clear unique concept of a community in Cambodia. The social turmoil of the last decades resulted in villages with different social structures. In these social structures the notions of hierarchy and

---

[11]A woman in Prok Da, Ponhea Leu district, was abandoned by her *Boramey, her spirit, when we came to see her for another visit. Her spirit had been the spirit of a two year old child, who helped her heal people for about one-and-a-half year. This woman had many problems herself, and the spirit had asked her to act as its medium in return for helping her. The *kruu chool ruub, the medium herself, had become well known in the past months, and had seen hundreds of clients who often came from far to see her. But now she was tired of being a medium, and wanted the spirit to find someone else. She begged the spirit to leave her alone, and indeed the spirit agreed to move to another medium. The woman knows who the new medium for this spirit is, someone in a village not very far from hers. Others in the village told us that the women stopped being a medium after she had had some problems with patients, who were not satisfied by the results of the treatment received.

importance of order prevailed in many of the more traditional villages, while in others different groups would have different access to local resources.

This meant we had to adapt the composition of intervention teams in different types of communities. We also had to adapt the selection mechanisms for participants in group sessions, and we had to adapt the logic of using different training modules in a different order in different communities. These elements are described below under 'community interventions'.

In a society 'on the move' rural communities are changing, and urban centres change even faster. The dynamics of fast modernisation and influence of global developments through the media requires new role models and mixes up traditional patterns of respect, obedience and social control. New 'roles' had to be defined for effective helpers, which would bridge the traditional requirements with the demands of change.

This meant that the relationship between the various people able to help others had to be studied in order to ensure productive referral. It also meant that especially in individual encounters such as counseling sessions a new role could only be defined by developing new skills, as is further explained under 'counseling'.

'Helpers' in Cambodia ask for assistance: healers as well as health staff need assistance, sometimes for their own problems, often in dealing with their clients. There is confusion among many of the healers about the appropriateness of traditional concepts for modern problems. The health staff cannot cope with the psychosocial and mental health problems of their patients. But most importantly, there are the obvious needs of many individual Cambodians, families and communities.

THE INTERVENTION APPROACH

In February 1995 a project was started on the assumption that the Cambodian people could be helped in coping with the past.[12] The project wanted to support individuals, families and communities in coping with trauma. The idea was to introduce community workers (teachers, health workers, and others) to basic theoretical and practical knowledge in the field of psychosocial interventions, and to develop psychosocial care as an aspect of community work and general health policy.

We formed a core group of Cambodians who were offered culturally appropriate and relevant training, monitoring and supervision, based on the

---

[12]The project was started by the International institute for psychosocial and socio-ecological research (IPSER). In 1996 the organization changed its name to Transcultural Psychosocial Organization (TPO). The project was funded by the government of the Netherlands, and ran until November 2000. Since that time, the project continues its activities as an independent Cambodian NGO: TPO Cambodia.

daily experience of assessing existing problems and identifying realistic solutions in the field of psychosocial problems in the community. We developed, tested and evaluated culturally sensitive guidelines and manuals for improved detection, assessment, management and prevention of psychosocial problems on the basis of the reached understanding with the core group.

Subsequently we extended the training to other community workers. After being familiar with the curriculum and the practical work in case management, the core group was trained in didactic skills and trained others, who were selected according to the results of the action research within the project.

In working close with the University of Phnom Penh, the project strengthened domestic action research capacity. Students participated in the community-based activities, and their activities were incorporated in their training. They were also involved in various types of action research.

Interventions

We found individuals in need of mental health services, and others in need to break their social isolation. We found families in need of moral and material. There are healers and monks who are looking for ways to understand what is happening to society, in order to be able to improve support to families in their community. There are communities struggling with psychosocial problems, and individuals and families who are looking for others for a sense of community. The program set out to develop interventions for these needs. In this section of the chapter we will describe these interventions and the difficulties we had in developing and implementing them. The interventions can be summarized in a matrix (Table 1).

Four elements are basic in this intervention model:

1. to create awareness concerning psycho-social and mental health problems, by producing appropriate materials and training local health workers and NGO staff in psycho-education;
2. to support community rebuilding and strengthen the existing sectors on the basis of information on the right match between problems and resources, by installing referral potential and collaboration between different sectors;
3. to better equip the existing resources, by offering training, based on an especially developed manual, to different groups such as teachers, health staff, healers and NGO community workers;
4. to add appropriate new resources at different levels, including mental health clinics at the provincial and district level; trained villagers in teams to refer families and provide psycho-education; self-help groups where women and men find a 'niche' in village life where they are allowed to talk about their emotions.

Table 1. Intervention Scheme, Showing Needs, Missing Links and Interventions

Levels of intervention	Identified needs	Missing links	Interventions
Individual and family	Individuals and families suffer psychological effects of traumatic events—and do not succeed in finding effective help. Individuals suffering mental disorders have no services available to them.	Change in structure of communities has affects availability of resources. Events and modernization affects appropriateness of local explanatory models. No mental health service.	Rehabilitation of traditional links between families in need and resources in the community. Facilitation of new interpretations and new explanatory models Installation of basic mental health skills in primary health care levels.
Groups and community	Addressing events of the past in a 'search for meaning'. Alternative interpretations of common problems—to create alternative solutions.	There is no 'niche' that allows discussion of emotional burdens. In this fragmented society trust needs to be build to reinstall structures for social interaction.	Psycho-education (awareness) sessions at group and community level. Psycho-education through traditional resources. Organization of self-help groups.
Society	A need to come to terms with the past, and a better understanding of the effects of the events of the past decades for society. Psychiatric and psychological skills are needed for treatment of individuals.	There is no institutionalized knowledge, no implementing capacity. Central potential for reflective work on Cambodian history.	Enhancement of awareness of psychosocial effects through broadcasted psycho-education (newspapers, radio and television). Curricula development and central level training.

Before we discuss these different interventions we have to elaborate on what was the essential method of the program: training Cambodian people. The original intention was to find a group of people with a clear interest in doing psychosocial work and to start practical work with these people as soon as possible. Our daily experience would then give us sufficient material to build on in working towards culturally relevant and appropriate interventions. Training and the development of interventions was to feed in to each other. However, this turned out to be a gross underestimation of reaching shared understanding about the scope of our program: the introduction of a concept of 'psychosocial work' on all levels.

The agony of Cambodian history is often illustrated by the near extinction of educated groups under the Khmer Rouge regime. But to understand some of the issues in training, developments before 1975 and after 1979 are also important. Traditional education in pagoda schools was replaced throughout the 1950s and 1960s by a government installed educational system. Historians (e.g., Chandler, 1993) have described the weaknesses of this system before 1970. Whereas the main role of education in the colonial era was preparing people to take up roles as 'fonctionnaires', for which little technical know-how or analytical skills were needed, throughout the 1960s the gap between the content of education and the demands of society became clear. Some schoolteachers in Phnom Penh recognised this in the 1950s and 1960s, and this actually marked the beginning of the movement of which these teachers were to become leaders, the Khmer Rouge.

But also these teachers were firmly imbedded in the previously discussed hierarchical roles in Cambodia, and the traditional position of importance of the teacher was never questioned. This strict hierarchy made exchange of ideas or discussions between teacher and pupil unlikely if not impossible. Critical questions were seen as not polite—they were potentially embarrassing.

What could have gradually developed into a more modernized system of education and adapted teaching and learning skills was stopped short by warfare. In the civil war years (1970–75) many people were barred from education for very practical reasons, and after April 1975 the rice fields became the University for the whole of the population, according to Pol Pot.

The subsequent presence of the Vietnamese caused fear which, however irrational or unjustified it may have been, had a paralyzing effect on society. The educational system had to be rebuilt amidst lack of material, lack of trained staff, and a deep sense of insecurity about what would happen next in Cambodia. New teachers as well as students at the time found that the best way to avoid danger was to accept what was offered without skepticism. The traditional importance of playing the given role in society to perfection was now turned into a caricature. Curricula were followed strictly. The teacher would write texts from his textbook on the blackboard, and students would copy. The teachers would speak, the students would repeat. Teaching became a ritual based on the experience of the old traditional religious schools: the copying and chanting of texts. After the texts were being used this way, they became instantly meaningless. Pages from notebooks would be torn out at the end of the day to wrap food or roll cigarettes. Only empty pages represented some value: they had still to be used in the training ritual, for one day.

One of the consequences was that many people kept using the same coping style which had helped them to survive the Khmer Rouge era, characterized by quiet, low-profile, non-confrontational acceptance. The bureaucratic system in all levels of government encouraged reserved behavior, where one would do as was told, follow rules and regulations, forms and protocols to the letter. Initiative was discouraged, obedience the norm. The educational system in the 1980s was constructed in a situation where strict communist bureaucratic rules came on top of traditional hierarchy and the experience of Khmer Rouge authority. This strengthened the already existing tradition of non-critical acceptance in educational settings.

The status of texts is a complex matter in Cambodian society. Secular texts are mainly seen as administrative tools of control. The detailed documents produced in torture centers (Tuol Sleng most notably) and the role of the press are two examples on different ends of a continuum (Chandler, 1999; Mehta, 1997). Written confessions quite obviously held no truth but functioned as the justification of immediate killing, and the newspapers were mainly used—and tolerated—as channels for provocative and phony accusations. In both examples, the written word does not mean much. The spoken word is much more important. Truth and meaning are in the words people speak, not in the words people write. The chanting of Pali texts is important—not reading them. And this has consequences for training programs as well as action research in Cambodia.

In doing action research in Cambodia, language is an important tool of communication, but is by no means the only aspect of it. Language itself reflects some of the aspects of social life that are important in Cambodia, and it also reproduces these aspects. In every-day life Cambodia, the presentation of what is said, or '*how* things are said', is at least as important as the content of the message.

The role people have according to status, which shapes the conversation, can easily lead to misunderstanding. Roles of people change: a woman can be an employee, and employer, a mother, a wife, and a daughter, and has to act accordingly at different times of the day. People talk in accordance with the role they take at a specific time and place. This role influences not only what they say, but also how they say it. The westerners 'obsession with truth', and the methods used in finding, or creating a version of, the truth, are often incompatible with specific culture-bound ways of communicating.

When questionnaires are done about the needs of people, the answers can easily be misinterpreted without anyone being aware of it. People may say yes when they mean no, and everybody may understand—except the interpreter-researcher at the end of the line, who feeds the answers into the computer, and reduces all meaning to digital information. Too often one finds examples of assumptions based on superficial understanding, not only of what has been said, but also on how it has been said. Examples are studies concerning reproductive health (the reports say that women report an overwhelming need for contraceptives, but in practice most women refuse to use means even when offered free in their own house); the selection of trainees for NGO programs (incentives offered make it attractive for a patron in the phum to ensure that his clients benefit from these—although they may not be the implementers looked for); medical misinterpretation (the patient-doctor role does not allow a patient to report complaints which she or he could, and would, easily discuss with the same doctor outside the medical space). Answers given to questionnaires are a mix of politeness, curiosity and specific interests. Everyday in the newspapers there are examples of how confusion exists about the meaning of what has been said. Not only the content, but the show-element of talking, the rhetoric of repetition, the 'chanting' of messages is often not picked up by the foreigner, or the Cambodian researcher who follows 'orders' from the methodological textbook.

Issues of meaning and traditional learning styles have played a huge role in the pilot phase of the project. The initial exchange of information between Cambodian and expatriate members of the team took much more time than expected. The expatriate trainers noticed an inability to read with comprehension, to access information, poorly developed skills in analyzing and synthesizing, a lack of concepts and perspective, a fear of not being right, and an expectation that there were strict rules to be found which would tell the core group what to do in any circumstances. The core group members noticed a lack of language skills, a fuzzy set of ideas about what should be done exactly, a disregard for the classroom as the proper venue for training, and a confusing desire of wanting to be colleagues and employers at the same time. The notion of supervision was difficult to distinguish from control, and especially the idea of a 'cybernetic loop of information', fine-tuning interventions or creating new interventions on the basis of experience, was difficult to implement.

Thus we learned that the insights slowly gained in aspects of Cambodian society could immediately be applied to our own work. The general lack of trust, the silence about emotions in hierarchical situations and the extreme carefulness in avoiding unpleasant comments in an unsafe setting were all having their effect in our daily work. It took a long time to establish the trust that allowed for internal evaluation in a constructive manner.

With hindsight one easily sees the reasons for this. Basic skills such as report writing or planning work schedules can be taught and learned. Much more difficult and time-consuming is to first adjust to the idea that some knowledge is not, and cannot be, precise, in the sense of technical factuality or political correctness.[13] Then was has to feel comfortable enough with this idea to use accumulated experience and self-written reports as a basis to change interventions.

---

[13]Some trainees were disappointed when there were no straightforward answers to questions such as 'how many times does a woman with four dead children need counseling, as compared with a woman who has two dead children?' Some took the reply that there is no definite, context-free answer to this as a sign that a better teacher was needed: someone who would know.

In the end, we managed to bridge the gap by applying the age-old way of learning that seems universal: role modeling—which is how traditional healers have always been trained. The core group became more confident as they slowly familiarized themselves with casework, and especially as they helped writing the manual (see below). After basic trust had been established, we found common ground in the exchange of opinions and experience that led towards new initiatives, and the development of new interventions. We used well known elements in culture, such as stories, the traditional relations between people, and we worked with various traditional healers. The challenge was in deliberately creating something new by combining older and newer elements.

In the first four months of the program, the focus was on an exchange of information: the core group was introduced to mental health and psychological concepts, while the expatriate team was informed on the social context and personal experience of problems of the *heart-mind*—the Cambodian expression closest to psychosocial problems. The core group started working in clusters of villages in the provinces of Kandaal, Kampong Speu, and Battambang. Practical training was done in the field. The work in the villages offered new material for discussion and learning sessions every day. It was in this stage that mutual understanding was beginning to grow.

Production of Culturally Competent Materials. One of the challenges in the project was the production of teaching material. Next to posters, videos, radio and television appearances and verbal modules, the way to reach trainees, health authorities, and other organizations was to develop a curricula and texts on community mental health. Curricula for health staff were developed for the Ministry of Health, according to the guidelines of the 'minimal and complementary package of activities' under the health reform plan. In these curricula we could use the experience gained in endless discussions on community mental health, in combination with international expertise on primary mental health care. The most time-consuming and complicated work was in the development of a community mental health manual.

The UNHCR/WHO Mental Health for Refugees Manual (De Jong & Clarke, 1996) was used as a source of inspiration for a new manual, especially developed for the situation in Cambodia. The structure includes the most common and important part of the community workers responsibility and offers a complete range of possible psychosocial interventions to be chosen according to the needs of the client. Although theoretically, academically and to some extent clinically, the demarcation between major (psychosis) and minor mental disorders (psycho-social, for which the Khmer term 'wrecked heart-mind' or *khooc cet is appropriate) is not all that clear cut, the distinction is helpful for teaching about mental illness at a basic level. Subtle psychological concepts had to be introduced for the first time and the need was for simple and clear lessons that could be easily understood.

Specially given the lack of skills and material in the western sector, it was felt to be important to include lessons learnt in co-operation and research into the traditional sector in the manual. Thus throughout the manual there is special attention for local idioms of distress, the locally used taxonomy of mental disorder, and there is a special unit on local resources to fit the local context. In the chapter about relaxation exercises it was thought appropriate to introduce the age-old Buddhist practices of mindful breathing (Ana Pana Sati) and meditation, as well as local massage techniques.

The manual has been titled Community Mental Health in Cambodia, and exists in a Khmer and English version (Somasundaram, D. J., Kail, K., Van de Put, W. A. C. M., Eisenbruch, M., & Thomassen, L., 1997). The contents of the manual include units on helping skills, the community and its resources, stress and relaxation, psychosocial problems, major mental disorders, children, alcohol and drug problems, and epilepsy and head injury.

There were many technical problems in translating from English to Khmer and vice-versa. Many English psychological words had no equivalent in Khmer. A whole Khmer vocabulary for psychological terms had to be created. Part of this effort resulted in and benefited from the Psychology Dictionary brought out by the Department of Psychology, University of Phnom Penh. Some terms had to be literally coined and short explanations included in the text.

Training using this draft was first given for the program team, who then used the draft for training a variety of trainees, who were then followed-up to ascertain what they were doing with the training. The feedback from the team, the trainees, their follow-up assessment and comments from experts in the field were used to prepare the pre-final draft. Before the core group started the first batch of training for village workers a preparatory session of the material was organized. In these sessions the units were reviewed word-by-word, and the core group had many suggestions on the appropriate terminology, and added examples based on their own experience in the villages. Back-translation was checked again. In this process the core group made the last steps to becoming familiar with the units of the manual.

Field-testing the manual involved several topics. First, the selection of the trainees is a test in itself. By follow-up and monitoring the core group checks how the villagers saw the training, how they use this new knowledge, and how this effects their communities. Another point for field-testing is how to match the content of the manual with the different levels of education of the trainees. Different levels of understanding call for fine-tuned didactic skills and training styles. Specific training in didactic skills for the core group helped them to adapt the training to the groups selected.

THE CAMBODIAN EXPERIENCE

On the basis of this manual the core group has been training a total of some 1600 people up to 1999. Training is still ongoing. The trainees are various health staff, NGO staff, ministerial staff, traditional healers, formal and informal village leaders, other villagers and students.

We shall now turn to the interventions these people were trained in. We will begin at the community level, and descend to the level of the individual. Thus we can describe the work of the program in a natural order: we enter a village, identify problems, and apply interventions. When relevant we will refer to the characteristics we have identified in the first part of the chapter, and show how we tried to overcome difficulties and be complementary to existing resources.

Community Interventions: Entering the Village

First contact in any community was with the local authorities, respecting the importance of hierarchy and order. The team explains the ideas of trying to collect information about the problems of the 'heart-mind' (*paññyeahaa plav cet) families are facing. The history of the particular village is discussed with some of the leaders at the house of one of them, and anyone standing around quickly joins in. Soon demarcation lines in the social structure of the *phum are clear. Especially vulnerable groups are identified, and the *phum will be one of the three types mentioned above.

If a tight group is encountered, it is easy to contact healers and other resources for help, and organize group sessions where the problems of the 'heart-mind' are discussed. Materials for psycho-education have been developed, and the posters, videotapes and presentations on special modules allow people to shift the angle of interpretation of their daily problems. Building on the existing relations in the village, the team can begin organizing training for interested helpers in the community, and group work (see below) comes almost automatically.

In mixed villages the approach has to be more careful. The different groups are best approached separately, and the team finds out through interviews of key informants (teachers, village leaders, monks) what the local history is. In these phums building individual relationships between healers or helpers and people in need meant building up a sense of mutual trust that is the basis for group sessions. In 'new *phum' the most effective approach is for the team to start individual casework and identify individuals who have common interests. Once they are brought together, psycho-education is given for various groups, and relationships begin to be possible.

In all villages, people tell the team about the problems in either their own family or direct relatives, and usually agree with the suggestion of the team to go to the house where the problems are. These initial discussions about the project in the beginning phase of the program helped to develop material for psycho-education later on. At the house of one of the identified families, the discussion about the problems and their causes is continued. The family is asked what was done to find solutions, and if possible, the informant is asked to come along to the house, market, or hospital where help was found. There the healer, health worker or any other resource is asked to comment upon the problem and give her/his views about the causes and potential healing chances. Since the overall majority of people have visited several of the health sectors, it is often possible to reconstruct the health-seeking path and see a number of the helpers involved in the reported problem.

If possible, the next step in help-seeking behavior is followed. Sometimes suggestions are made. This involves the team actively in the help-seeking behavior of some patients, and allows them in other cases to be part of the search for help. These visits provide documented information on help-seeking behavior and current beliefs in the individual, family and healer.

The next step is thus defined by the type of village entered, and can consist of either psycho-education for anyone interested, and/or individual case work aimed at strengthening local resources for help, or individual case-work that builds a basis for a group approach.

We will discuss these related interventions separately, but will first present an example of how the teams were able to successfully break through culturally mediated patterns of expectations and dependency.

Breaking the Cycle of Poverty and Depression: the 'Isolated Woman'. To give an example of how this works in practice, we present a case example of a pregnant woman whom we shall call Somaly, living in extremely poor conditions with four children at the edge of a *phum where her husband was born. He had left her after the fourth child was born. He now lived with another woman, but every now and then he would come back, and Somaly always hoped he would stay. Problems would start within a few days, however. The last time the man left, he had taken the last valuables and left her pregnant and beaten up. The malnourished and weak children did not go to school. They had scabies. The woman did not have any relatives in the village. Her mother lived about 10 km away, and would sometimes visit her. The mother was in no position to offer material support, since she hardly had enough for herself.

This woman was one of the many widows, *mee-may, a term also used for abandoned women in Cambodia. Living isolated in a village where she was not originally from, she belonged to a group we had come to see as one of the most vulnerable in rural areas. She seemed to be in really hopeless situation. In the first flowchart, put together in the course of discussion with the team after they had seen the woman, one sees how the problems are all related, and how it would not help to suppose that one problem solved at the time would not come

THE CAMBODIAN EXPERIENCE

back quickly afterwards. The related problems are like a downward spiral, which needs to be stopped.

1. Problems.

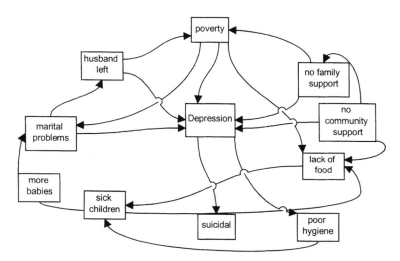

Figure 1. Problems.

At first the team found it difficult to get away from the expectations given with the roles they felt they had in this community. As people with positions, jobs, and therefore rich as compared to the villagers, they felt they should confirm this status by giving presents. Embarrassed and shy at first contact because they felt ashamed for having no material support to offer, they became somewhat more confident when they realized how happy the woman was when they returned for a second, and third visit. But what was to be done? One way to begin is to look for the simplest problem, and start there. One of the team showed the woman how she could treat the scabies by washing the children with water, boiled with the leaves of the tamarind tree.

The team was suspicious. Would one really have to teach the woman how to do things that were so common in Cambodia—and would she actually do them and keep doing them? If so, more women might be in need of this simple advice. The traditional birth attendant (*cmab*) would be the right person to do this, as we had found in our interviews with healers. In the same vein, the group realized that one could relate all the different problems to different resources in the community. There could be organizations working in the area in fields such as health education, health care, family spacing, food programs, income generation and small credit schemes. There is the pagoda, there are the traditional healers, the older people, teachers, the *phum* leaders. All these people can be seen as resources available—if one would just know what to ask them and how to stimulate them to help. The second flowchart shows the resources related to the problems.

2. Problems and resources.

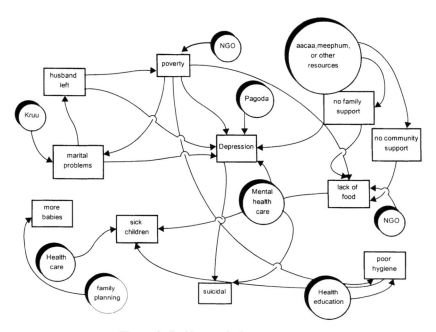

Figure 2. Problems and relevant resources.

For marital problems, one can go to the *kruu*. For the food situation one could look at the rice bank or other initiatives. An important part of facilitating interventions thus became mapping these various resources. The different sectors for help need to be localised, people need to be found and asked what one could do in a situation like this.

It is possible to find the traditional sector, the public health sector, the community development sector, but what is there for problems such as depression and suicidal behavior? Many problems can be referred, but that in itself was not seen as sufficient. Some part of the problem seemed to need new interventions. There was no referral option for mental health problems of this woman in this specific situation. Here was a role for the program—installing basic psychiatric skills in primary care (see below). Next to that, Somaly was a 'new person' in this *phum*, which meant no more than that none of the community leaders were related to her. But this severely affected her access to normal local resources. This was a typical situation of where traditional relations could be re-invented.

THE CAMBODIAN EXPERIENCE

3. Problems, resources, and interventions.

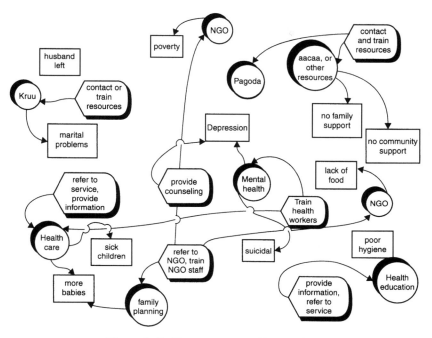

Figure 3. Problems, resources and interventions.

The above scheme shows the resources for the various interventions needed. Now it could be seen how the activities of the team relate to the problems of the woman. The team kept visiting Somaly, and listened to her. They were themselves impressed by the effect of this activity, which was seen as 'nothing' at first, but laid the first foundation for 'talk therapy'—a modest beginning of counseling skills, something very new in Cambodia (see below). The initial fear that Somaly would want to have nothing to do with them once she found there was no material support proved to be wrong.

The tip about the tamarind tree leaves worked well. The children were getting better. Somaly, in talking with the team, came to realize that she was not the only one in this situation. Shame, hopelessness and the conviction that help could only be expected from people who were far better of had prevented her form recognizing others in similar positions. Somaly began to talk to others, and took more care of her children. It seemed like the team had succeeded in finding a way 'in'—breaking through the cycle of causation.

One day, her mother was visiting when the team was there. The team asked the mother what she would have done if a similar situation had occurred when she was young, in the 1960's. The mother responded that a situation such as this would be unthinkable then. The chief of the *phum*, the older men, and especially the *aacaa* would not have allowed such behavior from a young man (the husband). Somaly would have found support from the community against a man who was clearly behaving out of bounds—and this would have been easier because she would have lived in her own village, where her husband had joined her. The team then asked why Somaly would not try to go and talk to the *aacaa*, but both mother and daughter said that this could not be done. When asked why, they said that they felt to be too poor to go to the *aacaa* and ask his help.

Later the team visited the *aacaa* and talked about his role in the phum. He was proud to have the team coming to the pagoda to talk to him, and complained that few people seemed to want his advise anymore. He felt his status as *aacaa*, which used to be a respected position only open for the best of the older men, had inflated since his father had been one. The team told him about the woman, and her hesitations to come to him for advise. The *aacaa* explained that he would be delighted to see what he could do, as long as the woman would respect his position as an *aacaa* and come to him—she could not expect a man of his position to go to her house to offer his support. The roles had to be played well. When this message was brought back to Somaly, she eventually gathered courage and went to see the *aacaa*.

This contact was a turning point in a process of re-socialization for Somaly. Not all her problems were solved, but her isolation had become less. She now had contact with other women, with whom she could share work and help in looking after the children. She was now known to the *aacaa*, and had better access to the pagoda and the monks. Village committees were helpful in getting the children to school. The vicious cycle had been broken, and was turned upward.

In this approach we made full use of the information on explanatory models used by people in distress. The explanatory models pointed the way to the right resources for help. Knowing these resources, and knowing what they did and how they could be approached, helped us bridge the gap between a woman in distress and the community around her. Knowledge on the role-play and hierarchy informed us about thresholds in accessing various resources for Somaly. The characteristics of a mixed phum helped in realizing why in this community a special intervention was needed to restore age-old Cambodian community relations.

The mix of problems Somaly had to cope with reflected what we earlier called the banality of psychosocial problems. Her problems seem no different from those of many women in other countries. Yet the context in which she had to cope with them was laden with the effects of war and the breakdown of social life. Her husband's behaviour is no longer as remarkable as it was in her mother's youth. Her social position in her village is a direct result of warfare. Her lack of access to a community and her depressed state counted for a loss of even the simplest folk treatments.

Flow charts as shown above, based on real experience, where used as a training device; as the beginning of a map of a district to show where problems and resources are; and as an inventory of intervention possibilities. Exploring social structures showed the most productive composition of teams of village volunteers for psychosocial work. Being offered a role as a helper for others further helped women like Somaly, and important villagers such as the *aacaa* felt recognized when included. Both had a keen interest in participating in training: the women because it helped them understand and act upon their own situation, the *aacaa* because it raised his status and gave him ideas on how to help others. The women were happy to do outreach work: visiting marginalised families brought them social contacts. They felt safe under the protection of their colleagues in the 'village team', important people such as the *aacaa* or village leader, who in turn enjoyed being consulted by families sent to them by the women.

Mapping local resources also brought the team to community workers involved in other programs. We co-operated with local and international organizations that implemented community development programs in many sectors. We managed to establish contact between these programs and the population who would benefit most of them via the local counterparts. In that way community development programs benefited from a motivated target group, while the most vulnerable people benefited from the development program. This way the project had a preventive impact on psychosocial problems by offering people real chances to improve their well being.

The experience with Somaly showed the team that talking and listening was helpful. This notion in turn helped the team to move away from more traditional ideas of helping, which consisted mainly of providing material aid and using the hierarchical role to order behavior change.

Psycho-Education

In the approach towards the total community, in group work and in sessions with individuals, psycho-education is essential. In the 'old *phums*' an initial discussion with the village chief and the crowd that would immediately gather around his house was enough to set a date for a village-wide session on psycho-education. People in these villages have easy access to their local resources for help. The interest in discussing the 'heart-mind' problems was nevertheless enormous.

One important aim of psycho-education was to help people see their problems in a fresh way. The vicious cycle of depression and poverty leads to a series of problems as shown in the case of Somaly. Unraveling this knot was a process people highly enjoyed in group sessions. It helped to distinguish between the different aspects of a problematic situation, and made people think again about what kind of help might be available. An example is how women are affected by *toah*, which can only be healed by the kruu, but at the same time have abdominal problems that need medical care. Treatment offered by different sectors can easily be complementary.

A clear example of the need for complementarity is in perinatal and postnatal disorders. These are widespread across cultures, but little is known of indigenous taxonomies, explanatory models, or local treatment methods used to ameliorate or prevent them. The Khmer term *toah* means 'to be different', 'in conflict', 'incompatible', or 'to quarrel'. Perinatal disorders can be viewed as partial solutions to sociomoral predicaments. The illnesses provide women, who have few options over how they work, eat, and cohabit, with a socially acceptable 'way out' to signal their distress and to find partial support from the traditional healers. These disorders involve many symptoms, while the causes for these symptoms are seen differently by traditional and western healers. In order to heal the person, the symptoms as well as the cause need to be treated. Sometimes the traditional healer may not be able to treat the symptoms. Sometimes the doctor may not be able to treat the cause.

Using posters and video material in psycho-education sessions helped people look at their own problems from a slightly different angle. Domestic violence and alcoholism now became symptoms of underlying causes rather than unavoidable facts of life. An alternative idea of causality where abnormal situations caused normal reactions helped people think of alternative ways of coping, such as sharing experiences and finding help with local resources for special parts of their problems. Psycho-education helped people to make more effective use of available resources, and also facilitated new approaches.

Relaxation Techniques. As a practical part of psycho-education relaxation techniques were introduced. Promoting body-awareness and encouraging the use of body-oriented techniques like relaxation exercises and breathing exercises was also used in individual encounters in counseling. The following four methods were adapted to suit the culture and religion of the Cambodian community (see also the chapter on Sri Lanka):

- Breathing Exercises. Buddhist Mindful breathing or Ana Pana Sati.
- Muscular Relaxation. A variation of Jacobson's Progressive Muscular Relaxation, the technically similar Yogic exercise, Shanti or Sava Asana or the Buddhist Mindful body awareness was used.
- Repetition of Words. A meaningful word, phrase or verse is repeated over and over to oneself.
- Meditation. Various meditation practices known in Cambodia, such as *Samadhi and *Vipassana meditation were used.

Using traditional methods of massage like *Thveu Saasay* to produce profound relaxation is both culturally familiar and effective. Therapy with relaxation methods, being non-pharmacological, is safe, cheap, non-toxic and has no side-effects.

The benefits to these practices are not confined to producing relaxation. When methods are culturally familiar, they tap into past childhood, community and religious roots and thus release a rich source of associations that can be helpful in therapy and the healing process. Although these techniques do no formal psychotherapy, they may accomplish what psychotherapy attempts to do by releasing cultural and spiritual restorative processes. One way is by teaching the traditional practices to large groups in the community, in pagodas, community centers, and as part of the curricula in schools. This is be promotive, preventive and curative. When people come together to learn and practice these methods in a Pagoda under a senior *aacaa or monk, the atmosphere is therapeutic and socially healing. Apart from the actual practice of the methods, people interact in a healthy way, support each other, find meaning for their problems and suffering through the *religious* doctrines on Karma and suffering.

Staff of ministries of rural development, women's affairs, and social welfare and NGO staff are trained in organizing psycho-education sessions. Some of the monks are eager to use parts of the manual in their chants at funerals and at other occasions. The core group members themselves directly reach some 5000 people per year in psycho-education sessions for groups. The numbers reached by ministry and NGO staff and monks are not easily available, but should be many more.

Psycho-education was used as a means to reach groups of villagers who gathered to hear about a different way to look at familiar problems. It was also used within self-help groups to open discussions, and as well as a tool in individual treatment. In the 'old *phums' one of the effects of psycho-education is an interest in self-help groups. In the 'new *phums' individual case management builds relationships and leads to group work.

Group Work

The group approach is not only appropriate because so many people require help, but is necessary to facilitate a joint process of coming to terms with the past. Since problems people face are often related to a process of finding some kind of meaning, or at least an acceptable explanation, for the events of the past and the present, and this calls for discussion, exchange of opinions, and mutual reinforcement. The fact that people actually help themselves, prevents an extra layer of 'psychosocial workers' and facilitates (re)building social networks.

In the composition of groups and the gradual transition from facilitated group work to self-help groups, it is important to know the local history and the type of village. According to Kinzie (1997) group therapy is a 'professionally led therapeutic activity occurring in a group setting employing techniques varying from educational to those in which specific interactional and dynamic issues are

Ancestral Spirit Illness—Violations of Moral Hygiene in the Family

The transition from childhood to early adulthood is the critical period when the person's upbringing will be tested—not only in terms of how they will respond to the developmental pressure to become sexually active, but also whether their choice of marriage partner will be the most propitious. Any community misfortune can be traced to the couple's miscreance, so parents have to guard their daughters for everyone's sake. This belief helps to explain the elaborate marriage ceremonies that inform the ancestral spirits that a particular couple are properly together and that no offence should be taken when they begin to have sex. The fit between the partners shapes the sort of descendants they in turn will raise, so naturally their ancestors keep a watchful eye during his phase. It is also a testing time for the parents who, after all, were accountable for rearing the children and for their character development.

The most common general term for family lineage is 'family line' (*puuc*). Families in which an illness run are designated 'leprosy family', tuberculosis family' or simply 'illness family'. Another popular related term is 'family line' or 'family tree' (*trakool*) which refers to the race or the clan. Another widely known term is 'mum-dad ancestral spirits' (*mee baa*) which designates, too, the parents and the representatives of the bride and groom during the marriage ceremony. This term is reserved to delineate close relationships within two generations of the person. Healers have an additional vocabulary. The 'line of the family lineage' (*cuə cambuə*) takes in assumed ancestral links to a person.

In 'wrong to the ancestral line' (*khoh cue cambue*), the illness stems from the remote ancestral line some generations removed from the patient. The victim can be any direct descendant of the culprit, in any generation, with no implication that the patient has done wrong. And the preliminary illness can be arrested when the victim apologizes on behalf of the family line and offering propitiation in apology to the ancestral spirits. In the second taxon, the illness stems from an ancestral spirit one generation removed from the patient and their still-living forebears and known in Khmer as 'mum-dad ancestral spirits' (*mee baa*); the victim was the wrong-doer or their parent, spouse, or sibling. The group covered domestic conflicts.

The preliminary stage of illness can be divided along several lines:

- The origin of the illness, or punishment: remote generations of the ancestral spirits of the family line, or the immediate ancestral sprits
- The identity of the violator of the code of conduct
- Whether the victim, or the patient, was necessarily the culprit who had committed the infraction
- The clinical features of the illness
- Whether there was a time limit during which the culprit could admit guilt or perform the necessary propitiatory offerings to the ancestral spirits
- Expected course and outcome (death, recovery, or chronicity).

The ancestral spirits, in their capacity as moral policemen and in withdrawing protection, leave the descendant open to the depredations, such as sorcery attack, initiated by the aggrieved family against him. In this way, the person's ancestors act in concert with the community.

There are three components to the diagnosis of illness from ancestral spirits. One procedure, 'augury with the chicken egg', was used to detect who in a family group had committed the offence, a critical question when 'wrong to the mum-dad spirits' was suspected, but irrelevant when the patient was afflicted by 'line of illness' because the culprit, one of the patient's forebears, was long dead. Astrological prediction, known as (*tiey*) or literally 'seeing divination' (*tɔəh tiey*), was a method used to determine which ancestral spirit had been wronged and offended and had caused the illness, but the healer did not disclose his logical steps to the patient. In another procedure, 'examining the healing manuals', also employed to diagnose which ancestral spirit was angered, the patient's personal history was important, and the patient followed the logical deductions used by the healer. If a person was already ill, the manuals could help explain why; if they were in good health, the manuals warned of their proneness—everyone had their Achilles heel.

Treatment

The spectrum of ancestral spirit disorders can be treated by a ritual sequence that follows roughly this order:

General vaccination of the whole community. The calendrical ritual offerings to the ancestral spirits, performed on behalf of the whole community, in a ritual known as 'erecting the pavilion' (**laəŋrɔən*). This ceremony, rather than curing an individual patient, helps everyone.

Before the patient has been cured of first-stage illness. Treatment focuses on the clarification of the problem and with appeasement through dialogue of ancestral spirits. Ritual offering to the ancestral spirits, known by the general term (**saen*): these rituals include calling the protective ancestral spirit to possess the medium and reveal the nature of the patient's offence (**bañcoan ʔaarak*); and 'feasting the ancestral spirit' (**lieŋ ʔaarak*).

Immediately after the cure of the first-stage illness. Treatment focuses on termination of issues to do with the ancestral spirit. The patient, if a promise has been made to the ancestral spirit, must discharge it and announce that it has been discharged (**lie bamnan*). Treatment then focuses on minimizing the sequelae of the illness caused by invading wild spirits unconnected to the ancestral line.

Follow up. Defensive manoeuvres to prevent attack by wild spirits unrelated to the ancestral spirits: these include the use of magical yantra designs.

examined'. He notes that in group therapy with Cambodian people cultural values such as respect for authority, the need for smooth relationships and the traditional interdependent family relationships are important in the psychotherapeutic relationship, and would pose difficulties for a positive outcome (Kinzie, 1997). There would be no cultural analogue to the type of self-disclosure required in individual psychotherapy in any of the Asian healing ceremonies. Asians would be reluctant to speak about themselves publicly. Group processes may be less straightforward than in the West.

We found that a group approach to deal with problems was not only possible and effective, but also embedded in culture itself.

By taking the social structures of the communities in account, and organize groups accordingly, we could prevent some of the constraints Kinzie found. Once people have been selected from the same social strata, being in comparable positions, we find that sharing emotions turns out to be an enormous relief. People have to feel safe in this new setting, and begin to talk about the daily problems everybody shares. The facilitator helps to create an atmosphere of trust, and uses modules of psycho-education to start a discussion about problems of another order, the problems that cause much more emotional discomfort then the usual daily things.

The group sessions in Cambodia proved to provide a setting where, for the first time ever, people have an opportunity to talk about their emotions. Groups of women or men need a safe setting, a facilitator who can introduce the topic, and not much more to begin a process of finding out what actually happened to them, and why. This cannot be overestimated: in a society where any attempt to come to terms with the past has been frustrated by a complex knot of socio-cultural and political reasons, organizing group talk about the events of the past simply offered an excuse that was eagerly used by many to finally 'just talk'. In group sessions people often repeat stories from the past. It is as if the stories need to be repeated until they start making some sense.

Group members start offering each other very pragmatic mutual support. They help each other find work, look after each other's children, or simply comfort each other. This works well as long as no label is used to describe these activities, such as solidarity, group-work, friendship, brotherhood, or social support. These terms have all been abused by one or another totalitarian system in the past.

The group setting, which allows its participants for the first time to talk freely about their daily emotional problems, is seen by most of them as too precious to be risked by the potential problems related to communal business. The repetition of life stories serves the purpose of finding meaning for what has happened, and, of course, the process of rebuilding mutual trust requires time. Some of the self-help groups slowly create new networks of friends that stretch much farther than the *phum. And once they are connected, introduced to each other, these networks develop quickly and start functioning as communities with mutual support. Some 2000 people are reached per year in groups facilitated by team members. Some of these groups quickly require no more facilitation and turn into self-help groups. Others function for some time and then dissolve, but not without having at least given people an opportunity to start building supportive relationships. And these are used to find practical solutions leading to additional income, shared responsibilities, and a sense of belonging.

Counseling

One of the most common interventions in psychotherapy and psychosocial work is the supportive verbal contact between the helper and the client, of which counseling is one type. Supportive verbal contact takes place in the sessions with mediums (kruu chool ruub), and although the client contacts a supernatural entity through the medium, the idea of verbal healing already exists in the Cambodian context. The team found people also appreciated talking and listening about problems without the supernatural context, and we set out to see if counseling techniques could be used in Cambodia.

There are reasons to question the potential use of these techniques (Van de Put et al., 1998a). People do not talk easily amongst each other about emotional distress. The general feeling is that one should not think, and certainly not talk about traumatic events. They should be forgotten. Talk would open up old wounds in the listener, and the result would just be more pain. Even in the 'old *phums*' relatives avoid to discuss traumatic events.

In counseling sessions the client is invited to talk about her/his personal life. As said before, the quality of a life has much to do with the perfection of playing ones role according to now it should be'. Legends and stories provide a mold to shape reality in communicable ways, and are important for constructing role models. Truth is constructed in a careful process where hierarchy and role-expectations are respected or even cautiously mocked, in order to present the often chaotic reality in a polished way.[14] To the western listener who compares notes of various counseling sessions with one client, this results in confusion about what actually happened and sometimes outright frustration.

Another difficulty is related to the importance of regulated behavior and communication, and helps to explain the success of the mediums. Open discussion aimed at solving conflicts is usually avoided. The strength of the mediums is in their ability to allow people to communicate directly with spirits who are beyond conventional limitations in communication. Problem solving without supernatural assistance is different. When heads of families used to meet in order to find ways to prevent escalating conflicts they would not aim at taking away the cause of the conflict. Finding acceptable ways for all parties to let the conflict rest, in other words, defining the proper way to behave in a crisis situation is more important to than 'tackling the roots of the problem'. Finally, the social hierarchy tends to rule out the emphatic relationship required for counseling.

Nevertheless, contacts as described in the case of Somaly made the team see that verbal contact had effect. People actually liked contact with 'strangers' such as the team, because, they said, they could not talk about emotions and problems in the village. As we went along, we learned to respect that in counseling sessions people were actually reconstructing their lives, as they did in group sessions (see below). The positive results helped the team accept a new role, where empathy was not prevented by hierarchical expectations.

In describing common factors in brief psychotherapeutic approaches, Garfield (1997) lists the following basic general therapeutic factors: helping the client to understand his problem, the therapeutic relationship, emotional release, reinforcement of client responses, helping clients to confront a problem, giving information, reassurance of the client, promoting successful coping, and

---

[14]In Cambodian culture, stories, including life-stories, are not expected to simply reflect what happened. People tend to reconstruct the story of their own lives until it fits in a culturally and socially desirable standard story. This tendency was reinforced by the communist ritual of creating false autobiographies: in self-criticism sessions, or worse, in prisons under torture.

emotional involvement of the client. These factors actually do apply in Cambodia, but were not easily transformed in practical counseling skills.

The two biggest barriers taken in installing counseling skills were related: the new role a counselor has to assume in order to be effective, and the ability to improvise. They are related in, again, the tension between fixed roles and potential loose behavior. The team initially wanted a clear protocol, prescribing in detail what to do under which circumstances. It was difficult to accept the theoretical concept of counseling as a skilled improvisation in unpredictable, unique situations, where the aim is not to offer clear-cut solutions but helping people think about their problems.

Working on counseling skills is at the same time highly relevant, because it attempts to find answers to this tension between rigid answers to new problems, a given fact in a modernizing society as Cambodia. And it also turned out to be a very productive area to build mutual understanding between the Cambodian and international members of the team. It was a basis for developing a common language for describing helping activities.

After four years, the efforts to introduce counseling as a skill to the members of the core-group were successful. Core-group members are functioning as adequate professional helpers. Counseling techniques include problem analysis, situation analysis, incident exploration, detailed discussion of a traumatic memory, and giving reassurance through psycho-education (cf Van der Veer, 1998b). The team is effective in supporting clients with a variety of complaints, symptoms and problems, such as physical complaints without an identifiable physical cause, post-traumatic symptoms, depressive complaints, marital problems, substance abuse and so on. Also, they have been able to share their knowledge with others. Last but not least, all team members seem to be better equipped to deal with their own problems related to traumatic experiences in the past.

Core-group members today are involved in counseling contacts up to about 15 sessions, with frequencies varying between twice a week and once a month. Clients can be referred for medication or a second opinion. Cases are discussed in regular team meetings. Some team members have specialized in attending special categories of clients, including landmine victims, terminal aids-patients, homeless women and so on. It must be noted, however, that they achieved these skills after a prior education ranging between nursing school and a completed study in medicine or psychology, followed by three years of training within the program. We have not found a shortcut to create counseling skills in 'crash courses' in Cambodia.

In the coming years the needs for counseling are huge, for example due to the continuously growing amount of land mine victims and the explosive AIDS epidemic. It is clear that counseling offers a valuable additional resource for many in Cambodia. But training counselors is a complicated process that should not be underestimated. The program works closely with the Royal University of Phnom

THE CAMBODIAN EXPERIENCE 147

Penh, where introductory courses in counseling were introduced at the department of psychology, where they are now regularly taught by department lecturers.

Psychiatric Services

It was no surprise that at the start of field work the first problems presented by villagers to the teams were patients with psychotic disorders, causing considerable distress to themselves and their surroundings. Faced with many who were severely deteriorated, sometimes chained up, the program had first to attend to these, which were seen by communities as a priority and a test for the new workers' credibility.

Examples of Mental Illness in Cambodia: Madness of Wrecked Brains and Nerves

The most common term for this illness is 'madness of the nerve tubules' (*ckuǝt saa say prasaat). It arises from any condition in which the brain and nervous system are injured. Women often were anxious about a sick child, or because the husband had run off with a 'second wife'.

The patients spoke, sometimes to themselves, in a disorganized and careless way about things that weren't true, a condition termed (*pdeɛh-pdaah). They spoke deliriously (*rɔvǝǝ-rɔviey). There were persistent headaches. There is a fear among Cambodians of abnormal sensations around the temples; the temple is literally 'wearing a flower in the ear'. People are also terrified of problems around the back of the neck, as it is believed that this is the junction of the nerve tubules ascending to the brain and, if injured, the brain will be damaged too. There were other somatic sensations, such as tightness in the chest, a sense of 'weak' respiratory movements, heat in the chest, and the heart raced.

Damaged or disrupted nerve tubules needed direct treatment—the most direct was to apply a burning wick to the skin in the method of moxibustion. Since the disease is believed to stem from overheated nerves, some healers prescribe 'cooling medicine' followed by ritual pouring of lustral water.

There was no existing psychiatric care within the public health care system in Cambodia at the start of the project. The public health system itself was weak in terms of skilled staff, funding, and utilization. In view of the efficacy of the traditional sectors in dealing with common psychosocial stress and eventual rehabilitation of mentally ill patients, the program set out to interfere as little as possible with existing traditional healing networks and sought to encourage their use while offering its own treatment. Western biomedicine is capable of recognizing and effectively treating severe neuro-psychiatric disorders such as schizophrenia and major affective disorders as well as epilepsy. Primary health workers can be given basic training to manage the majority of mental health problems with a few inexpensive drugs (De Jong, 1987, 1996; WHO, 1990).

Well aware of the weaknesses of the Cambodian public health system as described above, we decided to begin mental health clinics in the District Hospitals in the areas we worked in (Somasundaram et al., 1999). Implementation of the health coverage plan designed by the Ministry of Health requires a clear definition of the services at each level within the health system. The MOH defined a 'minimal package of activities' for health centers and a 'complementary package of activities' for referral hospitals, which were finalized in 1998 and 1999. The TPO project provided the mental health material for these, and the staff at local hospitals was trained accordingly. In each hospital, 10 medical staff was given training in basic mental health care. Psychiatric specialist supervision, support from the TPO team and supply of psychotropic drugs were provided. The clinics opened one day a week, under supervision. It proves difficult to offer psychiatric services on an integrated basis in the outpatient clinics. The motivational problems of staff, who receive no extra salary or other incentive, is the biggest constraint in installing regular and reliable service. As we mentioned above, the average salary of a health worker amounts to about 10% of what is needed to reach an income which can sustain a small household. Not many staff are interested in giving more time without extra pay. Most of the clinics so far keep offering psychiatric services on a one-morning-per-week basis. But in some clinics staff shows a personal interest and enthusiasm. Here the number of people seen keeps growing steadily over the months—incidentally proving that health workers attitude is one of the main constraints in utilization of health services in Cambodia. On average, each clinic sees about sixty patients every day they open. The clinics staffed by enthusiastic health workers see over a hundred each day they open. Patients often travel from far to reach the out-patient in district or referral hospitals. The catchment area of the four clinics officially covers some 350,000 people, but patients come from far beyond the catchment area. There are no beds available for psychiatric care in Cambodia. The four clinics set up by the team attracted 1524 new cases in 1999, and managed some 10,000 follow-up visits.

From the point of view of western nosology, the most common psychiatric conditions treated in the clinics were anxiety (26.1%), depression (19.8%) and schizophrenia (16.6%).[15] Psychosis was diagnosed in 12.9% of patients, and this included both acute psychosis and many cases later re-diagnosed as schizophrenia on long-term follow-up. Those receiving the diagnosis of schizophrenia had obvious chronic symptoms of self-neglect, deterioration in functioning, loss of touch with reality, withdrawal or grossly abnormal behavior, hallucinations in the auditory or visual modality and strange beliefs of persecutory or religious nature. The hallucinations and delusions were often related to local events and culture but with bizarre twists and clearly not shared by others. Much of the paranoia involved traumatic events in the past.

---

[15]Based on the diagnoses of 9.950 patients seen in 1999, when diagnostic skills of staff were deemed sufficient to yield data for monitoring purposes.

There was a high number of epileptic patients (14.8%), mostly generalized tonic clonic seizures.

Pig Madness—Epilepsy as a Psychosocial, Even Mental Disorder

The rural patients generally prefer traditional healers to treat epilepsy. This was partly a reflection of the cost of attending the clinic, and that the clinics until recently were not stocked with any form of anticonvulsant medication. Everyone knows about 'pig madness', the local idiom for epilepsy, in which the person has a sudden seizure. Given the presumed brain disorder, healers used moxibustion in an effort to reverse the disturbance—to get the pig out of the patient. The ritual transformed the pig into an image of the patient, and the patient metaphorically became the pig. After performing moxibustion, the healers gave medicine, sometimes to cool the febrile patient.

Therapeutic interventions for major mental disorders in the clinics included pharmacotherapy, crisis intervention, counseling, behavioral-cognitive methods, relaxation techniques, psycho-education, and emotive methods. When possible families were referred to selected traditional resources, group therapy or family therapy. Psychological forms of treatment like counseling, relaxation exercises and other non-pharmacological forms of therapy were encouraged to be used for the appropriate conditions, particularly the minor mental health disorders (Somasundaram, 1997).

The majority of patients received medication. Chlorpromazine, haloperidol, amitriptyline and imipramine covered most serious mental disorders, while benzhexol was needed for side effects. As epileptic patients also came in large numbers to the mental health clinic, phenobarbitone and phenytoin were added.

The interventions were often used in combination as the following case illustrates:

Theary, a 44 year old married lady with 6 children complained of having headaches for the last ten years due to 'thinking too much (*kit craBn)'. When asked what she thought too much about, she recounted an incident that happened in 1973. She had been carrying food for combatants when she had suddenly seen 'big' tanks coming towards her. There had been heavy shelling with death and destruction all around her. Many of her relations and friends were killed. She saw corpses, body parts such as hands and fingers, blood and people crying out in pain. Heavy bombing had followed and she had taken shelter in a bunker, which collapsed under the bombing. She had been buried under the sand, suffered head injury and lost consciousness. She came to in the hospital but could not remember for how long she had been unconscious. She had difficulty in remembering many of the details of what happened. She tried not to remember and often suppressed her memories ('forced them out of her mind'). Sometimes she could not remember anything, while at other times she had vivid recollections of the scene, particularly when she saw military personnel or heard loud explosions. At these times she became very

> frightened. She had frequent nightmares of the event both at night and when she slept in the day.
>
> She became markedly distressed when recounting her past experience, her hands shaking visibly. She resisted trying to remember, saying she didn't want to remember. She had been given a responsible position during the Khmer Rouge regime, being in charge of the Children's unit in her area, and had been unusually harsh. She admitted during subsequent counseling sessions that she feared retributions from those who had been affected in her village. She did not wish to talk about this time.
>
> In 1979, Vietnamese soldiers had come, fired some shots in the air, and taken her husband away. She had become severely frightened, her body shaking terribly. Now her appetite is poor and she is not able to work as before. She has attacks of fainting lasting two hours or more, a few times every month. She often has chest pain, with a heavy pressure as if a heavy weight is on her, making it difficult to breathe (she said this started after she had been buried in the sand). She started neglecting her self-care, sometimes crying and feeling sad.
>
> She was started on imipramine, counseling, relaxation exercises and participation in women's group was arranged. She improved quickly, her appetite and sleep returning to normal and frequency of re-experiencing decreased markedly. However she remained very sensitive and vulnerable to reminders of the trauma, and becomes distressed whenever it was brought up. Attempts are made to gradually desensitize her to the trauma using a behavioral-cognitive technique.

It is difficult to evaluate the effect of introducing basic psychiatry. The preliminary results suggest that after the first flush of treatment, most patients improve to the extent that they can lead reasonably productive lives (Somasudaram et al., 1998). One evident outcome of starting western psychiatric clinics with the objective of providing a source of medication for the more severe mental illnesses in the community was that the clinic soon outstripped this basic function and began to attract all types of psychosocial problems.

In a country without any psychiatric inpatient or outpatient services patients often are a severe burden to their families and their community, not to mention their own suffering. Basic psychiatry proved to be helpful to alleviate these situations. The challenge is in installing these services in a sustainable and user-friendly way. Motivation of health staff running the clinic, follow-up options in the community, and the awareness of the local population are equally important determinants for the effective use of these services. As we mentioned above, motivation levels connected to low salaries limit the effect of training efforts in general on behavior change and increased skills in health workers. But recent experience in introducing health financing schemes in Cambodia has now shown results in increased utilization of public health services (Soeters & Griffiths, 2000). The combination of this effect with growing awareness within the population and increased options for follow-up within the community allows basic psychiatry to be installed properly—and the experience of the project shows how this can technically be done.

CONCLUSIONS

The experience gained in the TPO program reaffirms the reality that people undergo a series of traumas as they either move from war to border camps, to resettlement, to repatriation, to internal displacement, or are exposed to a series of traumatic episodes in their home country. Resettlement, even from the awful conditions of the camps, does not necessarily bring relief (Muecke & Sassi, 1992). The work of the program runs consistent with the findings that people in chronic- or postconflict situations do best if they keep a grip on their cultural identity (Cheung, 1995; Berry, 1991; Moon & Pearl, 1991; Eisenbruch, 1986). Our findings underscore the need for public mental health programs to give careful consideration to the long-term consequences of post-war adjustment, and how people show cultural as well as personal losses (Schindler, 1993; Lipson, 1991; Lipson, 1993). All this has implications for trauma theory and also for public mental health interventions. The program in Cambodia strives for culturally competent clinical management, for it is known that the right treatment in the wrong cultural garb, with the best of intentions, may further undermine identity and might exacerbate signs of PTSD (Schreiber, 1995).

Local resources should be utilized. The experience in Cambodia supports the growing literature attesting the value of traditional healers as 'trauma therapists' in countries recovering from war (Gibbs, 1994; Wilson, 1989; Taussig, 1986; Bracken, Giller, & Summerfield, 1995). It seems that they provide a means that for some is more agreeable than the methods brought by the classical public health and psychiatry. People need to have access to their local resources. Different circumstances, from closed areas like refugee camps and open situations where the displaced population has more access to its own local resources and ecosystem, have pointed out the hazards of adopting any single preconceived blueprint.

At the same time there was a need to introduce new interventions, and this need was seen both by Cambodians in general as by healers of different sectors. Drawing lessons from the initial interventions of the program as well as the contextual studies done, it was clear that any sustainable intervention technique had to be fully imbedded and complementary to existing explanatory models, and be installed in the right group of helpers. This chapter has attempted to present a general amalgam of work done in these different contexts, and the case examples serve to demonstrate how local culture and history stamps the training and the interventions.

The experience shows that it is not enough to come and train local staff. Like all foreign programs, this one runs the risk of leaving the research in the hands of foreign experts at the expense of the local staff. By involvement of local staff as far as possible, the program has sought to minimize this inevitable hazard. More information is now gathered about the outcome of interventions, to differentiate types of mental distress and their attributes with reference to their predicted time course and healing without intervention.

The psychosocial problems found in communities, families and individuals in Cambodia are often not recognized and have a paralyzing effect on social rehabilitation. Although mental health clinics are helpful for individuals that need medical treatment and their families, their coverage is limited and the solution they offer does not match the overall majority of the problems people have. The essential question remains how certain characteristics of Cambodian society are causes as well as effects of what has happened—and the challenge—as shown by this chapter—is how this knowledge might be harnessed to develop interventions aimed at reconciliation and rehabilitation.

REFERENCES

Berry, J. W. (1991). Refugee adaptation in settlement countries: An overview with an emphasis on primary prevention. In F. L. Ahearn Jr. & J. L. Athey (Eds.), *Refugee children: Theory, research, and services* (pp. 20–38). Baltimore, MD: Johns Hopkins University Press.

Boehnlein, J. K., Kinzie, J. D., Ben, R., & Fleck, J. (1985). One-year follow-up study of posttraumatic stress disorder among survivors of Cambodian concentration camps. *American Journal of Psychiatry, 142*(8), 956–959.

Bracken, P. J., Geiller, J. E., & Summerfield, D. (1995). Psychological responses to war and atrocity: The limitations of current concepts. *Social Science and Medicine, 40*, 1073–1082.

Brody, E. B. (1994). Psychiatric diagnosis in sociocultural context. *Journal of Nervous and Mental Disease, 182*, 253–254.

Chandler, D. P. (1991). *The tragedy of Cambodian history: Politics, war and revolution since 1945*. New Haven, CT: Yale University Press.

Chandler, D. P. (1993). *A history of Cambodia* (2nd ed.). Chiang May, Thailand: Silkworm Books.

Chandler, D. P. (1999). *Voices from S-21: Terror and history in Pol Pot's secret prison*. Chiang May, Thailand: Silkworm Books.

Chandler, D. P., & Kiernan, B. (Eds.) (1983). *Revolution and its aftermath in Kampuchea: Eight essays*. New Haven, CT: Yale University Southeast Asia Studies.

Choulean, A. (1986). *Les êtres surnaturels dans la religion populaire khmère* [Supernatural beings in the folk religion of the Khmer]. Paris: Cedoreck.

Collins, S. (1982). *Selfless persons: Imagery and thought in Theravada Buddhism*. Cambridge, England: Cambridge University Press.

Davenport, P., Healy, J., & Malone, K. (1995). *Vulnerable in the village: A study of returnees in Battambang Province, Cambodia, with a focus on strategies for the landless*. Phnom Penh, Cambodia: UNHCR, Lutheran World Services and Japan Sotoshu Relief Committee.

De Jong, J. T. V. M. (1987). *A descent into African psychiatry*. Amsterdam: Royal Tropical Institute.

De Jong, J. T. V. M. (1996). A comprehensive public mental health programme in Guinea-Bissau: A useful model for African, Asian and Latin-American countries. *Psychological Medicine, 26*, 97–108.

De Jong, J. T. V. M. (1997). *TPO program for the identification, management, and prevention of psychosocial and mental health problems of refugees and victims of organized violence within primary health care of adults and children*. Amsterdam: Transcultural Psychosocial Organization. Internal document.

De Jong, J. T. V. M., & Clarke, J. (Eds.) (1996). *Mental health for refugees*. Geneva: World Health Organization.

Delvert, J. (1961). *Le paysan cambodgien* [The Cambodian peasant]. Paris: Mouton.
Desjarlais, R., Eisenberg, L., Good, B., & Kleinman, A. (1995). *World mental health: Problems and priorities in low-income countries*. New York: Oxford University Press.
Ebihara, M. (1968). *Svay, a Khmer village in Cambodia*. Unpublished doctoral dissertation, Columbia University, New York.
Eisenbruch, M. (1990a). Classification of natural and supernatural causes of mental distress: Development of a Mental Distress Explanatory Model Questionnaire. *Journal of Nervous and Mental Disease, 178*(11), 712–719.
Eisenbruch, M. (1990b). *Report of preliminary study of mental health in Cambodia*. Document submitted to UNHCR Geneva.
Eisenbruch, M. (1991). From post-traumatic stress disorder to cultural bereavement: Diagnosis of Southeast Asian refugees. *Social Science and Medicine, 33*(6), 673–680.
Eisenbruch, M. (1992a). The ritual space of traditional healing in Cambodia. *Bulletin d'École Français d'Extrême-Orient, 79*(2), 283–316.
Eisenbruch, M. (1992b). Towards a culturally sensitive DSM: Cultural bereavement in Cambodian refugees and the traditional healer as taxonomist. *Journal of Nervous and Mental Disease, 181*(1), 8–10.
Eisenbruch, M. (1994a). *Resources and limitations in meeting the health needs of the Cambodian population*. Paper presented at the conference Mental Health Education for Medical Doctors in Cambodia, Phnom Penh, Cambodia.
Eisenbruch, M. (1994b). *The taxonomy of the psychoses in Cambodia*. Paper presented at the Geigy Transcultural Psychiatry Symposium, 1–3 December, Perth, Australia.
Eisenbruch, M. (1996). The indigenous taxonomy of psychiatric disorders in Cambodia. In H. Vistosky, F. Lieh Mak, & J. J. López-Ibor, Jr. (Eds.), *X World Congress World Psychiatric Association, Madrid, August 23–28, 1996: Addendum* (p. 22). Amsterdam: Elsevier Biomedical.
Eisenbruch, M., & Handelman, L. H. (1989). Development of a culturally appropriate Explanatory Model Schedule for Cambodian refugee patients. *Journal of Refugee Studies, 2*(2), 243–56.
Evers, H. D. (Ed.) (1969). *Loosely structured social systems: Thailand in comparative perspective* (Cultural report series no. 17). New Haven, CT: Yale University Southeast Asia Studies.
Evers, H. D. (Ed.). (1980). *Sociology of South-East Asia: Readings on social change and development*. Kuala Lumpur, Malaysia: Oxford University Press.
Geertz, C. (1983). *Local knowledge*. New York: Basic Books.
Gibbs, S. (1994). Post-war social reconstruction in Mozambique: Re-framing children's experience of trauma and healing. *Disasters, 18*, 268–276.
Greve, H. S. (1993). *Land tenure and property rights in Cambodia*. Report to UNTAC, Phnom Penh, Cambodia.
Kiernan, B. (1996). *The Pol Pot regime: Race, power and genocide in Cambodia under the Khmer Rouge*. New Haven, CT: Yale University Press.
Kim, U., Triandis, H., KâgitÇibaş, Ç., Choi, S., & Yoon, G. (1994). *Individualism and Collectivism: theory, method, and applications*. Thousand Oaks, CA: Sage Publications.
Kinzie, J. D. (1990). The 'concentration camp syndrome' among Cambodian refugees. In D. A. Ablin & M. Hood (Eds.), *The Cambodian agony*. Armonk, NY: M.E. Sharpe.
Kirmayer, L. J. (1996). Confusion of the senses: Implications of ethnocultural variations in somatoform and dissociative disorders for PTSD. In A. J. Marsella, M. J. Friedman, E. T. Gerrity & R. M. Scurfield (Eds.), *Ethnocultural aspects of posttraumatic stress disorder* (pp. 131–163). Washington, DC: American Psychological Association.
Kleber, R., Figley, C., & Gersons, B. (Eds.) (1995). *Beyond trauma: Cultural and societal dynamics*. New York: Plenum Press.
Kleinman, A. M. (1980). *Patients and healers in the context of culture*. Berkeley, CA: University of California Press.

Lipson, J. G. (1991). Afghan refugee health: Some findings and suggestions. *Qualitative Health Research, 1*, 349–369.

Lipson, J. G. (1993). Afghan refugees in California: Mental health issues. *Issues in Mental Health Nursing, 14*(4), 411–423.

Marsella, A. J., Friedman, M. J., Gerrity, E. T., & Scurfield, R. M. (Eds.) (1996). *Ethnocultural aspects of posttraumatic stress disorder.* Washington, DC: American Psychological Association.

Martel, G. (1975). *Lovea, village des environs d'Angkor: aspects demographiques, economiques et sociologiques de monde rural cambodgien dans la province de Siem Reap* [Lovea, neighboring village of Angkor: Demographic, economical and sociological aspects of rural Cambodian society in the province of Siem Reap]. Paris: L'Ecole Française d'Extreme-Orient.

Mehta, H. C. (1997). *Cambodia silenced: The press under six regimes.* Bangkok, Thailand: White Lotus.

Ministry of Planning (1996). *Demographic survey of Cambodia—1996.* Phnom Penh, Cambodia: National Institute of Statistics.

Mollica, R. (1994). Southeast Asian refugees: Migration history and mental health issues. In A. J. Marsella, T. Bornemann, S. Ekbald, & J. Orley (Eds.), *Amidst peril and pain: The mental health and well-being of the world's refugees* (pp. 83–100). Washington, DC: American Psychological Association.

Mollica, R., & Jalbert, R. (1989). *Community of confinement: The mental health crisis in Site Two (displaced persons camp on the Thai border).* Alexandria, VA: World Federation for Mental Health.

Moon, J. H., & Pearl, J. H. (1991). Alienation of elderly Korean American immigrants as related to place of residence, gender, age, years of education, time in the U.S., living with or without children, and living with or without a spouse. *International Journal of Aging and Human Development, 32*(2), 115–124.

Muecke, M. A., & Sassi, L. (1992). Anxiety among Cambodian refugee adolescents in transit and in resettlement. *Western Journal of Nursing Research, 14*, 267–291.

Myslewiec, E. (1988). *Punishing the poor: The international isolation of Cambodia.* Oxford, England: Oxfam.

Nepote, J. (1992). *Parente et organization sociale dans le Cambodge moderne et contemporain* [Kinship and social organisation in contemporary Cambodia]. Nantes, France: Edition Olizane.

Ovesen, J., Trankell, I., & Ojendal, J. (1995). *When every household is an island: social organisation and power structures in rural Cambodia.* Stockholm: Swedish International Development Cooperation Agency.

Ponchaud, F. (1978). *Cambodia year zero.* London: Alien Lane.

Porée-Maspero, E. (1962). *Étude sur les rites agraires des cambodgien* [Study into Cambodian rural rituals]. Paris: Mouton.

Project Against Domestic Violence (1996). *Household survey on domestic violence in Cambodia.* Phnom Penh, Cambodia: Ministry of Women's Affairs.

Schindler, R. (1993). Emigration and the black Jews of Ethiopia: Dealing with bereavement and loss. *International Social Work, 36*(1), 7–19.

Schreiber, S. (1995). Migration, traumatic bereavement and transcultural aspects of psychological healing: Loss and grief of a refugee woman from Begameder County in Ethiopia. *British Journal of Medical Psychology, 68*(2), 135–142.

Schriever, S. H. (1990). Comparison of beliefs and practices of ethnic Viet and Lao Hmong concerning illness, healing, death and mourning: Implications for hospice care with refugees in Canada. *Journal of Palliative Care, 6*(1), 42–49.

Shawcross, W. (1985). *The quality of mercy.* Glasgow, Scotland: William Collins Sons.

Somasundaram, D. J. (1996). Post-traumatic responses to aerial bombing. *Social Science and Medicine, 42*(11) 1465–1471.

Somasundaram, D. J., Kail, K., Van de Put, W. A. C. M., Eisenbruch, M., & Thomassen, L. (1997). *Community mental health in Cambodia.* Phnom Penh, Cambodia: Transcultural Psychosocial Organization.

Somasundaram, D. J., & Sivayokan, S. (1994). War trauma in a civilian population. *British Journal of Psychiatry, 156*, 524–527.

Somasundaram, D. J., Van de Put, W. A. C. M., Eisenbruch, M., & De Jong, J. T. V. M. (1999). Starting mental health in Cambodia. *Social Science and Medicine, 48*, 1029–1046.

Taussig, M. (1986). *Shamanism, colonialism, and the wild man: A study in terror and healing.* Chicago: University of Chicago Press.

Thion, S. (1993). *Watching Cambodia.* Bangkok, Thailand: White Lotus.

United Nations Development Programme. (1996). *Cambodian human development report 1997.* Phnom Penh, Cambodia.

United Nations Research Institute for Social Development (1993). *Rebuilding war torn societies: Report of the workshops on the Challenges of Rebuilding War torn Societies and the Social Consequences of the Peace Process in Cambodia, Geneva, 27–30 April 1993.* Geneva.

Van de Put, W. A. C. M. (1992). *Empty hospitals, thriving business: Utilization of health services and health seeking behaviour in two Cambodian districts.* Amsterdam: Medicines sans Frontières Holland.

Van de Put, W. A. C. M., Hema, N., Sovandara, S. C., Renol, K. K., & Eisenbruch, M. (1996). *Psycho-social problems and the use of community resources in Cambodia.* Paper presented at the International Conference on Khmer Studies, Royal University of Phnom Penh, Cambodia.

Van de Put, W. A. C. M., Somasundaram, D., Eisenbruch, I. M., Kall, K., Soomers, R., & Thomassen, L. (1997). *Facts and thoughts on the first years 1995–1997.* Phnom Penh, Cambodia: Transcultural Psychosocial Organization.

Van de Put, W. A. C. M. & Van der Veer, G. (2001). Counseling in Cambodia. *Mind & human interaction* (University of Virginia, Center for the Study of Mind and Human Interaction).

Van der Kolk, B. A., McFarlane, A. C., & Weisaeth, L. (Eds.) (1996). *Traumatic stress: The effects of overwhelming experience on mind, body, and society.* New York: Guilford Press.

Vickery, M. (1984). *Cambodia: 1975–1982.* Boston, MA: South End Press.

Wilson, J. P. (1989). *Trauma, transformation and healing: An integrative approach to theory, research and posttraumatic therapy.* New York: Brunner/Mazel.

World Health Organization (1975). *Organization of mental health services in developing countries.* (Technical report series no. 564). Geneva.

World Health Organization (1981). *Report from the WHO collaborative study of strategies for extending mental health care.* Geneva.

World Health Organization (1990). *The introduction of a mental health component into primary health care.* Geneva.

World Health Organization (1994). *Primary health care concepts and challenges in a changing world: Alma Ata revisited.* Geneva.

World Health Organization (1996). *Diagnostic and management guidelines for mental disorders in primary care—ICD-10 Chapter V Primary Care Version.* Geneva.

3

Community Based Psychosocial and Mental Health Services for Southern Sudanese Refugees in Long Term Exile in Uganda

NANCY BARON

INTRODUCTION

The southern Sudanese refugees living in northern Uganda suffer from the consequences of long-term exile. Lost lives, homes, properties and experiences of horror fill their memories. Day by day they experience the erosion of their identities living as guests, sometimes wanted, most times not, on someone else's land, in some one else's country confronted by someone else's culture and values and ambivalent hospitality. Adults, helpless to care for the children they adore, watch as their children depend on the good will of others. They are caught in a cycle of violence in which they feel powerless; victims of a war that is supposed to be for their benefit yet without a voice. Many try to hold onto the memories of the touch of their soil yet when they close their eyes home becomes harder to recall (Box 1).
Rangaraj (1988) describes

> Refugees who have been in the camp for a long time—five, six, or seven years sometimes—seem to die internally. Outwardly, they have lost everything—family, country, culture and suddenly they are nobody. Everything is done for them—they are not left to do anything for themselves: and there is no future for them—nobody wants them. Decay seems to set in and they seem to disintegrate day-by-day.

> **Box 1. Examples of Psychosocial Problems Among Sudanese Refugees**
>
> *Suicide*
> The family gazed in shock at John's hanging body. He hung himself and no one seemed to know why. He became a refugee in 1994 after his home and property were burned. Like most of the refugees he lived first in a transit camp in poor crowded accommodation and now in a family compound on a small piece of land given to him to farm by the Ugandan government. He avoided family life, returning home only to eat and sleep. His wife and sons worked their land while he spent his time drinking with his friends. His life was just as miserable as the others, therefore, it was unclear what drove him to suicide.
>
> *Family Breakdown*
> Michael beat his wife. He felt ashamed when confronted by his wife's uncles. The family went into exile six years ago and since that time there has never been enough of anything. Not enough food, poor shelter and inadequate school fees for the children. At home he supported his family but in exile they became totally dependent on the United Nations. His wife complained he should do more to help the family but he did not know what to do. He beat her to make her stop complaining.
>
> *No Future Possibilities*
> A boy is searching for someone to pay his boarding school fees. He was abducted by the Ugandan Lord's Resistance Army (LRA) rebels last year and released after 3 months. During his time in captivity he was forced to participate in murders, watch as other children starved to death and witness torture. Since returning home he has nightmares and feels fearful because the LRA threatened to find children who escaped and kill them and their families. He wants to go away to boarding school but has no money to pay the fees.
>
> *Excessive Family Responsibility*
> Sara is concerned about her husband since he has heart pain and drinks excessively. Last year his brother died and he inherited his two wives and 11 children. There is no other adult male in the family so the responsibility is solely his. With two wives and ten children of his own, he now has 25 dependents. He feels miserable since he cannot feed them well nor afford to send the children to school.
>
> *"Vulnerable" People*
> A widow struggles to care for her three years old severely retarded child. She works in the field to feed her family but the child is too big to carry on her back. She has constant headaches and worries about leaving the child at home all day unattended. Her family members are all dead and she had no one to help her.
>
> *Mass Spirit Possession*
> A community complains that a spirit is coming each evening and entering various huts. While in the hut it appears like fire to the women and the children defecate in their sleep and wake up screaming.

There is little question that emotional distress and psychosocial problems can be related to being a victim of violence and displacement (Marsella, Bornemann, & Orley, 1994). Even though the research about the intensity and duration of psychosocial and mental health needs of refugees and the effectiveness of interventions is still minimal, in recent years there has been an upsurge of services attempting to help people during and after war and organized violence. Brody (1994) states "the mental health of any individual can be understood in terms of optimal function, well-being, and capacity to cope and adapt. All these variables reflect the interaction of innate personal characteristics with the socio-cultural context." Understanding the natural resilience and methods for recreating life used by long-term refugees and the degree of mental distress, post-traumatic stress disorder, psychiatric disturbance and social dysfunction is essential to determining when outside interventions are necessary.

The Transcultural Psychosocial Organization (TPO) began its psychosocial and mental health assistance utilizing a culturally sensitive community based approach to assist southern Sudanese refugees living in northern Uganda in 1994. This chapter will include discussions about the need for psychosocial and mental health work in long-term refugee situations and the TPO philosophy and interventions utilized to assist the Sudanese refugees.

BRIEF HISTORY OF THE SUDANESE REFUGEES IN NORTHERN UGANDA

In 1988 and again in 1994, waves of 1000s of refugees fled from Sudan into northern Uganda.

They were fleeing from a war between the Muslim Sudanese government and a Christian rebel group called the Sudanese People's Liberation Army (SPLA). The government and the rebels were both accused of burning civilian homes, looting property, raping women and torturing and killing civilians. Such events are not new to this corner of Africa since Sudanese refugees also entered Uganda in the 1960s and the now hospitable Ugandans fled their country's war and were welcomed guests into southern Sudan in the 1970s. Due to the unpredictable currents no one knows when the tide may turn again so hospitality has been a wise plan.

Homes Controlled in Sudan by the SPLA Rebels

At present the SPLA controls those areas of southern Sudan that were once the homes of the refugees. These areas are just over the border from the refugee settlements. Over the years some refugees have returned home but 156,374 continue to wait (UNHCR Statistics, 1999). Of these 49% are male, 51% are women, while 62% are children under 18 years old. Even though the SPLA encourages them to return, the ongoing bombing by the Sudanese government and the minimal education and health care available in their war-torn country discourages repatriation. Peace talks and agreements are not long lasting so no return home is eminent.

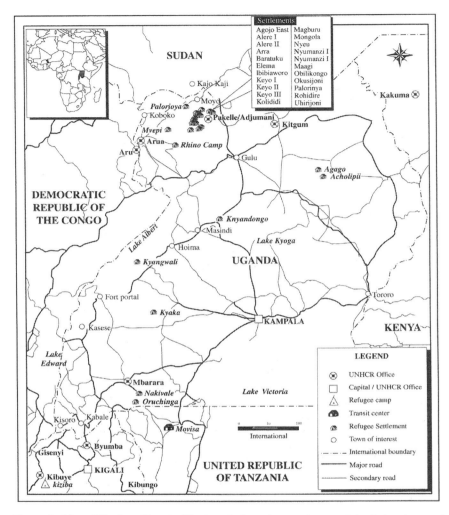

Figure 1. Map of Northern Uganda. (The boundaries and names shown and the designations used on this map do not imply official endorsement or acceptance by the United Nations).
Sources: UNHCR, ADC WORLDMAP.

Welcome in Uganda

The Government of Uganda and the northern Ugandan population welcomed the refugees because they recognized the advantages of allowing them to settle on their land. This vast land in northern Uganda has a minimal population, mostly farmers. There are no industries, no manufacturing, no telecommunications and no regular markets.

The refugees arrived with financial support from the United Nations High Commission for Refugees (UNHCR) and other helping organizations committed to not only assist the refugees but also those nationals living in the refugee hosting areas. Due to the refugee presence, infrastructure was developed and roads, bore holes for drinking water, government buildings, schools and health centers were built. The districts got more protection from the military and some jobs and money spent due to the United Nations (UN) presence in the towns. Refugees, therefore, have been a boost to the economy of the north of Uganda.

Poor Physical Security in the Refugee Settlements

The areas in which the refugees settled in the north of Uganda have ongoing rebel activity by local Ugandan rebel groups. The mission of these rebels is to de-stabilize the Ugandan government. Periodically, the rebels loot homes and abduct Ugandan nationals and Sudanese refugees and force them to carry their supplies for many miles, rape and abduct women and girls to be their "wives" and abduct boys as future recruits for their force of rebels. It is alleged that the SPLA in Sudan receives support from the Ugandan Government and the Ugandan rebels receive support from the Sudanese Government. The ongoing rebel activity restricts the willingness of the government, private business and community development organizations to make or implement plans for socio-economic growth to the north of Uganda.

Plan for Refugee Self-Reliance in Northern Uganda

Initially, the Sudanese refugees were moved into transit camps with cramped substandard living conditions. While living in transit camps the refugees were dependent on full support: food, shelter, water, sanitation and health care. All their survival needs were provided by the UNHCR. Never enough of anything but the hope of returning home seemed to be vitamins for survival.

Over the years, however, it became obvious that the refugees return home was not eminent so the Government of Uganda and UNHCR revised the plan. The Ugandan Government generously agreed for the refugees to move onto arable unused farmland. Most landowners were eager for the refugees to be their tenants since the unused land was not used due to rocks, lack of roads, physical isolation, no schools, no medical care, and worst of all, active rebel activity. The refugees and their United Nations caretakers took on the task of developing this land.

Most of the refugees were moved from transit camps into *settlement sites*. The UNHCR and all its partners re-focused their activities on a highly publicized innovative program to encourage refugee self-reliance and integration. The plans are for the refugees to grow their own crops and feed themselves. The hope is that as the UN pulls out community development organizations will move forward with assistance for further income generation. The Sudanese, people with the same religion and languages as the northern Ugandans, will be integrated with their Ugandan neighbors, sharing land, health care and education facilities and joining together to develop the area.

Self-reliance is not only a physical activity requiring hard work but also a mental and emotional activity. Years of refugee life seems to have promoted "learned helplessness", a position from which people feel little power to control or influence their own lives (Seligman, 1975). After years of dependency, the switch is complicated especially when self-reliance is attached to the refugees' recognition that the soil presently beneath their feet is bequeathed by people believing their return home is not eminent.

PSYCHOSOCIAL NEEDS ASSESSMENT

TPO plans to begin work in northern Uganda began in 1993 when the Ugandan government and UNHCR recognized the psychosocial suffering of the refugees and initiated a request for an assessment of psychosocial and mental health needs and determination of the viability of establishing a helping program.

The psychosocial needs assessment included:

1. *Consultation with the authorities* responsible for the refugee population including UNHCR and Ugandan government officials.
2. *Focus groups and key informant interviews with refugee leaders* to understand the population's perceptions of the causes of psychosocial problems, the usual traditional methods of assisting people and the effectiveness of these traditional methods.
3. *Focus groups with refugee subgroups* including: health staff, teachers, and the general population of men, women, youth, elderly and children to determine the prevalence of psychosocial problems.
4. *Observations of the refugee communities* to confirm the data from the interviews and to better understand the way of life.
5. *Discussions with local authorities and staff* directly assisting the refugees (including local government officials, camp and settlement officers, UN and NGO organizations) to learn their perceptions of needs and discuss how to coordinate with existing services.
6. *Discussions with donors* about possibilities of funding a psychosocial program.
7. *Design of psychosocial program.* Utilizing the information from the assessment culturally sensitive intervention strategies were designed.

Over the years of operation TPO has recognized that the psychosocial problems of the refugees keep changing so that intervention strategies are regularly reassessed and altered to meet the present needs.

PSYCHOSOCIAL PROBLEMS OF REFUGEES CHANGING OVER TIME

Initial Response to Exile

The quality of life and life's usual psychosocial balance is altered after becoming a refugee. Relief assistance provides for survival but this only nourishes the body. Due to their experiences of war and displacement the Sudanese refugee population experienced some psychosocial losses immediately after their displacement. The initial losses reported in focus groups included:

Security. Incidents of bombing, rape, torture and death were terrifying. Running away and losing the security of home and country and entering an unknown life in exile caused fear and emotional distress.

Independence. Prior to the exile most Sudanese were farmers and independently cared for their families. Producing, feeding, caring and educating children were the goals and responsibilities declared by most adults. As refugees, the independent ability to provide for their children was lost. The adults reported that they felt ashamed by their lack of ability to care for their families and the children reported a loss of respect for fathers and mothers who could not care for them.

Property. Having material possessions, like nice clothes, household goods and radios are important to the Sudanese. These possessions represent the success of the family, therefore, the loss of properties was profoundly felt.

Wealth. Cattle represented wealth and are used to pay dowries. Most of the cattle were either stolen or died. Due to tradition most men are polygamous and families try to have as many children as possible. They feel it is their responsibility to enlarge the numbers of their extended family and clan. Without a dowry, arranging for wives was difficult and without wives there was the serious risk of not having children.

Land. Land is not only essential for crops and survival but also provides a stable homestead for the family, clan and tribe. Ancestors are buried on a family's land and the Sudanese want to live amongst the spirits of their ancestors and be buried with them. They want to have their children till the same land and be buried alongside them. The loss of land was felt profoundly.

Leadership. Community, clan and tribal elders are relied on to make decisions and establish law and order. As refugees this system was disorganized due to the premature death of many adults and estrangement of the natural communities of clans and tribes who always lived in close proximity and were now split apart.

Initial Feelings of Distress

Many refugees ran away with only a bundle containing the memories of horrific experiences. Dead, dying, lost and suffering family members alongside the loss of home and property were predominant recurring memories. Feelings of fear seemed to prevent sleep and limit activity. Entering a new land controlled by others with the ability to care for self and family stripped away, many of the new refugees felt helpless and humiliated by their new status. Once proud and self-sufficient and now, despite how hard they worked all of their lives, they had nothing and appeared to the world as paupers. They saw pity in the eyes of those who helped them. They felt ashamed because it felt like the helpers thought that they wanted to be refugees and wanted a life of handouts.

Theodore and Elioto's (1990) description of Afghan refugee men is reminiscent of Sudanese refugee men in Uganda "the tragic psychopathological consequences of proud men becoming dependent on others for things they once handled well themselves. As a group, the men felt helpless, frustrated, angry and anxious. Their sense of helplessness in the face of brutality toward them and their families, coupled with the vulnerability they felt due to the destruction of their traditional self-reliance and pride, left many of them depressed, helpless, anergic, and demoralized" (Marsella et al., 1994).

The Sudanese refugees feelings of shame and despair seemed to increase as the aid structure was established. They sat and waited for the distribution of life, queues for water, queues for food and health care; none of it enough. No one asked their opinions about how to lead their lives. Survival was given to them stripped of dignity and they felt they were, expected to be satisfied, even grateful. Yet, most people only wanted to go home and have life as it was before but there was nothing they could do about it.

Initial Post-Traumatic Stress Symptoms

Though some Sudanese refugees needed immediate mental health treatment after exile apparently due to their reaction to their tragedies, the majority of people did not express severe symptoms that warranted treatment. In fact, some of those exposed to extreme stress even responded positively and may have had personal growth and increased self-respect (McFarlane & Yehuda, 1996).

Though there were relatively few people with extreme symptoms, at one time or another most Sudanese refugees felt miserable and reported experiencing some mental health symptoms in various degrees of severity and complained of some loss in ability to function. The complaints included: feelings of fear and anxiety, physical pain (head, neck, back, chest, stomach, joints), shortness of breath and tightness in chest, loss of energy and motivation, change in temperament, estrangement from friends and family, disturbed sleep or nightmares, inability to make decisions, concentrate or remember, lost faith and spirituality, inability to work, loss of interest in care of family and self and change in interest in sex, food or pleasure.

Most refugees were unaware of the normal emotional and physical stress reactions that could follow displacement. Some were distressed by their feelings of stress and became further distressed by the fear of not understanding their symptoms. Speaking of emotional distress is not culturally acceptable so as a result it is not surprising that some developed psychosomatic aches and pains. They feared that these pains were associated with life threatening disease or injury and felt further stressed when health professionals refused them treatment.

There was no standard individual response to the initial distress. Levels of intensity of trauma and levels of intensity of distress were not clearly related. A rape or a family death or loss of property could all cause low or high levels of distress seemingly dependent on the individual and family protective factors and capacity to cope. Some people responded without a problem to the initial displacement and had symptoms of stress later while others had symptoms at the beginning and they later disappeared.

1–4 YEARS AFTER EXILE: REPORT OF PSYCHOSOCIAL PROBLEMS

As the years in exile progressed there was a wide disparity in response. Though many refugees continually felt miserable about their ongoing status, the ability to cope seemed to differ. Some coped adequately and created a new life while others were unable to re-organize and re-stabilize their lives. Some refugees had previous psychosocial problems that were exacerbated while others had psychosocial problems caused by their displacement and exile. Some people developed somatic symptoms. The vulnerable members of the society, those who were disabled, mentally ill, mentally retarded, elderly or widows without family had the most difficulty surviving.

Ongoing Post-Traumatic Stress Symptoms

Individual Adult Response. Most of the research conducted on refugees and displaced populations found rates of serious individual psychopathology higher than in the average population.

TPO research found that 29% of the Sudanese refugees reported experiencing five traumatic events and 20% reported seven traumatic events during their escape. Despite having experienced traumas during their escape the study found that a "a high level of daily hassles and feelings of hopelessness in the camp instead of traumatizing experiences during their escape caused most of the refugees' problems." Reactions such as feeling you have no future, spending time thinking about why these events happened and feeling there is no one to rely on were all experienced as hurtful. The study found that desiring a higher social and economic status and not being accustomed to poor conditions predicted a higher level of PTSD symptoms (Sieswerda, Komproe, Hanewald, & de Jong, 1999).

Youth and Children's Response. Due to the longevity of their exile many children were born in Uganda or arrived at a young age and have little memory of life in Sudan. These children only know the struggle of their present lives. For most, protective factors in the family and outside of the family in the schools and communities assist their capacity to cope.

Family and Community Response. Most completed research studies examined individual reactions and resultant pathology. No studies clearly examined the family or community response. In African culture the extended family and community are an integral part of life and no individual suffers alone or is expected to solve his or her problems alone.

Importance of Meaning to a Traumatic Event

Victims react to extreme trauma in accordance with what it means to them, their families and their communities. Generating these meanings is an activity that is socially, culturally, and often politically framed (Summerfield, 1995). The differences found in response to traumatic events seemed to be caused by differences in personality, effectiveness of coping style and family or community support.

The meaning of an event is not only an impetus of change for an individual but it can also change the overall tone or personality of a family or community. The following example describes two Sudanese mothers who lost a child.

> **Susan** was sad and grieved for about a month. She had three other children. Her husband and family reassured her that the death was God's Will and not her responsibility. Community members were compassionate. After a month she returned to her usual chores and though sad was functioning within her normal range.

> **Jesca** was sad and continually grieved. This was her only child. During the first month her crying never lessened and by the second month it intensified. Her husband, mother-in-law and community blamed her for the child's death. They said she was negligent and the husband threatened to leave her. She could not sleep, did not bathe or eat regularly, her head always hurt and she sat in her house day after day alone.

This is especially relevant in Africa where individuals rarely act alone and life is strongly influenced by family and community. Sudanese communities often shared experiences of violence and in reaction to these traumatic events not only did individuals suffer and change but people reported that the overall personality of the family and community changed. Some reported that as an overall group they were now less trusting and more fearful of each other and less motivated to help each other. Feelings of hopelessness and helplessness pervaded some families and communities. Some blamed their neighbors or other tribes and wanted revenge or to remain distant from them. Families and communities reported changes in culture, traditions, faith and spirituality due to their shared experiences. Some communities strengthened their belief in God and/or Spirits; others believed less. Some believed that they caused the traumatic events to occur due to their lack of adherence to traditional rituals or lack of faith, others felt it was God's will.

Coping Ability

Those who coped with their displacement and established a new life structure minimized their feelings of stress. "Coping with stress implies coming to terms with the new reality and trying to fit new assumptions about the world with its harsh facts and with ourselves" (de Jong, 2000).

Though the entire population suffered from many traumatic experiences prior to their displacement once in exile most coped. In a reasonable amount of time they were doing their daily chores, playing with their children, making new babies and occasionally laughing. The determination of who copes best, under what conditions and why is not yet clearly understood. Here are two examples of coping within the community:

> After a massacre by rebels in one community the Elders met to discuss the reasons it occurred and to decide how to ritually cleanse their community. Goats were slaughtered and drums beat out songs of contrition to appease the spirits as the people danced until dawn. The next morning the people reported that they felt cleansed.
>
> In another community, the Religious Leaders called the people together to pray. They proclaimed their faith in the will of God and prayed and beat drums until dawn. The next morning these people reported that they felt cleansed.

The refugees' mechanisms for coping were further challenged as the cumulative stress continued to grow as the years in exile progressed.

5–15 YEARS LATER: CONTINUING PROBLEMS OF LONG TERM EXILE

After many years in exile the cumulative effects of the stress of their living situation seem to outweigh the memories of the initial traumatization. "For refugees, traumatization is usually not a specific traumatic event in the sense of an isolated incident or a set of events that have left painful scars. More often, it is an enduring, cumulative process that continues during exile because of distinct new events, both in the native county and in the country of exile. It is a chain of traumatic stressful experiences that confront the refugee with utter helplessness and interfere with her or his personal development over an extended period of time" (Van der Veer, 1995).

Cumulative Stress

Certain cumulative stressors seem to lead some people to suffer from psychosocial problems:

Loss of Hope. After years in exile, many refugees feel that Uganda may be their home for an extended time. Recognizing this is the cause for many to feel anxious, depressed, stressed, and to lose hope. Those placed in settlements that are safe and with good farmland seem to be the best adjusted. Those in insecure sites and poor land seem to have increased emotional distress.

Poverty. First as refugees dependent on handouts of insufficient food and now as subsistence farmers with small plots of land in areas of unpredictable weather these southern Sudanese are some of the world's poorest people. Relative poverty in Europe or America where there are social welfare nets to assist people is very different from the poverty of Africa where starvation and disease pervade (Desjarlais et al., 1995). Poverty is found to be one of the prime indicators of mental illness. An individual's economic situation seems to be a better indicator of well-being than any social change that one might undergo. Employment status is a clearer indicator of psychiatric morbidity than residential status (Desjarlais et al., 1995). For the refugee "low socioeconomic status is a major risk factor for failure to adapt, cope, and achieve well-being in the new living environment" (Brody, 1994).

Dependency. Refugee experts believe that dependency on UNHCR and NGOs diminished the refugees' self-esteem and the future UNHCR self-reliance plan assumes that the renewal of self-esteem will accompany self-reliance (UNHCR-Uganda, 1999). Experts continually find that dependent refugee environments promote "learned helplessness". People in situations in which they feel they have no control give up the little control they do have. Seligman (1975) reported that a low level of perceived control over their lives resulted in high levels of frustration and chronic depression in refugees. Becoming "overinstitutionalized" causes refugees to lose self-confidence and become numb and apathetic (Von Buchwald, 1994).

In the aid system it is not the giving and getting that is destroying the people's self-esteem because people are accustomed to giving and getting. It is more likely that it is the *method* of giving assistance that causes the destruction of self-esteem. The system of aid established for the Sudanese and known in many aid situations not only creates a type of dependency but in the process of giving assistance demoralizes people. Aid is initially organized to be efficient and keep people safe and alive; emotional, social or family needs are not considered first. Rather than work in partnership with the refugees the caretakers set up a hierarchical model of assistance that in short term refugee care, in the midst of a new crisis, is felt to be the most efficient means of ensuring survival. As the UNHCR recognized that northern Uganda required long-term refugee care, the methods used in the short term are now being dismantled and a sustainable refugee led infrastructure established.

Philosophically, the Sudanese refugees prefer self-reliance. They prefer it since depending on a system that is often not dependable has caused them much distress. Surviving in a world that often has famine, natural disasters, rebels and war is frightening, however, and many worry about their ability to sustain their survival without help. The refugees despair because in Sudan they could depend on a traditional structure of family, clan and community support that could assist them with problems but that is now less available.

Overwhelming Family Responsibilities. Sudanese, like most Africans, feel strong responsibility for the care and maintenance of their nuclear and extended families. Denial of this responsibility is rare. AIDS, war, health conditions caused by the poor living conditions and lack of good health care are prevalent and cause large numbers of deaths of adults and children. The living adults are burdened by these deaths and must take full responsibility for the care and education of all related adults and children. It is not unusual for a living adult to have the full financial responsibility for up to 40 relations.

The vulnerable populations (including the disabled, mentally ill, mentally retarded, abandoned or orphaned children, physically ill, elderly without families and widows without families) struggle to cope within the settlements. With substandard living conditions and the need for caretakers to spend large amounts of time struggling with daily survival tasks like fetching water and wood, the vulnerable become a burden to their families and communities (Desjarlais et al., 1995.)

New Traumatic Experiences. The refugee settlements continue to be plagued by rebel attacks. Each incident directly effects from a few to fifty people. With a history of previous trauma these continuing incidents have a traumatic effect on the victims and the overall population.

Many of the refugees do not feel safe in the settlement environment that was set up for their protection. The continuing rebel insecurity triggers the fears caused by the original exile. Every incident of insecurity, even though it only directly effects a small portion of the population, has a strong ripple effect throughout the extended refugee community and 1000s of refugees leave their homes to run to the bush to sleep. Many live in a heightened state of hyper vigilance that seems to increase stress related and psychosomatic illness. An example of a new traumatic event:

> The armed rebels entered the camp. Everyone was terrified. The women were lined up and thirteen chosen. Some had children clinging to their breasts. The rebels took turns raping them. One husband resisted and was beaten and killed. Some of the women were abducted and men were chosen to help carry the food and medical supplies that they looted. After they left the people in the settlement ran away; some into the bush some to family in other camps. Over the next week, the people living in all of the settlements within 20 miles of that camp left their homes at night to sleep in the bush. They felt safer in the wild.

Secondary Consequences of Long-Term Exile

There seem to be secondary consequences of long-term exile that cause an additional set of problems. Rates of suicide attempts and deaths are high and alcohol abuse increasing.

Suicide. Increased risk of suicide seems related to the apparent elevated rate of depression among refugees (Orley, 1994). In 1999 in this refugee population, 17 adults (10 males/7 females) committed suicide or 11.3 suicides per 100,000 people; an average number according to world standards. Within this population in 1999 only adults committed suicide. If we count only the adult population it becomes 25.2 suicides per 100,000 adults.

Compared to known worldwide statistics this result in a small adult population is potentially one of the highest known rates in the world (Desjarlais et al., 1995). In much of the western world professionals are concentrating on methods to prevent youth suicide, yet in this refugee population the adults are at greatest risk.

In an effort to understand the life of the deceased, TPO completed a post-mortem study utilizing psychological autopsies with 15 families. All were found to be married adults with children and despite the usual African sense of responsibility for family these victims chose suicide. Levels of poverty were average for the population but family problems were pervasive perpetuating anomie, estrangement and despair. All of the male victims drank alcohol excessively and seven of them physically abused their wives and children. Eleven of the victims had possible diagnoses of mental illness immediately prior to death, which included nine with major depression, one with schizophrenia and one with a first psychotic episode (Baron, 2001).

Alcohol Use. Generally, refugees report that the incidence of alcohol overuse throughout the settlements is on the increase. In particular, it is reported to affect men of all ages including youth and the elderly. These are groups who often feel particularly disenfranchised and without hope for their futures due to their displacement. Refugees belonging to a TPO Alcoholics Anonymous group report that drinking excessively was their way to try to reduce or escape their feelings of depression and hopelessness.

It is a cyclical problem made more difficult because the women, with little means to make a living, brew alcohol within the camps in order to earn money to feed their families. This readily available cheap alcohol is drunk by the men. An example:

> Jack came home late in the evening stumbling, singing and smelling of alcohol. His wife sent the children to sleep and served him his dinner. While eating Jack became angry due to the lack of meat. He blamed his wife for wasting money and not caring for him. His wife became angry and accused him of buying alcohol and leaving her without food. They grabbed sticks and beat each other.

The increase in alcohol use seems to be a causal factor of other problems i.e. domestic violence, marriage break-ups and child abuse or neglect.

Loss of Culture—Changing Morality. The elders complain of a loss of culture and despair that the youth are not respecting or adhering to the traditions.

There is an increase in youth pregnancy. In Sudan girls are encouraged to wait for marriage to have sex usually by the age of eighteen. In the camps, the opportunities for constructive activity, education and employment are limited. Youth are bored and searching for excitement, life meaning and purpose. Procreation gives purpose so many youth choose to move into early adulthood. In Sudan, the usual community response to a youthful pregnancy would be marriage. However, in exile due to lack of resources the young men often have no means to pay the dowry so many families prohibit the young couple from marrying. To these poor families their daughter is a bank account for future income so they are unwilling to relinquish the girl until there is adequate compensation. Increased numbers of young men, over eighteen years of age, who impregnate underage girls are being imprisoned for defilement. Though sex was consensual and the couple within a couple of years of age the family will refuse the marriage if the man has no dowry payment and have him charged with a crime and imprisoned. The hope is that his family will raise funds for a dowry to have him released from prison.

The cumulative effect of these factors causes symptoms of distress of various levels of intensity throughout the refugee population. In Sudan, traditional methods of helping were used to assist people with any problem. The current problems are a challenge to these traditional helping methods.

TRADITIONAL HELPING METHODS

Prior to displacement the refugees lived in rural traditional communities with limited transport and communication with the contemporary world. For centuries, families internally managed their psychosocial and mental health problems through the help of family members, traditional healers, elders, community leaders, and church leaders.

Elder Leadership

Traditionally, the Sudanese have elder groups from each clan that make decisions and solve most conflicts. In Sudan, most rural villages had no government legal system so these elder groups were expected to mediate conflicts and provide punishment for offenses against family or community. For example:

> John, 11 years old, lived with his cousin's family in order to attend school. One morning Rose, his four year old cousin complained of pain in her vagina caused by John. Her mother realized that she had been sexually molested. Her father contacted the available clan elders in the settlement who arranged for John's family to come from Sudan. The elder men met to discuss the issue. John's mother and other relatives from Sudan brought the ingredients with them for a special fish soup. After much negotiation it was decided that John would return to Sudan and his family would pay two goats to the cousin's family. John's family would be responsible to pay the girl's school fees and medical bills until adulthood. If she had problems finding a husband or conceiving a child then John would marry her. After the negotiation, the fish soup was fed to the girl's family to appease any bad feelings and prevent future curses.

Due to exile many clans were split apart due to death and dislocation and the usual elder circles were often disconnected. The placement of refugees into settlement sites by authorities was random, thereby, further splitting the clans and tribes. A western idea to improve tribal relations was to randomly mix everyone together. This choice had repercussions. In usual African communities, clan members care for their vulnerable without question. In the present settings a neighbor of a different clan or tribe is not going to easily change generations of tradition and assist in caring for an unknown neighbor's blind mother or retarded child especially not when the traditional beliefs are that the disability might be caused by angry spirits.

Local Healers

Historically, local ('traditional') healers were the mainstay of treatment for mental health and psychosocial problems. Some of the reasons they seem to no longer be as effective include:

1. Many people are following the tenets of the Christian church so they *no longer believe in the value of healers*. The churches are treating people with

problems through prayers. It is effective for some but people and church leaders report it does not cure all.
2. Healers charge their patients and many people have *no financial means* to pay a healer or pay for rituals. A $15 US dollar goat for slaughter is a major expense.
3. Some settlements *do not have local healers*. The Ugandan rebel group that is the greatest threat to the refugees is a Christian fundamentalist group so many of the healers have hidden.
4. Healers believe that problems are caused by spirits. The spirits become angry and punish people when they are neglected and/or traditional rituals are not performed. Resolution always involves performing rituals. Unfortunately, the healers are *not as effective as in the past* since psychological distress due to trauma and poor living conditions are not always resolved by the usual traditional healing methods.

The refugee population contains many tribes that share common traditional beliefs about the causes of psychosocial and mental health problems. They refer to these problems as "misfortunes". There are very clear traditional beliefs about the causes of misfortune (Box 2).

Box 2. Southern Sudanese Traditional Beliefs About the Causes of Misfortune

Spirits
- Meeting a spirit of the dead while awake.
- The spirit of a dead person comes to you in your sleep.
- Not visiting the burial place of a dead family member.

Unperformed Rituals
- The proper rituals are not performed at birth.
- Someone dies away from home and the proper ritual of bringing a stone or soil from a river or stream in the direction of where the person died is not followed.
- Someone is not buried in the proper way, on the left side for a female on the right for the male.
- Certain big trees that were the previous site of rituals cannot be chopped.
- Your mother dies and you do not pay a cow to your uncle.
- After the death of a family member, the rest do not discuss the cause or slaughter a bull.
- Upon killing an animal elders are selected to eat the most important parts including the testes, kidney and liver. If the parts are destroyed, so the elders cannot eat it, the cook or his family may have misfortune.

Curses
- In anger or spite one person can bewitch or put a curse on another.
- Buying charms from a healer it is possible that the charm can backfire and turn on you.
- Fighting with another person in a stream or river or lake.
- You murder someone and do not lick the blood.

For centuries, in the evenings, elders would sit around a fire and tell the children stories to teach the importance of following traditional rituals since not following certain cultural rituals and traditions is believed to provoke misfortune and as a result the consequence can be mental or physical illness, childlessness, accidents, social problems or sudden death. After displacement complaints of psychological, social and physical symptoms seem to increase. There was no history for understanding that these present feelings of physical or emotional pain or distress might be caused by the existing living situation. Rather, heart palpitations or head pain or whatever ailed them was explained as being caused by not adhering to certain traditional rituals.

Certain traditional methods are believed to be useful for treating any of these misfortunes. They include: consultation with a healer and performing rituals and ceremonies, use of herbs, witchcraft, sacrifice of domestic animals, drum beating for many days and specific songs with drums.

The healers continue to effectively treat those people who believe in them especially for disorders explained as spirit possession and curses. Healers report limited success with severe mental illness, mental retardation or epilepsy. If people believe in the healer then some community or family problems, psychosomatic complaints and general feelings of despair and discontent can also be assisted through ritual as shown in the following example:

> At 14 years Pascalina was abducted by rebels and forced to live as a "wife". She was initially beaten and raped after which she consented to sex. During her two-year stay with the rebels she was forced to participate in killings and looting. Finally, during one raid she escaped and returned home. Her parents welcomed her but the community feared her. A traditional healer offered to cleanse her. He slaughtered a bull and performed rituals. The community believed these cleansed the evil spirits within her so she was no longer dangerous. She was forgiven and accepted by the community.

Influence of the Church

In present times, the following of traditional beliefs are influenced due to the strong teachings of the churches. Most of the Sudanese refugees are Christians who practice their faith. Many are Born Again Christians or belong to Christian sects i.e.: Pentecostals, Jehovah Witness and Seventh Day Adventist. The religious beliefs help people to accept their life circumstances. "Religion fulfills the critical function of providing a sense of purpose in the face of terrifying realities by placing suffering in a larger context and by affirming the commonality of suffering across generations, time and space (McFarlane & Van Der Kolk, 1996).

The churches preach in opposition to the traditional beliefs and preach that traditional healers are heathens and their traditional rituals useless. The churches teach that mental illnesses and other misfortunes are caused by evil spirits who harm people who do not have strong beliefs in the church. They teach people to believe strongly and pray so they will not have misfortune. Prayer is used as the treatment for all distress and ailments, therefore, the people come together for long sessions of fervent prayer, drumming and singing:

> Joan felt tortured by evil spirits. She reported that they burned her clothes and threw rocks at her children. She was awakened one night with her roof on fire. The Pastors told her that she must pray and strengthen her Christian faith in order to deter the spirits. Joan became Born Again and prayed over and over with the Pastors and church members. Eventually, the evil spirits disappeared.

Integration of Tradition and Church

Some people are hesitant to give up the traditional beliefs despite the teachings of the church and integrate traditional rituals including animal slaughter with prayer to cover all the possibilities to appease God, spirits and ancestors in order to find relief.

Prior to determining if a program should be initiated TPO explored the traditional methods of helping to determine their effectiveness and gaps. The displacement and ongoing stresses of refugee life seem to have caused an array of symptoms that are not easily managed by traditional methods so TPO decided to initiate a helping program.

OVERVIEW OF TPO-UGANDA PROGRAM

The strength of individual resilience and the support of family and community have allowed most of the Sudanese to cope with their refugee status. Though many refugees believe that their fate is in the hands of God or Spirits they still believe that their actions can help to direct elements of their fate. Many of their problems are resolved by following traditional laws and the rules and advice of their elders, traditional healers, community and religious leaders. TPO-Uganda was designed to assist those refugees who had psychosocial or mental health problems that were not resolved through traditional helping methods.

TPO-Uganda Program Philosophy

The overriding philosophy of the TPO-Uganda program has remained the same through its years of operations. The model was designed to empower the refugee population to treat the unmet psychosocial and mental health problems of their members utilizing a community based culturally appropriate approach.

In the context of the Sudanese culture TPO assists individuals to find relief from their distress and resolution of their problems within the structure of their families and communities. It encourages them to be proactive in leading their lives. "The initial response to trauma needs to consist of reconnecting individuals with their ordinary supportive networks, and having them engage in activities that reestablish a sense of mastery" (Van der Kolk, 1996).

TPO-Uganda Program Goals

TPO developed a series of psychosocial and mental health interventions that not only assist the people with immediate crisis response and solving problems but also aim to strengthen the communities, families and individuals in long lasting sustainable self-help. According to a World Bank Study "Most successful strategies to improve basic social and economic conditions that contribute to well-being often involve work at the level of communities. ... programs that pay heed to local traditions and cultural values are usually more successful than programs that neglect local realities and concerns" (Desjarlais et al., 1995; see also chapter 1).

The goals of the TPO-Uganda program include:

- Culturally sensitive community based interventions utilizing an indigenous staff.
- Provision of curative psychosocial and mental health assistance through crisis intervention and mid and long term supportive problem solving assistance.
- Prevention of psychosocial and mental health problems through psychosocial education and community, youth and child activities.
- Increase community awareness and sensitization of psychosocial and mental health issues to assist in preventing problems and empowering communities and families to help their needy members.
- Encourage empowerment of individuals to help themselves within the context of family.
- Work cooperatively with all community, NGO or government leaders and helpers.
- Promote human rights, peace and reconciliation.

Overview of the Program

TPO-Uganda has an administrative office in the capital city of Kampala. In three northern districts with large Sudanese refugee populations there are base offices for the field operations. In the field each counselor has an office of a mud hut with thatched roof and an open building to hold groups.

TPO provides a range of preventive and curative psychosocial and mental health services. These interventions include individual and family psychosocial counseling, community sensitization and psychosocial awareness education, group activities and counseling, community, youth and children's cultural and recreational activities, community mediation for conflicts and crisis intervention. The TPO psychosocial counselors are mostly Sudanese refugees. All are required to live in the settlements in which they work and are members of the settlements and live in mud homes with thatched roofs alongside their clients. Most counselors have motorbikes that give them the mobility to visit their clients at home.

Psychiatric nurses lead mobile mental health clinics in each field site. They provide psychiatric assessments, medication and crisis intervention for people diagnosed with mental illnesses or epilepsy. The counselors work with the nurses to educate and provide counseling for the families of the mentally ill or epileptic.

Staff Structure

Over the years of operation much has been learned and many program and management changes have been made. Initially, TPO-Uganda was directed by an international staff person assigned to implement the program according to a flexible protocol established by the central TPO office. This international person was assigned since there were no Ugandan or Sudanese nationals with the education and skills needed to facilitate the program.

Management Staff. After much training and team building, after a few years TPO-Uganda decided to alter its management structure and move from a hierarchical to a cooperative team approach in which the international person was a team player along with national staff. Group decision-making improved morale and the staff reported feeling more empowered. Their capacity to work effectively seemed to grow with the change in structure. "The most important role that expatriates can play, more important than delivering services, is helping refugees run their own programs" (Martin, 1994). Program sustainability is dependent on having a responsible skillful local management. International staff is expensive and only available for a limited number of years so local staff must be capable of managing independently.

Five professionals divide the management responsibilities and combine their skills to manage the program:

Ugandan Administrator: Responsible for finance, administration and personnel.
Sudanese Field Coordinator: Responsible for field operations in the settlements.
Sudanese Training Coordinator: Responsible for staff and community training.

Ugandan Program Coordinator: Responsible for the integrative program with the national population.

International Psychologist: Responsible for program development, overseeing clinical supervision, training, proposal writing and fund raising.

All efforts are made to work cooperatively and each team member is encouraged to make decisions within his or her realm of responsibility.

Field Staff. The staff includes:

Psychosocial Program: 2 Assistant Field Coordinators/15 Full Time Counselors/3 Field Supervisors

Mental Health Program: 1 Psychiatric Nurse Supervisor/3 Psychiatric Nurses/1 Psychiatrist (part-time)/5 Mental Health Clinic Managers (part-time for drug distribution). As well as 3 Office Managers and 20 Support Staff (driver, watchmen, cleaners and messengers).

International Staff. International psychosocial programming is a new field and finding qualified international staff is difficult. TPO employs internationals to live and work long-term within an assigned country. In and out short-term or holiday consultancies are not part of the framework. These consultancies may be a boost to the consultant's cv and career but our experience shows that most offer little sustainable benefit to the field program. Field staff needs ongoing training, supervision, support and monitoring in low-income countries in the same way that it is needed within western social service and psychological systems.

As the field of international psychosocial programming evolves it is clear that training for internationals is essential. Cross-cultural work requires more than just awareness and sensitivity. Western trained professionals cannot merely enter a foreign culture and easily transfer their knowledge and skills. These western professionals need to be trained and assisted in combining their western ideas with those appropriate to the new culture in which they will work.

The role of the international person is complicated. His or her time is least effectively used in direct field work with the clients. National staff with the knowledge of culture, tradition and language can be trained in the psychosocial and mental health skills to do effective field work. Internationals need to be involved in programming as trainers, advocates and others who can identify needs and develop strategies for creating effective programs (Martin, 1994). TPO finds that internationals are most useful as supervisors, trainers, program developers, program advocates, proposal writers and fund raisers. These activities often require the professional education of the international. Additionally, in low income countries the bureaucracies that control funding are often more easily entered by the internationals "who have greater freedom to protest government policies that may undermine refugees' ability to operate their own services" (Marsella et al., 1994).

TPO-UGANDA PROGRAM IN OPERATION

Core Group of "Psychosocial Counselors"

When TPO began there were no mental health or psychosocial counselors, social workers, psychologists or psychiatrists in northern Uganda. A first core group of "psychosocial counselors" was hired and trained as full-time paid staff in 1994. Over the years, TPO educated counselors about psychosocial and mental health issues and treatment and used this educated group to bring awareness of these issues and treatment to the general population.

Counselor Selection. The criteria of selection of new counselors altered over the years as the characteristics of successful staff were identified. The present selection criteria for psychosocial counselors include:

- Commitment to help, genuine compassion and empathy for people is essential.
- Counselors with strong assertive personalities fare best.
- Staff must live within the camps or settlement sites.
- Capacity to work as a team member with people of different ethnic groups and mixed ages and gender is essential.
- Physical health is important.
- Flexibility is necessary since counselors are responsible for immediate crisis response.
- Counselors work alone in a settlement site and must be motivated to work independently.
- Completion of secondary school is preferred since counselors need to understand English in order to participate in the training program. Since English is an official language in Uganda and Southern Sudan it is not difficult to find these staff.
- Previous community development workers, health care workers, nurses or teachers have transferable skills and knowledge that can make them good counselors.
- Many of the counselors are strong Christians. Their faith seems to provide a strong base for a moral commitment to help others.
- Some of the counselors have had psychosocial problems, others have not. This does not seem to be an important criteria for selection. Some of those with previous problems seem to develop personal insight through their training that can help them to empathize with their clients while some were overwhelmed with personal problems and unable to help others.

Psychiatric Treatment

As the TPO-Uganda program evolved the initial people brought for treatment most often had serious mental health problems or epilepsy. The counselors were unable to treat these cases effectively so it was essential to add a drug treatment component to the program.

Within the northern Uganda districts in which the refugee settlements are located there are few medical doctors, limited health and hospital facilities and inadequate drug supplies. Uganda has less than a dozen psychiatrists and none of them is based in the north. The only psychiatric hospital in Uganda is based in the capital city and there is minimal access to this hospital from the north. Even though Ugandan psychiatric nurses are based in most of the hospitals, including the north, due to a general shortage of nurses and lack of psychiatric drug supplies most end up doing medical nursing. Little transport is available so they are unable to work in the rural health centers and are restricted to outpatient hospital based treatment.

Even though plans are underway to integrate services, presently, separate medical services are available for refugees and Ugandan nationals. The Ugandan government supports medical care for nationals and the UNHCR does the same for refugees.

TPO employs four Ugandan psychiatric nurses. Each Ugandan nurse has a two years degree in nursing and an additional eighteen months specialization in psychiatric nursing. It is hoped that in the future a group of Sudanese nurses can be trained to specialize in psychiatric nursing.

Influence of Traditional Beliefs on Staff

The TPO counselors and nurses are members of communities with traditional beliefs. Prior to working with TPO, most counselors had little contemporary knowledge about psychosocial and mental health identification and treatment and were only aware of traditional methods of healing. The role of a counselor was unknown and needed to evolve to find a place within the traditional structures. The nurses had medical training but no psychosocial or counseling training. One counselor in training reported:

> I remember when I was young. A relative became mentally ill. He was locked in the house and the meat of an elephant was burned. The smoke successfully chased away the demons.

Prior to beginning training, discussions were held to understand the future staff members' beliefs about psychosocial and mental health problems. Their responses show a combination of traditional and religious beliefs and are similar to the belief structure and explanatory models of the general population.

Prior to training the future staff members believed that the best treatment for emotional distress included: "advice by an elder, building individual self-esteem, the words spoken during a ritual not the goat slaughter, church can send the evil spirits away with prayer, love from family and solving the problems that caused the distress."

The future staff members were able to identify the seriously mentally ill or "mad people" prior to training. They believed the best treatment for mental illness included: modern drugs, herbs, beating drums, offerings of domestic animal sacrifices, consultation with a diviner or healer, performing rituals for the dead and other traditional rituals and strong prayer to chase away the evil spirits (TPO-Uganda Counselor Training Manual, 1998).

Training was needed to help them to integrate their traditional beliefs with useful western ideas. The maintenance of tradition is important since they must continue to be members of their communities. Also, some of the traditional beliefs are helpful. Those traditional beliefs that may prevent effective helping, however, need to be changed. For example, ostracizing people with epilepsy because people believe they are cursed rather than providing western medication is damaging. Often when western ideas are introduced societies grab them and forfeit that which is important to their own culture. One of the advantages of using refugee staff is that they are part of their cultures and can work with the people as insiders. To accomplish this an integration of ideas and techniques was critical to the training.

Counselor Training Format

Staff training is an important basic element in successful implementation of the TPO-Uganda program. Needs are immediate so staff must be trained quickly. There is little availability for counselors to refer to other helpers so training must be comprehensive and prepare staff to work with a wide array of problems.

TPO is asked to assist with all sorts of problems each of which has an effect on the mental health of individuals, families and communities. Problems rooted in the everyday structure of society, can take as great a toll as problems of mental health. To think about mental health we must consider a range of interrelated forces that, at first glance, might not appear to be 'mental health' problems" (Desjarlais et al., 1995). Some of the examples of requests for help to TPO-Uganda include:

- Help a family find a confused, naked man who had run into the bush talking to himself and threatening to harm anyone who stood in his way.
- Rebels stole a family's food supply and the children are starving.
- Calm a violent quarrel between a drunken man and his wives.
- Find a home for an abandoned child.
- Speak to a parent who is not paying a child's school fees.
- Advocate to the United Nations for a community whose seeds for planting did not germinate.
- Rush to a home where a child is dying.

- Help a widow with seven children and no extended family.
- Assist a suicidal childless woman.
- Assist a man charged with defilement locked in prison without a trial.

The counselor training program is intensive and uses a practical hands-on approach (Box 3).

Future counselors and nurses are trained to identify, assess and treat people with psychosocial and mental health problems as well as prevention techniques. In addition to classroom teaching and field experience all of the information taught is given'to each participant in writing to increase the chance that it will be remembered. Each trainee is given a small library of reference materials. After the training supervisors, who are more experienced counselors, provide weekly individual supervision in the field sites. They also coordinate ongoing group supervision and regular refresher training.

Curriculum for Training Counselors. The initial six weeks of intensive training is a combination of classroom lectures and discussion, field

---

Box 3. Framework for Training Counselors

1. *Intensive 6 weeks of training: 288 hours*
   Training is held six days a week, eight hours a day, during 6 weeks.
2. *Written and oral trainee evaluation: at the end of the intensive 6 weeks*
   Trainees are evaluated and only those deemed competent move onto field training.
3. *Field training: 80 hours over 2 weeks*
   Trainees live and work in the field for two weeks with an experienced counselor.
4. *Probation contract and begin independent work*
   New counselors are placed on three months probation and assigned to a work site.
5. *Supervision: weekly*
   Counselors and nurses receive weekly supervision at their field sites.
6. *Refresher training: additional 72 hours of training over 10 days.*
   This training is held after the new staff work in the field for two months.
7. *Certificate of completion as Psychosocial Counselor:*
   Trainees are given certificates saying they completed a course of 440 hours of classroom and field training as a Psychosocial Counselor.
8. *Team building and ongoing training:*
   After five months in the field: additional 32 hours of training over 4 days.
9. *Contract of six months:*
   After six months each trainee's skills are assessed and strengths and weaknesses discussed with a supervisor. Those found capable are given a year contract while others have their probation extended.
10. *More refresher training:*
    Staff meetings for case reviews and for problem solving difficult cases are continued monthly. Refresher training courses are held quarterly for 3–5 days.

training and reading of relevant materials. The curriculum includes:

- Role of the TPO Counselor
- TPO Philosophy of Helping
  - Focus on Empowerment
  - Community and Family Orientated
  - Practical Problem-Solving
  - Utilizing Outreach Strategies
  - Integration of Traditional Healing and Problem-Solving
- Promotion of Personal Growth and Awareness of Counselor
- Understanding of Psychosocial Problems: Identification, Symptoms, Causes and Treatment
- Knowledge about Mental Health Problems: Identification, Symptoms, Causes and Treatment
- Management of the TPO Mental Health Clinics
- Epilepsy Symptoms, Causes and Treatment
- Review of Trauma and Stress and Methods of Treatment
- Assisting the Mentally Retarded
- Basic Counseling and Support Skills for Individual, Family and Groups
- Crisis Intervention Skills/Suicide Prevention
- Community Organization, Mediation and Peace Building Skills
- Skills for Community Training
- Understanding Youth and Child Problems and Provision of Interventions
- Skills in Stress Reduction
- Counseling Alcoholics and their Families
- How to Write and Use a Plan of Action
- TPO Monitoring and Reporting System
- General Health Knowledge: Family Planning, STDs, AIDS and Common Diseases
- 11 Spiral Steps for Helping (Box 4)

Psychiatric Nurse Training

The nurses' university training provides them with an adequate knowledge of drug treatment but they receive little practical training. It is our experience that the recent graduates need at least two months of supervised field work with an experienced nurse prior to working independently. In the western world, drug treatment is usually supervised by medical doctors. Without the availability of doctors, the nurses learn to prescribe utilizing a limited array of drugs. It is usually found that psychiatric nurses can adequately provide mental health care after appropriate training courses (de Jong, 1996).

Each psychiatric nurse also completes the TPO psychosocial counselor training so that each can also provide counseling and other psychosocial assistance.

> **Box 4. 11 Spiral Steps for Psychosocial Helping**
>
> *Step 1*: Direct all help toward self-help. Empower a person to help him or herself within the context of family and community. (Continuous Process.)
>
> *Step 2*: Involve a network of potential support including family, friends or community in the helping process. (Continuous Process.)
>
> *Step 3*: Build a trusting helping relationship between the person asking for help, his or her family or support network and the helper. (This is a prerequisite for all helping).
>
> *Step 4*: Listen attentively to all of the involved people. (Continuous Process.)
>
> *Step 5*: Probe for all necessary information. (Continuous process.)
>
> *Step 6*: Encourage expression of all feelings by the involved people. (Continuous process.)
>
> *Step 7*: Offer compassion, empathy, emotional comfort and support to all without bias. (Continuous process.)
>
> *Step 8*: Assess the problems thoroughly. (Important as a step to build the initial plan of action.)
>
> *Step 9*: Develop a Plan of Action with all of the involved people in compliance with context, culture and capacity. (Essential to update the plan throughout process of helping.)
>
> *Step 10*: Step by step implementation of the Plan of Action toward problem solving.
>
> *Step 11*: End the helping when the process is complete and evaluate the effect of the helping.

The nurses receive training and supervision bi-monthly by a Ugandan psychiatrist. This psychiatrist is flown to the north by TPO. She supervises the nurses by reviewing cases, visits unresponsive or difficult cases and helps to devise effective treatment regimes.

Training of Trainers (ToT)

Programs cannot remain dependent on international trainers and administrators due to expense and the need for long-term commitment. Training an indigenous group of trainers is essential to the sustainability of a program. These trainers need to have the capacity to educate the community and other helpers as well as train new TPO staff. These trainers also need to learn skills for future program development. Though essential it is not easily accomplished. In the TPO-Uganda program none of the counseling staff had prior education, training or experience in mental health prior to beginning work with TPO. It is impossible to be trained as a counselor for a few weeks and then immediately become a trainer without any field experience. Initially, out of necessity TPO-Uganda tried to do this but it was not effective. Without practical field experience a trainer merely memorizes information and tries to teach it to others, which is mostly ineffective. To become an effective trainer most people first need to have field experience so that the knowledge they were taught is combined reasonably into their traditional beliefs and integrated into practical skills. Once counselors can do this themselves they can be trained as a trainer to teach it to others.

A small select group of TPO-Uganda staff, employed since 1995, was trained in 1999 for three weeks as psychosocial trainers. They learned a wide variety of skills including how to assess the needs of a future training group, participatory training techniques, the use of role play in training and how to build a curriculum. This enabled them to provide community education workshops and awareness and skill training to groups like teachers, health workers, peace educators, and community service workers. TPO counselors in Uganda were always trained by international staff. To become sustainable it was essential that local staff also build the needed skills to train counselors. Additional training was provided to prepare them to work as a team to train new counselors with the assistance of a written training manual. All new counselors are now taught by local staff which is a major milestone toward having the program independently managed and sustained.

PSYCHOSOCIAL AND MENTAL HEALTH INTERVENTIONS

TPO psychosocial counselors and psychiatric nurses provide a full range of psychosocial and mental health interventions. They include a combination of psychological and social initiatives since collective recovery requires reconstruction of psychological, social and economic networks. The following interventions used in Uganda are all framed within the model of the inverted pyramid described in the first chapter.

Psychosocial Interventions

TPO-Uganda has an indigenous group of counselors helping their own people. The counselors have created a new role within their traditional systems. Soon after TPO began the counselors found it difficult to appreciate the value of what they had to offer. They felt inadequate and wanted to give a quick fix through something concrete. They gave money out of their own pockets, fed the people and asked to start mental health clinics in the hope that drugs would help everyone. Over time the counselors' appreciation of the value of their own work improved. As the refugees gave them the feedback that having someone to talk to, listen to their pain and suffering and help them to solve problems was beneficial the counselors' relaxed and felt confident at what they had to offer. As the community respect grew their roles expanded beyond the usual psychosocial and mental issues and they are also asked to assist with all levels of decision-making and act as advocates for the refugees to government and UN authorities.

Psychosocial Approach. The TPO counselors utilize a family and community focused approach. An individual's problem is understood within the context of family and community and support and resolution is found within the family and community. Western psychology theories that promote intrapsychic dynamics seem to be of limited use within this culture.

Counselors provide the basics of good counseling by giving understanding, compassion and support to their clients. They work with an individual and his or her family to empower them using an action oriented problem-solving approach. Additionally encouragement, advice giving, cognitive and behavioral interventions and stress reduction techniques are used. For example:

> Joan was married for two years and had not conceived a child. Her family and her husband's family were concerned and blamed her. She explained in detail to the families and elders that the problem was her husband's nightly alcohol use and impotence. The elders met the husband and demanded he stop drinking. The man felt ashamed. He joined a TPO Alcoholics Anonymous group. Soon after he stopped drinking his wife conceived.

Plan of Action. Counselors are trained to develop Plans of Action with each client (Box 5).

Numbers of Psychosocial Clients. Each year the number of people coming to TPO for help increases as the communities become more aware of the usefulness of the service. In 1998, 1279 new cases came to TPO for help and in 1999, 1656 cases requested help. The numbers listed are per case and since

---

Box 5. A Helping Plan of Action

John is 55 years old. His neighbor finds him preparing a mixture of battery acid to drink to commit suicide. The neighbor stops him and immediately informs the community leader. This leader notifies the TPO counselor. The TPO counselor goes with the leader and neighbor to speak with John. John is depressed and explains that an abscess treated at a health facility many years ago never healed. The health center staff is unable to assist him and he is in constant pain and the abscess has a putrid odor. His wife recently moved away complaining of his smell. The TPO Counselor listens closely to John and offers him emotional comfort and support.

The counselor assesses the problem:

Problem	Goal	Action	Timetable
Depressed	Re-establish hope	Advocate for medical care	Now
Lonely	Re-establish marital relations	Counsel wife	Now

Based on the assessment the counselor develops an initial Plan of Action:
- The counselor and leader interview John, assess the problems and compassionately give him emotional support and encouragement.
- The neighbor offers to have John stay with his family and keep him safe from immediate harm.
- The counselor advocates to the health center for treatment.
- The neighbor accompanies John to the health center.
- The leader meets the wife to regain her support of John.
- The Counselor and leader met with John and his wife.

the families are also assisted the numbers of people assisted are considerably higher. Forty-two percent of the clients found TPO by self or family referral, 25% by the community, 9% by other organizations and 24% were found by the counselors through exploration in the communities.

The frequency, style and goals of psychosocial services vary according to the needs of the clients. Clients come with problems and want concrete resolutions, therefore, the approach is usually short term and directed at problem solving. The data show that 72% of all clients are assisted by counselors from 2–10 times, 19% once, 8% 10–20 times, and 1% more than 20 times.

Psychosocial Problems Prevalence Rates. In the early days people came to TPO asking for financial assistance and food but with greater awareness they now come primarily with family problems and problems related to emotional feelings [Table 1].

Counselors also provide support to people with mental health problems. They refer those with severe psychopathology or epilepsy for whom individual, family or community counseling is not sufficient to the TPO mobile mental health clinics. The nurses provide the psychiatric treatment and the counselors continue to provide psychosocial support to people treated at the clinics.

Table 1. Psychosocial Complaints Presented by Southern Sudanese Refugees to TPO (Average N = 695 Cases Per Month)

Rank	Problem	n	%
1	Family Problem	128	18
2	Health Problem	84	12
3	Feel Stress	69	10
4	Alcohol Overuse	55	8
5	Economic Complaints	53	8
6	Child Problems	50	7
7	Depression–Sadness	41	6
8	Traumatic Event	37	5
9	Mental Retardation	29	4
10	Lack of Food	25	4
11	Domestic Violence	23	4
12	Spirit Possession	19	3
13	Community Relations	16	2
14	Drug Use	16	2
15	Psychosocial Education	13	2
16	Psychosomatic Complaints	12	2
17	Sexual Complaints	9	1
18	Suicide Attempts	8	1
19	Torture	6	1
20	Rape	2	<1

Counselor Burnout. The job of the psychosocial counselors is very difficult because so many of the problems presented to them have no resolution and are beyond the scope of what the client and counselor can do. Often the counselor's job is to help people to create a life that is tolerable within daily inescapable misery. It is difficult to treat depression, fear, anxiety and stress when there is not enough food, rebels attack indiscriminately, children are dying due to limited health care and the future looks realistically bleak. It is a challenge to help people to find the courage and strength to persevere. Counselors center their work on support, sincere encouragement and problem solving for those issues that can be improved.

Counselors cope with the difficulties of their jobs well. Most maintain a positive pragmatic attitude believing that the service they provide is useful and few succumb to the type of burnout that is seen in the west. There is minimal employment available to refugees so the counselors feel fortunate to be employed. Due to their salaries and knowledge their families and communities view them as important community members. Families give the counselors emotional support and encouragement. Despite the difficulties of their jobs this helps them to maintain positive self-esteem. The counselors and the communities accept the limitations of what they can and can not provide. Most want to help people but helping is not the only reason for their employment so that they are not so easily frustrated when they are unable to succeed with their clients. They are performing a job and do so to the best of their abilities and do not feel driven to help as some helpers feel in the west. Most maintain a clear distinction between what they can and cannot do. Many have devout religious beliefs and believe that things happen according to God's will which seems to give them solace (Box 6).

Community Participation in Psychosocial Helping Workshops

To be effective community education needs to flood the entire community. TPO counselors developed a community education approach that reaches throughout the settlements. They designed a one-day community workshop entitled Community Participation in Psychosocial Helping (CPPH). The workshops target community leaders and the overall goal is to increase community sensitization and awareness and mobilize community leaders to help their vulnerable members and activate their communities to help themselves and know when and how to make referrals to TPO and other helpers. Each counselor learned basic training skills and is responsible for training the leaders and selected community members in the settlements where they live and work. Counselors use short lectures, discussions and roleplays to train the community leaders (Box 7).

Some counselors are better trainers than others so they form teams to facilitate the workshops. Training the community that they serve has increased the trust and respect between the community and the counselor.

Box 6. A Day in the Life of a TPO-Uganda Counselor

The counselor awakens in the home of her family within the refugee settlement. After preparing breakfast, she sends her older children to school and turns over the care of her baby to her sixteen years old niece.

It rained during the night so the roads are muddy and she drives her motorbike over the slippery, rutted roads to her field office. She arrives at 8:30 A.M. to find a client's mother waiting for her. The mother is frantic. Her son refused to take his medication for the past couple of days and has relapsed. He was shouting and running about all night and this morning threatened to harm a neighbor. The counselor tries to calm the mother and get the details of what has happened to determine the seriousness of the problem.

Using her radio hand set the counselor contacts the larger field office and speaks to her supervisor. She explains the situation and it is agreed that she will try to stabilize the family until a psychiatric nurse can arrive. The settlement is about an hour drive from the field office. The nurse is responsible for a clinic that day and must be found at another location. With bad roads, it might be afternoon before she arrives.

The counselor accompanies the mother to her home. Neighbors report that the man ran into the bush. The counselor meets with the camp chairman and some of the man's relatives. They arrange to go and look for him and will report to the counselor when he is found.

The counselor returns to her office and spends 30 minutes completing her case notes from yesterday. She then begins the field visits arranged for that day. She drives by motorbike to a client's home about 30 minutes away. The client is a woman who was raped by rebels in an attack to the settlement last week. Immediately after the incident, the counselor went to the settlement and found the victims. She assessed their needs and decided to offer some supportive counseling to this woman and her family. The woman is appreciative that she has come again. They talk alone for about an hour. The woman cries and talks of the incident and her feelings and her husband's reaction. The counselor meets the couple together and discusses their feelings. The husband is fearful that his wife might have contracted AIDS and refuses to have sexual relations with her. The wife feels frightened that he might leave her. The counselor encourages them to talk and tries to assist their problem solving. There is no easily available testing for AIDS but the counselor agrees to try to arrange testing. She teaches them about condom use and leaves after two hours.

The counselor drives half an hour to the home of a family with a four years old retarded child. The child is severely retarded and unable to sit. Last week the counselor and father talked about how to build a seat for the child since the mother was burdened by having to carry the child on her back. The counselor was pleased to see the father had followed through. The child was sitting and the mother able to perform her chores. The parents talk to the counselor about their eldest daughter. She wants to marry but the boy's family is hesitant due to the retarded sibling. They fear that retardation is a family trait that will be passed to future grandchildren. The counselor explains that since the child's brain damage appeared after having a high fever it is not hereditary. The family invites the camp chairman to discuss the problem. It is agreed that a meeting with the boy's family will be held to discuss the problem. A local traditional healer will also be consulted and invited to the meeting to discuss ways to prepare the family so that the marriage can take place.

The counselor returns to the home of the mentally ill man. He is found and some of the relatives are sitting with him inside a hut. He is shouting and appears to be delusional. The counselor uses her hand set to call the field office and learns that the nurse is on her way. When the nurse arrives, he meets the client and assesses the problem. He decides to medicate him with a quick acting psychotropic injection. The counselor and nurse speak with the family and develop a plan for maintaining the client safely at home. The nurse and counselor will return the next day to follow-up on their treatment.

It is now 6 P.M. and the sun is setting so the nurse and counselor return to their homes.

> **Box 7. Community Participation in Psychosocial Helping Training**
>
> The content of this training includes:
> 1. Basic explanation of causes, symptoms and treatment for psychosocial problems. Discussions about trauma, stress, alcoholism, suicide, psychosomatic illness, family and child problems using case examples.
> 2. Basic description of causes, symptoms and treatment for mental illness, mental retardation and epilepsy.
> 3. Promotion of compassion toward people with psychosocial and mental health problems and importance of involving families and community in helping.
> 4. Teach basic helping skills including listening, empathy, attending and problem solving through role play.
> 5. Discuss methods the participants can use to assess psychosocial needs.
> 6. Teach how to design a plan of action that empowers family and community to assist a person in need.
> 7. Discuss when and how to make a referral to TPO, UNHCR or other NGOs.

In 1998 and 1999 using the Community Participation in Psychosocial Helping Workshops (CPPH) counselors held 360 training sessions in which they trained 8180 settlement based community leaders, religious leaders, teachers, health workers, youth leaders, women leaders, traditional healers, government officials and NGO workers.

Integration of TPO with Traditional Helping

Interventions integrate traditional, religious and community methods with TPO helping (Box 8).

Responses to Mental Illness

Why Mental Health Treatment? The north of Uganda, especially the refugee settlements, struggle to provide adequate health care. Some would question why TPO encourages the spending of money on psychiatric care when the most basic health care is not adequate? In a refugee society to survive the members must struggle and work hard. If a family has a mentally ill, retarded or disabled member this person can become a serious drain on the family's ability to survive. The family's meager resources are often consumed in search of care, and enormous time and energy are diverted from other domains of life (Desjarlais et al., 1995). The disabled person can become a burden and out of necessity neglected. A dignified quality of life is an international human right. Mental health care is relatively inexpensive; medication costs an average of $9 a month for the most seriously mentally ill and half a dollar for people with

	Box 8. Integrative Helping
Problem	*Preferred Provider of Treatment*
Serious Mental Illness	Psychiatric Clinic Drug Treatment—Psychosocial Counselor—Mental Health Education—Traditional Healers—Religious Leaders
Epilepsy	Psychiatric Clinic Drug Treatment—Health Center Assessment—Health and Safety Education—Psychosocial Counselors
Mental Retardation	Psychosocial Counselor—Community Leaders—Relatives
Family/Community Problems	Elders—Community Leaders—Relatives—Traditional Healers—Psychosocial Counselor—Religious Leaders
Alcohol Problems	Elders—Traditional Healers—Relatives—Psychosocial Counselor—Alcohol Group—Alcohol Education
Spirit Possession/Curses	Traditional Healers
Unmet Survival Needs	Psychosocial Counselor Referral—United Nations—Other Helpers
Health Problems	Psychosocial Counselor Referral—Health Center Treatment
Security or Legal Issues	Psychosocial Counselor—Police—Government officials—UNHCR

epilepsy. With proper treatment many of those who were once a burden on their families can become productive.

TPO advocates strongly to the Uganda health ministry, United Nations and aid donors to understand the importance of treatment for the mentally ill. They are encouraged to build their capacity so that in the future this treatment can become their responsibility.

Depression. If one assumes that some of the people listed as suicide risk, alcohol abuse, headaches and other problems on Table 2: Prevalence of Mental Illness Diagnosis may also be depressed, then depression would rank as the most prevalent problem.

A World Bank Study estimates that depression ranks fifth among other diseases in disability burden among women and seventh among men in the low income countries (Desjarlais et al., 1995; compare chapter 1).

Schizophrenia. Prior to TPO services in the refugee camps, a typical case of schizophrenia and the course of traditional treatment would resemble this:

> Steven is 25 years old. After finishing primary school, he apprenticed as a tailor and set up his own business in his village. When the war surrounded him, he ran with his family into exile. Though unhappy with the living conditions and the limited food and fear of further violence, he coped okay. He had taken his sewing machine with him

into exile and re-established a small business. Steven began to have headaches and his mother noticed that he was daydreaming frequently. One day, Steven was missing from home. He was found miles away, confused, wandering naked and talking to himself. He was brought home but did not respond to his family's demand that he behave properly. The family brought him to a traditional healer where he stayed for two months. The healer gave him many herbs and performed many rituals. He explained that Steven was suffering since his brother had died in Sudan years earlier and the family had not adequately performed the rituals during his death. After two months, Steven returned home, unchanged. He continued to run naked and disappear and the family feared that he would harm himself. The family elders held a meeting and decided that Steven must be tied to a tree in the family compound for his own safety.

TPO provides extensive sensitization and awareness workshops within the communities to promote referral of mental health cases. The counselors live within the communities, provide outreach home based visits and clinics are easily accessible with a proven track record of success. In 1998 TPO treated a total of 1106 patients or 0.70% of the population for mental illness or epilepsy. Sixty per cent of the patients were male, 40% female, 60% adults, and 40% children. About 24% of the population of people with mental illness are diagnosed with schizophrenia, i.e. 274 people or 0.175% of the overall population which is low by world standards. The numbers of people attending our mental health clinic program increase every year. It is possible, however, that the prevalence of mental illness is lower in the camps than in the general population. Either because these vulnerable people were left in Sudan since they were difficult to

Table 2. One Month-Prevalence of Mental Illness Diagnosis of Southern Sudanese Refugees Treated at TPO Mobile Mental Health Clinics (N=157 Patients Per Month)

Rank	Diagnosis	n	%
1	Major Depression	38	24
2	Schizophrenia	38	24
3	Organic Brain Syndromes	31	20
4	Major Anxiety	13	8
5	Non-Mental Health Problems	8	5
6	Psychosis	7	5
7	Manic-Depression	7	5
8	PTSD	5	3
9	Childhood Disorders	5	3
10	Headaches	3	2
11	Alcohol Dependence	2	1
12	Drug Dependence	0	0
13	Sleep Disturbance	0	0
14	Psychosomatic Complaints	0	0
15	Suicide	0	0

move during the exodus, or that due to their vulnerability and disruptive behavior they did not live long lives. Other explanations are that families still prefer to take their patients to healers only, despite our health education, or that the geographic accessibility of our services is low. Further study will examine these issues.

Prevalence of Epilepsy

Within the refugee population the incidence of epilepsy is high due to illness, fever, infection, accidents, poor obstetric care and injuries. Prevalence of epilepsy can be as high as 3.7–4.9% in Africa and Asia (Adamolekum, 1995). Out of a total of 280 patients with epilepsy per month seen by our mobile clinics, 58% is male and 43% female, whereas 65% are children and 35% are adults.

Due to their seizures people suffer many accidents particularly falling into fires or drowning. The health centers do not treat people with epilepsy since they diagnose epilepsy as a mental illness. The TPO clinics provide assessment and drug treatment for people with epilepsy as well as education and support for the person and family. The TPO psychiatric nurses and psychiatrist are leading seminars for health center staff about the causes and treatment of epilepsy. Our goal is to educate health services staff in order to transfer the treatment of the people with epilepsy to the health centers.

Mental Health Interventions

TPO-Uganda provides what is believed to be the most effective treatment; a combination of medication and community or family based psychosocial interventions. In addition to the use of drugs, most of the TPO treatment depends on the support and good will of the families.

Mobile Mental Health Clinics. TPO's psychiatric nurses and counselors facilitate mental health clinics in different locations each day. They are assisted by clinic managers trained in drug distribution. All of the refugees needing assistance assemble at the clinic on the assigned day in the morning and each is given a number to order the treatment. The clinic begins with a 15 minutes educational workshop about some aspect of mental health taught by the nurse. Clinics range in size from 10 to 75 patients and may be staffed by 1 or 2 nurses. There are many languages spoken so often the nurse requires a translator. The patient is interviewed by the nurse in the presence of the TPO counselor. The nurse provides medication when needed and refers patients needing psychosocial support to the counselors.

Frequency of Visits. Educating patients about the importance of maintenance treatment remains difficult. People frequently move or stray from treatment. It is most difficult to sustain treatment with patients who have no families or caretakers. TPO statistics show that 60% of people come for treatment from 2–10 times, 17% come 10–20 times, and only 1% more than 20 times. This seems too little when such a large percentage of patients are diagnosed with epilepsy and schizophrenia. Many stop coming when they begin to feel better despite all efforts to have them continue. Continued efforts to educate people about the importance of continuing treatment are essential.

Hospitalization. It is remarkable that the TPO nurses manage their large numbers of patients without being able to admit them to a hospital. Occasionally, a patient who is at suicide risk or a danger to others is confined in a police station. Most of the time the nurse, family and community must work together to develop a plan of treatment for even the most dangerous and seriously mentally ill patients.

Drugs. The nurses work with a limited drug supply. At present the drugs are provided to the clients for free but a system of minimal payment is being organized. The program uses the psychotropic drugs of WHO's essential drug list.

Patients respond well to psychotropic drugs when they maintain their treatment.

> A man begged the TPO nurse to assist his son. He brought him to his mud hut and unlocked the door. Inside was a naked man of 25 sitting in his own excrement and chained to a log. He had been placed there two years earlier during an apparent psychotic episode in which he attacked a neighbor and burned a house. He was immediately placed on psychotropic drugs. Within months he was dressed, released from his confinement and beginning to assist his family in the fields.

Assistance to the Mentally Retarded

Families frequently bring their retarded children to the mental health clinics desperately searching for assistance. Many of the children appear to have brain damage, which seems to have occurred after high fevers before five years old, and frequently they also have ongoing convulsions. Often the families have been to healers and spent a great deal of money trying to find a cure for their children. The problems for a retarded child and the family are many. Often the child is neglected and few retarded youth or adults are found within the settlements. Fathers often desert the mother of a retarded child believing she is cursed and fearful that she will give birth to more retarded children. Communities often shun the family and child, therefore, many are locked away so no one can see them. Single mothers often have to leave the retarded child unattended in a hut all day in order to tend their fields.

The TPO counselor completes a needs assessment of each retarded person and his or her family and an individualized plan is developed. Counselors provide a range of services from emotional support to families, education about mental retardation, encouragement to families to provide love, compassion and care to the child and training to show parents how to educate their children and teach them basic self-help skills. Ongoing support and education groups for parents are held in some settlements.

Since many parents complained that the care of this child restricted them from being able to care for the rest of the family TPO initiated a special income generation project. When this project began more families with retarded children appeared than TPO realized existed in the settlements. Each child was given two goats with the plan that the goat milk could be drunk and as the goats multiply they can be sold for income. It was a surprise to many families to see how responsibly their retarded child handled their goats.

> Steven is 10 years old. He developed normally until he was two years old when late one night he had a high fever and convulsions apparently due to cerebral malaria. The family lived far from a health clinic so no treatment was given. After that he began to have convulsions a few times a week and never learned to speak fully. The family realized he was different from their other children and brought him to a traditional healer for a cure. The healer believed that the problem was caused due to the family not performing a proper burial ritual for an uncle who died in Sudan. Much money was spent to perform this ritual but the child did not improve. The father left the family for fear having more retarded children. Steven's mother sought help from TPO. The counselor explained that the retardation was caused by damage to the brain probably due to the fever. She explained that there was no cure but that with perseverance the family could teach the child self-help skills. The mother felt relieved and was eager to educate the child. The counselor also educated the father and he returned to the family. The child was taught to assist in household tasks. When the goats were given to the child, he was delighted. The father asked for money rather than goats and the child declared, "No, these are my goats." Steven responsibly cares for the goats and is eagerly waiting the birth of the first offspring.

Crisis Intervention

TPO staff members respond immediately to any crisis and are often the first respondent since they are the only NGO staff living within the refugee settlements. UNHCR and the Ugandan government often rely on the staff to assist in response to any crisis. TPO trained a team of three community leaders in each settlement as a Community Crisis Intervention Team (CCIT).

It is believed that the initial response to trauma needs to consist of reconnecting individuals with their ordinary supportive networks, and having them engage in activities that reestablish a sense of mastery (Van der Kolk, 1996). TPO counselors provide psychological first aid similar to schemata set up by Raphael (1986) including comforting and consoling; protection from further threat; immediate care for shelter and other needs; goal orientation and support for reality based tasks; facilitating reunion with loved ones; if there is a trauma, facilitate telling of the trauma story and ventilation of feelings; linking the person to systems of support and ongoing help; facilitating some sense of mastery and identifying need for further counseling (Van der Kolk, 1996).

Crisis intervention was originally recommended by Kaplan and Sadock (1985) as a preventive technique to lessen the likelihood of unfavorable outcomes after stressful life events. Research has not proven that this technique is effective in actually minimizing future stressful responses or PTSD (Van der Kolk, 1996). However, according to the refugee communities the counselor's quick response has the effect of immediately calming the victim and community, supporting the victim and family, assisting in quick referral for assistance and activating community and family support for the victim. It seems to help to minimize the victim's immediate symptoms of trauma and stress but it is hard to judge if this has a long-term effect of reducing the risk of more serious symptoms.

A typical month of crisis responses as reported in April, 1998 for the TPO-Uganda counselors and nurses included: 2 suicide attempts; 18 persons abducted and 8 killed by rebels; 5 psychiatric emergencies; 1 epilepsy emergency; 1 health emergency; one situation of domestic violence; 1 incident of violence in the extended family; 2 pregnant teens in crisis; 2 situations of excessive alcohol use and a fire displacing three families.

Suicide. Large numbers of suicide attempts and deaths prompted the counselors to begin a suicide prevention initiative. TPO staff led workshops to educate government, UN and NGO staff. Health workers received training in identification and treatment. The Community Crisis Intervention Team (CCIT) responds to each crisis and when needed requests the assistance of TPO. The Community Crisis Intervention Team and TPO co-lead special workshops for community members to explain suicide risk and encourage prompt assertive community response.

> The TPO counselor trained a CCIT and encouraged them to make the community aware they were available to help in a crisis. About one month after the training a community member rushed to the team asking them to assist her neighbor. The neighbor is a woman of 32. She had a misunderstanding with her brother. He accused her of leaving a plate unwashed and beat her. She became very upset and purchased 25 chloroquine tablets. She took all of the tablets and at that time was sick shaking and unable to speak. The CCIT ran to the woman's home and brought her to a health center. She was treated successfully. The next day the CCIT held a meeting with the suicide victim, her brother and parents and resolved the conflict. Afterward, they informed the counselor. He will continue to follow-up the case with the CCIT.

Group and Community Interventions

Counselors report the effectiveness of group and community interventions. Group treatment modalities are molded according to the counselors' preferences and the methods most appropriate to the group or community's purpose, context and membership. The counselor usually facilitates the organization of group meetings but encourages self-help and promotes members to interact and help each other. Psychosocial support from counselors is not a long-term sustainable option. The formation of groups in which people with similar problems help each other is a more sustainable framework. Problems will exist forever, as can community self-help groups.

Curative and Preventive Groups. Martin (1994) suggests that too much focus has been placed on curative care and not on preventive care with refugee health systems. Too little attention has been paid to the environmental aspects of what creates physical or mental health problems. Also, too little attention has been paid to preventive measures that build on community resources since on the return home a curative approach may not be affordable. TPO groups are both preventive and curative. The curative groups are usually formed with people with related problems and provide support, counseling and problem solving. Groups are encouraged to be self-help and members often give each other advice and offer support in and out of the group setting. Curative groups include: support groups for alcohol abusers, widows, mothers of retarded children, children who experienced recent traumas, ex-rebels, returned abductees, families of unreturned abductees and mothers for children at malnutrition centers.

Preventive groups include psychosocial and mental health education classes and discussion; and peace and community building through activities. Efforts are made to understand the causes for certain problems and to prevent their exacerbation. Preventive groups include psychosocial education on alcohol and epilepsy for communities, youth and children; sport leagues, drama groups and traditional dance for children and youth and sports competitions.

Alcohol Self-Help Groups. Special groups are arranged by counselors according to community needs. Many communities complain about the increase in problems that stem from excessive alcohol use. In response, TPO initiated a campaign to educate people about the risks of excessive alcohol use and to help those with alcohol problems.

Counselors include alcohol education as part of their community workshops. They teach about the problems of excessive alcohol use and use role play to practice how to SAY NO to drink. Educational groups are led with children in which song, dance and drama teaches about alcohol use.

Individual counseling has proven to be of little use to the heavy drinkers. Throughout the world, Alcoholics Anonymous (AA), which uses self-help groups with a strong spiritual component, has been successful in assisting drinkers and their families. AA programs have been successfully started in Kenya, Uganda and Tanzania. TPO arranged for an AA member from Kampala to work in the camps with the counselors to pilot AA styled groups. The first group began two years ago with 7 members, six of whom have remained sober. This group assisted the initiation of groups in other camps. The combination of spirituality and group support and peer pressure seems to be ideal so a more comprehensive program is planned. Some wives of alcoholics have also formed supportive talking and problem solving groups.

Youth Activities

Many youth feel frustrated and depressed by their life within the camps. Education and employment are often not available and many youth are frustrated by the limitations of their futures.

TPO counselors have initiated youth clubs throughout the settlements as a non-threatening way to meet the youth and become known as a supportive adult who can help in times of distress. The counselor encourages the youth to be self-motivated and after the initiation of the club the youth establish a leadership and independently organize activities like sporting leagues and traditional dance groups. The Counselors periodically meet with them for encouragement and psychosocial education.

> In a camp of people of the Dinka tribe, the counselor reported that there were usually 10 arrests for violence by male youth (aged approximately 15–25 years; a male is considered a youth until marriage) each month. Since the onset of the sport programs in this camp three months earlier there has been only one arrest.

There are no easy answers to ease the problems faced by the youth. TPO cannot solve these problems and advocates for the initiation of vocational training and special income generation for youth. The TPO groups are a small means for youth to feel some mastery over their life's activities.

Children's Activities

TPO-Uganda counselors observe that the Sudanese children are often resilient and with the help of supportive families and communities often cope with even the most stressful situations. Yet, life in the camp is often without much pleasure so the counselors provide recreational opportunities to the children for laughter and play.

In many camps, campfires in the evenings are not allowed due to fear of rebels. In the usual Sudanese communities it is around these campfires that children would learn through stories, riddles and rhymes about their culture, traditions and morals. Without the campfires, many children are apparently not getting this knowledge. Some of the organized play groups use dramas and story telling to make up for this loss and teach the children traditional values.

Community Building and Peace and Reconciliation Activities

A history of tensions between tribes in Southern Sudan continues within the settlements. Children and youth continue to be taught fear and hatred of other tribes as has been taught for centuries. It is often blind hatred and rarely based on present day real issues. TPO promotes activities to try to change attitudes. Sport leagues between tribes that hate each other yet do not really know each other are organized. Due to historical hatred the Dinka tribe lives in a camp in isolation from the other tribes. TPO has organized numerous activities in which Dinka youth are transported with some of their elders and parents to a neighboring settlement to play football, share traditional dance and dramas. At first the TPO staff were as anxious as the youth about the activities. Now, it has become an exciting monthly event with as many as 1500 community members watching the matches. A small step toward building peaceful relations. TPO offers a workshop to help community members especially youth entitled Bridging Tribal Conflicts. In the workshop a poster of warring tribes trying to kill a lion is used for discussion with familiar proverbs and metaphors related to peace. It seems that it is more difficult for children, youth and adults to maintain hateful stereotypes when they have had positive experiences.

Two years ago TPO reexamined its staff and added some members from tribes with whom relations had a history of tension. Initially the distrust and antagonism caused needed self-examination. The intensity of the struggle to build positive relations within its own staff highlighted the daunting task of doing this in the communities.

More and more TPO staff has become aware of the attitudes that maintain discord between tribes. Initially, TPO counselors, like the communities would search for a clansman whenever help was needed by someone. Recognizing the limitations of this within the present living context, counselors are trying to assist communities in organizing mixed elder councils that include members from various clans and tribes.

Referral

TPO counselors refer people to available resources in the community since many people do not know what services exist or how to access them.

A typical month would include approximately 170 people referred by TPO to other services: 55% to health care, 23% to social welfare, 8% to protection and 14% to other services. Health care is the most common referral with only a small percentage of the people that come to TPO for health care suffering from psychosomatic complaints. Many seem to be physically ill people searching for medical care within a system with few services.

Advocacy

As an organization and as individuals, TPO advocates for human rights, refugee rights and children's rights.

Research

TPO Counselors organize and participate in studies to understand the changing needs of the affected communities and assess the effectiveness of its interventions.

PROGRAM MONITORING

The program uses a comprehensive reporting system for monitoring the activities.

Field work files for each client and group. Confidential files are maintained by counselors on each case and group and kept in a locked box in the field locations. The client file includes a comprehensive intake form, case history, diagnosis, plan of action, ongoing notes on every contact and a discharge summary.

Internal program monthly reporting system. All of the counselors complete a monthly report that summarizes their work. It includes a day by day accounting of their activities, the statistics of types of cases seen and details of any crises or problems.

External program monthly reporting system. The field based supervisors review the counselors' reports and then combine them to write a monthly report. This report is submitted monthly to UNHCR, local Ugandan Government officials and the program donors.

Annual report to donors. A comprehensive annual report is provided to the donors.

EFFECTIVENESS OF TPO-UGANDA INTERVENTIONS

TPO-Uganda repeatedly asks consumers including clients and community leaders and its working partners from government, the United Nations and other non-governmental organizations for feedback about its services. These reports suggest that many of the TPO interventions are effective. Some of the feedback about specific services includes:

Crisis intervention. Consumers and working partners reported that the immediate crisis response system designed by TPO that includes Community Crisis

Intervention Teams working with the counselors, helped to prevent problems from expanding. Quick intervention for mental health emergencies and suicide risk has saved lives and responses to domestic and community conflicts often prevented violence. Immediate response after a rebel attack offered victims and their families support and problems solving that seemed to prevent future symptoms and secondary problems from developing.

Problem solving counseling. Consumers and working partners reported that supportive and problem solving counseling was beneficial to people in need. They believed that it offered encouragement and hope. Without this, they believed people might become more desperate and less functional.

Community awareness education. Consumers and working partners agreed that community awareness education had a positive effect on the communities. With increased awareness it appeared that a community's compassion and understanding for problems related to psychosocial and mental health increased which promoted the community to provide more direct assistance to the vulnerable and others in need.

Groups. Consumers reported that TPO facilitated support groups assisted people with similar problems e.g. families of the retarded, people with epilepsy, or elderly to develop useful networks of support.

Youth activities. The youth and their families reported that activities helped to build self-esteem and decrease anti-social behavior and alcohol use.

Alcohol groups. Members of TPO sponsored alcohol groups reported that these groups have assisted them to stop their overuse of alcohol. Many of these previously nonfunctional people reported that they now work and have positive family and community relations.

Family and community conflict mediation. Consumers and working partners reported that the TPO counselors provided needed support to community leaders to help to mediate the most severe family disputes and violence.

Treatment for mentally ill and people with epilepsy. Consumers and their families and communities reported that the medications provided by TPO often reduced the incidence of seizures and control mental illness.

Community Building Activities. Growing attendance at monthly community sport meets and cultural activities showed the enthusiasm for these events. Most importantly, there has never been an incident of violence at these events.

TPO activities some times seem small compared to what is needed. TPO cannot make peace and help the refugees return home, it has no food to feed the hungry, no money for schools, no jobs; none of the basics. Sometimes staff members wonder about the depth of what we do provide. Yet, when you speak to the refugees assisted by TPO they have no doubt. They say that TPO listens to them, talks to them, cares about them, advocates for them and in their world, a world of people who feel forgotten this listening and caring is highly appreciated and felt to be effective.

REFERENCES

Adamolekum, B. (1995). The aetiologies of epilepsy in tropical Africa. *Tropical and Geographical Medicine, 47*(3), 115–117.

Arcel, L. T. (Ed.). (1998). *War, violence, trauma and the coping process: Armed conflict in Europe and survivor response.* Copenhagen, Denmark: Rehabilitation and Research Centre for Torture Victims.

Baron, N. (1998). *TPO-Uganda counselor training manual.* Kampala, Uganda: TPO Uganda. Internal document.

Baron, N. (1998). *TPO-Uganda reporting system.* Kampala, Uganda: TPO Uganda. Internal document.

Baron, N., & Jurugo, E. (2001). *Comparing worldwide suicide rates to a refugee population.* Manuscript submitted for publication.

De Jong, J. T. V. M. (1996). A comprehensive public mental health programme in Guinea-Bissau: A useful model for Africa, Asia and Latin-American countries. *Psychological Medicine, 26,* 97–108.

De Jong, J. T. V. M. (2000). Psychiatric problems related to persecution and refugee status. In F. Henn, N. Sartorius, H. Helmchen, & H. Lauter (Eds.), *Contemporary Psychiatry* (Vol. 2, pp. 279–298). Berlin: Springer.

Desjarlais, R., Eisenberg, L., Good, B., & Kleinman, A. (1995). *World mental health: Problems and priorities in low-income countries.* New York: Oxford University Press.

Harrell-Bond, B. (1986). *Imposing aid: Emergency assistance to refugees.* Oxford, England: Oxford University Press.

Jablensky, A., Marsella, A. J., Ekblad, S., Jansson, B., Levi, L., & Bornemann, T. (1994). Refugee mental health and well-being: Conclusions and recommendations. In A. J. Marsella, T. Bornemann, S. Ekblad, & J. Orley (Eds.), *Amidst peril and pain: The mental health and well-being of the world's refugees* (pp. 327–339). Washington, DC: American Psychological Association.

Joseph, S., Williams, R., & Yule, W. (1997). *Understanding post-traumatic stress: A psychosocial perspective on PTSD and treatment.* New York: Wiley.

Kaplan, H. I., & Sadock, B. J. (1985). *Comprehensive textbook of psychiatry* (Vol. 4). Baltimore: Williams and Wilkins.

Kleber, R. J., Figley, C. R., & Gersons, B. P. R. (Eds.). (1995). *Beyond trauma: Cultural and societal dynamics.* New York: Plenum Press.

Marsella, A. J., Bornemann, T., Ekblad, S., & Orley, J. (Eds.). (1994). *Amidst peril and pain: The mental health and well-being of the world's refugees.* Washington, DC: American Psychological Association.

McFarlane, A. C., & Yehuda, R. (1996). Resilience, vulnerability, and the course of posttraumatic reactions. In B. Van der Kolk, A. C. McFarlane, & L. Weisaeth (Eds.), *Traumatic stress: The effects of overwhelming experience on mind, body and society* (pp. 129–154). New York: Guilford.

Martin, S. F. (1994). A policy perspective on the mental health and psychosocial needs of refugees. In A. J. Marsella, T. Bornemann, S. Ekblad, & J. Orley (Eds.), *Amidst peril and pain: The mental health and well-being of the world's refugees* (pp. 69–80). Washington, DC: American Psychological Association.

Mollica, R., Donelan, K., Svang, T. O. R., Lavelle, J., Elias, C., Frankel, M., & Blendon, R. J. (1993). The effect of trauma and confinement on functional health and mental health status of Cambodians living in Thailand-Cambodia border camps. *JAMA, 270*(4), 581–586.

Orley, J. (1994). Psychological disorders among refugees: Some clinical and epidemiological considerations. In A. J. Marsella, T. Bornemann, S. Ekblad, & J. Orley (Eds.), *Amidst peril and pain: The mental health and well-being of the world's refugees* (pp. 193–206). Washington, DC: American Psychological Association.

Orley, J., & Wing, J. K. (1979). Psychiatric disorders in two African villages. *Archives of General Psychiatry, 36,* 513–520.

Rangaraj, A. G. (1988). The health status of refugees in South East Asia. In D. Miserez (Ed.), *Refugees: The trauma of exile: the humanitarian role of Red Cross and Red Crescent* (pp. 39–44). Dordrecht, The Netherlands: Martinus Nijhoff.

Seligman, M. E. P. (1975). *Helplessness: On depression, development and death*. San Francisco: W. H. Freeman.

Sieswerda, S., Komproe, I., Hanewald, G., & de Jong, J. T. V. M. (2000). *Mental health and pychosocial problems of Sudanese refugees living in Ugandan camps*. Manuscript submitted for publication.

Summerfield, D. (1995). Addressing human response to war and atrocity: Major challenges in research and practices and the limitations of Western psychiatric models. In R. J. Kleber, C. R. Figley & B. P. R. Gersons, *Beyond trauma: Cultural and societal dynamics* (pp. 17–29). New York: Plenum Press.

Theodore, L., & Elioto, J. (1999). *Afghanistan in 1998: Stalemate* (Asian Survey and Monthly Review of Contemporary Asian Affairs). Los Angeles: University of California Press.

United Nations High Commission on Refugees. (1999). *Uganda statistics and self-reliance strategy literature*. Geneva.

Van der Kolk, B. A., McFarlane, A. C., & Weisaeth, L. (Eds.). (1996). *Traumatic stress: The effects of overwhelming experience on mind, body and society*. New York: Guilford.

Van der Veer, G. (1995). Psychotherapy with refugees. In R. J. Kleber, C. R. Figley, & B. P. R. Gersons (Eds.), *Beyound trauma: Cultural and societal dynamics* (pp. 151–168). New York: Plenum Press.

Von Buchwald, U. (1994). Refugee dependency: Origins and consequences. In A. J. Marsella, T. Bornemann, S. Ekblad, & J. Orley (Eds.), *Amidst peril and pain: The mental health and well-being of the world's refugees* (pp. 229–237). Washington, DC: American Psychological Association.

4

Psychosocial Consequences of War

Northern Sri Lankan Experience

DAYA SOMASUNDARAM and C. S. JAMUNANANTHA

BACKGROUND

History and Politics

Myth. The cause of the current ongoing 'civil war' in Sri Lanka has often been portrayed as a continuation of the racial (ethnic) conflict that has been raging between the Sinhalese and Tamils from the beginning of history (Table 1).

According to one dominant view based on myth, the Sinhalese are descendants of Aryans who migrated from Northern India in the hoary past. The Tamils are Dravidians from South India who invaded the island periodically, causing destruction and conflict. One source for the traditional antagonistic view of history is the Pali chronicle, '*The Mahavamsa*' (The great race or dynasty) (Greiger, 1964), which has been used to authenticate the view that Lanka is sacred to the Buddhist faith and to its guardians, the Sinhalese people. According to Mahavamsa the first king Vigiya (about 500 BC), son of a lion and a princess, was banished due to his unruly behavior from North India. He sailed southward with 700 friends and reached Lanka. Lanka was then said to be populated by the mythical Nagas and Yakhsas. Vigiya married a local queen, Kumini, and killed her relations. Later he got brides for himself and his friends from India. The National Lion flag is a manifestation of the Sinhalese belief in this myth.

The Tamils for their part believe that they came from Southern India and the dominant Tamil militant group, Liberation Tigers of Tamil Eelam (LTTE),

Table 1. Mytho-historical Events and Psychosocial Sequel

Year	Mytho-historical events	Psychosocial sequel
Proto History (?500,000–1000 BC)	Autochthonous inhabitants—Spirits: *Nagas* and *Yakshas*; *Veddas*	Devaluation of aborigines Absorption and extinction
480 BC	? King Vigiya comes from India	Mythic belief in Aryan origin for the Sinhalese
400 BC	Anuradhapura Period	Glorious past
250 BC	Reign of king Devanampiya Tissa (Introduction of Buddhism by Mahinda, son of emperor Asoka of India)	Buddhism as vital part of the Sinhala Buddhist identity
160 BC	Defeat of the Tamil king, Elara by the Sinhalese king, Dutugemunu Unification of country	Prototype for current ethnic problem & its solution
?500 AD	Mahavamsa written	Buddhist perspective of historical development in the island
1000 AD	Polonnaruwa period	Glorious past
1153–86	Reign of Parakramabahu the great	Ideal of Sinhala greatness
1200–1600	Repeated invasions from South India and successive moves of the capital south-westward	"Historical memory" of Indian invasions
?1100–1600	Jaffna Kingdom	Tamil memory of separate kingdom
1505 AD	Portuguese conquer coastal areas	Beginning of long period of Colonial subjugation; Western influence; religious (Christian) zealotry
1657	Dutch conquer	Introduction of Roman Dutch law; schools; economic primacy
1802	Ceded to the British	Imperial strategy; economical exploitation, socio-economic reforms; country unified through roads, railroads, communication, etc.
1815	Kandian kingdom captured by British	Last King—Tamil of Nayakkar dynasty from South India brought down by intrigue, a policy of divide and rule pursued by the British, perhaps resulting in the Sinhala–Tamil split

Table 1. *Continued*

Year	Mytho-historical events	Psychosocial sequel
1817, 1848	Rebellion in hill country	Example of Anti-colonial struggle suppressed brutally where the rebellious local patriots were pushed out of mainstream history (to the East) while those who collaborated with the Colonial powers were rewarded and their descendants are the present day ruling elite
1832	Colebrook Reforms	English speaking local elite; general education, voting and governance
1850	Arumugam Navalar	Hindu–Tamil revival (reaction to Christian proselytisation)
1900	Anagarika Dharmapala	Sinhala–Buddhist revival & identity; beginnings of ethnic consciousness
1911	First local, a Tamil, Sir Ponnambalam Ramanathan elected to the 'educated Ceylonese' constituency of the Legislative Council	Indication of harmony between Sinhala and Tamil community (Tamils were also 'sons of the soil'). Rift may have been created by British Governor Manning in 1921 for election to the same post to 'divide & rule'
1915	Anti-Muslim riots	First example of anti-ethnic violence
1927	Demand for federal state and regional autonomy for Kandyans	Indication of "up-country"–"low-country" identity among Sinhalese
1930's	Anti-Indian worker violence	Growth of anti-ethnic violence
1948	Independence (without national struggle)	Majoritarian politics (no common national identity)
1948	Citizenship act	Statelessness
1950	State–aided colonization of NE	Threat to Tamil territoriality
1956	Buddha Jayanthi—2500th anniversary of Buddhism	Resurgence of Sinhala-Buddhist ideology & populist politics
1956	Sinhala-Only Bill (making Sinhala the sole official language) passed in Parliament; violence against Tamils at Galoya	Threat to Tamil language (& hence, ethnic identity)
1958	Organized violence-race riots	Fear, terror, anxiety
1960	Anti-Christian conflict reaches climax	Christianity suppressed

Table 1. *Continued*

Year	Mytho-historical events	Psychosocial sequel
1970	JVP Crisis. Thousands of Sinhala youths were killed, tortured in detention camps	Precedence for large scale state terror and violence
1972	Ceylon becomes Republic, Buddhism given foremost place in constitution; standardization of University admission—restriction to Tamils	Discrimination
1976	Tamil Party—TULF demands a separate state—"Tamil Eelam"—as their election manifesto	Tamil extremism gains precedence
1977	TULF wins election overwhelming in the North-East on separatist platform; Anti-Tamil riots in the South and hill country	Expression of political dissatisfaction and desire for separation
1979	Army sent to Jaffna—arrests, assault & torture	Fear, terror, anxiety, suppression
1981	Jaffna Public Library burned by State forces and ministers	"Cultural Genocide"
1983	Large scale Anti-Tamil ethnic riots	Fear, terror, anxiety. Threat to ethnic identity. Clear message to Tamils to cow down
1984	Widespread Guerrilla attacks	Defiance, hope
1984–7	Militarization	Passivity, powerlessness, and aggressive behavior. Brutalization
	Attacks against Sinhala civilians	Counter–terror
1985	Internecine fratricide among Tamil militants. Ground control of Jaffna by LTTE	Internal divisions and terror
1987	Mass arrest	Helplessness
1987–90	Indian Army (IPKF) intervenes	Isolation from Indian support
1990	Transient peace	Hope and harmony
1989	JVP crisis in the South	Brutalization and terror extends into the south
1990–	Suicide attacks in South	Counter–terror
1994	Cease fire followed by 'Eelam War II'	Transient euphoria and hopes of peace followed by frustration, despair
1995	Mass exodus of 700,00 & hardship	Collective trauma
1996	People (500,000) resettle in Jaffna; 600 youths 'disappear'	Passivity, dependence

have a tiger in their emblem and flag from the past South Indian Chola kingdom. As a result, the current ethnic conflict is often symbolically depicted as being between the lions and the tigers (or as between the Aryans and Dravidians). The strong emotional beliefs in these "mythohistories" underpinning the ethnic conflict indicate that any step towards reconciling the two groups will have to address these misconstructions (see Table 1). As Hirsh (1995) explains, in most modern day mass killings a

> mythical and partially reconstructed past is used to create a pattern of identity that shapes behaviour and maps the future... People continue to hate and kill for the same reasons, and the memories of their attachments to ethnic, religious, racial, national, or regional identity continue as prime motivations... Memories, and the myths and hatreds constructed around them, may be manipulated by individuals or groups in positions of leadership to motivate populations to commit genocide or other atrocities.

Thus an important step towards reconciliation has been the recommendation that the standard but biased history books that are being used in the schools have to be rewritten to be more reflective of actual events. It would also mean persuading the island's 'scholars' to be more responsible in propagating histories.

Factual History. A deconstruction of the mythohistories reveals a more realistic account of past events (Social Science Association, 1985). The emerging dominance of the Sinhala dynasty from many others could be traced to support from Buddhist monks of the Theravada Mahavihara sect (as opposed to the Mahayana Abhayagiri sect) who received their patronage and to whom in turn they lent legitimacy. One event in the chronicle, which, through interpretation, has influenced modern day politics, is the epic battle between the 'Sinhalese' King Dutugemunu and the 'Tamil' King, Ellalan. Ellalan (or in Sinhalese, Elara) was a South Indian interloper who had conquered Anuradhapura, the seat of the 'Sinhalese' kings, and had ruled justly, as acknowledged by the Mahavamsa, for 44 years, giving his patronage to the Buddhist religion and organizing public works such as irrigation systems. In order to avoid needless bloodshed, the elderly Ellalan and the young Dutugemunu agreed to decide the contest in personal combat in which Ellalan fell. Ellalan was obviously held in veneration by the native people, for Dutugemunu ordered a shrine to be built for him, which should be revered for all time (Obeyesekere, 1988). It also reveals that there were several kings at that time and even families had divided loyalties. The Mahavamsa itself reveals that from the oldest times wives for kings and other prominent persons and artisans had been brought regularly from South India. Due to its geographical location and size, India has been a major influence in Lanka's developments, bequeathing the two major ethnic groups, Sinhalese and Tamil, which are in conflict today, and has been the source of their religions, Buddhism and Hinduism, as well as providing the stock of migrants who intermarried with the autochthonous inhabitants, the *Veddas*, to produce the current people and culture of the island.

Initially, the island was sparsely populated with small independent settlements separated by large distances and forest. Loose central control began with kingdoms being established first at Anuradhapura and then Polanaruwa. Later being moved south not only as popularly depicted, for security reasons, that is repeated invasions from South India, but also due to the fragmentation that followed the ambitious over-expansion of Parakramabahu's overseas ventures, the endemic malaria (originating in neglected irrigation tanks) which caused massive death, and economic reasons such as trade through Trincomalee (De Silva, 1981). Independent Tamil kingdoms appeared in Jaffna and the Vanni. The Sinhala Kings at Central Rajarata faced perennial separatist rebellion from the Southern Rohana (the most recent example being the JVP).[1] Later, Arabian merchants followed by their descendents from South India arrived to set up Muslim settlements at the sea ports.

All evidence points to the strong interconnections Lanka had with South India. The ancestors of the present day Sinhalese, Tamils and Muslims were essentially from the same stock (sharing the same genetic pool) from South India, and were generally dark complexioned. Language, religion and written scripts had no particular links with ethnic consciousness at that time. The historical development of this country was a rich admixture of many influences—ethnic, religious, cultural, trade and migrant workers who were assimilated, forming a large variety of blends in different places and in different times (Spencer, 1990).

The original autochthonous inhabitants have been progressively assimilated by the new arrivals. It is noteworthy that remnants of the authentic '*sons of the soil*', the *Veddas* are now facing extinction due to multinational development and encroachments on their traditional lands. As regards religion, Hindu temples co-existed with Buddhist temples throughout Sri Lanka and people approached different gods for different needs. This is still evidenced by the Hindu shrines as well as folk religious practices, such as the popular 'Pathini cult' (Obeyesekere, 1984) in Southern Sri Lanka that are integral to the local culture. Buddhism itself appears to have come over the years from South India, many of the influential missionaries like Buddhaghosa came from South India. Most Tamils had been Buddhist at an earlier time. The cultural differentiation apparent in present day Sinhalese and Tamils can be explained merely on the basis of divergence in spoken language and to a lesser extent, religious practices due to geographical separation over the years. Indeed, it has been pointed out that the North and to a lesser extent the East were more linked to South India until the turn of the twentieth century when British Colonial rule united the country by destroying

---

[1]Janatha Vimukthi Peramuna (JVP)—Armed insurrection by Sinhalese youth from mainly the rural south against government in Colombo in 1971 and 1987–90.

the intervening forests and building railroads and roads. Thus before this century, at least for people in the North, journeying to India took perhaps a few hours or days across the narrow Palk straits, while traveling to Colombo took months. The Sinhalese language developed as distinct entity from the Pali influence of the Buddhist religion, Tamil and Sanskrit. Interestingly, with the advent of "globalization", even these parochial differentiating should take a new turn towards more common concerns and needs.

Colonial Rule. The colonial history started in early part of 15th century. In 1505 Portuguese landed in this island and progressively captured the coastal areas except central hill country. They gave the island the popular name, Zeylon or Ceylon. They banned other religious practice, both Hinduism and Buddhism, and converted the people (some say on the point of the sword) to Christian Catholicism. Most of the fishing community converted to Catholicism. In 1657, Dutch conquered parts of the western sea coast and gradually took over from the Portuguese. The Dutch version of Protestantism was implemented while the Catholic Church was persecuted. Education was crucial to the new policy of conversion for the children had to be indoctrinated to the faith from an early age. In the change over to Christianity, first under the Portuguese and then the Dutch, different Christian saints replaced the various presiding deities of the Hindu pantheon. Churches were built over destroyed local temples. Stone images of Christ and Virgin Mary replaced Hindu and Buddha statues. However, local cultural influences continued to influence local Christian practices and a rich blend resulted. Dutch introduced the Roman Dutch law to this country.

By 1795, the island came under the control of English East Indian Company following developments in Europe. Then in 1802, the British were ceded the Dutch possessions in the island at the Peace of Amiens. All the emerging European powers after the industrial revolution, renaissance and reformation strove for expansion for economic and religious benefit. Later in 1815, British captured the central hill country, which was ruled by the Tamil Nayakar, King Rajasingan. The British established highways, railways, tea and rubber estates in this country. They had brought by a perilous land route, South Indian Tamils to work on tea and rubber estates on the central hills. Although suppressed socio-economically and politically, they have been the backbone for the Sri Lankan economy since then. As a by product of the colonial rule, education was introduced gradually to an ever widening group. Many, particularly the Tamils, found education a valuable avenue for social advancement and personal development. Lower castes and women were able to break out of their traditional state of bondage.

Independence. After independence was given ("on a silver platter" as the saying goes as there was no national struggle as in India) in 1948, the "estate" Tamils were made non-citizens by a series of parliamentary acts, voted for even by "Ceylon" Tamils. The creation of the new country, Ceylon, and the subsequent separation (by restrictions on travel, trade etc.) from Tamil Nadu (areas) in India, starting with the Portuguese, created a new Tamil identity within Ceylon. However, Tamil Nadu politics continued to influence local Tamil politics.

Though at Independence Ceylon started on a strong economic footing with a strong sterling balance, a thriving plantation economy and relatively contended population, increased population growth, welfare spending and poor economic development forced the Ceylon government to face the problems of unemployment. But under the majoritarian "democratic parliamentary system", the politicians manipulated the population for capturing votes in elections rather than work for economic stability. Thus it was the common ploy for politicians to woo the majority Sinhalese by whipping up communal emotions.

Anti-Tamil Politics. The communal politics began with state sponsored Sinhala settlements in the East and the passage of the Sinhala Only act in 1956. It was to later develop into discrimination in education opportunities and favoring employment for the Sinhalese. The elections of 1956 is said to have been a watershed in the emergence of Sinhala Buddhist control of the state.

The first organized violence against Tamils occurred in 1956 at Galoya. In 1958 communal riots against Tamils (Vitacchi, 1958) in the South made them flee as refugees to their homeland in the North and East. In the middle of the 1960's, economic instability and Malaria were the main problems in the country. The Cuban revolution inspired the youths in Sri Lanka towards a Red revolution. In 1970, following the short lived JVP insurgency, thousands of Sinhala youth were murdered after torture.

Ceylon became a Republic (breaking their last link to Colonial Britain) in 1972 as Sri Lanka. University admission for Tamils was restricted by the educational standardization passed in the Parliament. This created frustration for Tamils youth who then turned to fighting for freedom. In early part of 70's the Tamil Liberation movement started. A World Tamil Conference was held in Jaffna in 1974, during which Sri Lankan Police shot seven participants to death. In an election platform of 1976, the TULF put the motto "Tamil Elam" wanting a separate state and won the election in 1977 in the Tamil areas.[2] The second communal riots against Tamils occurred after the elections in 1977. Tamils who lived outside the North and East were again made refugees.

Ethnic War. The massive 1983 ethnic riots (Piyadasa, 1984) against the Tamils created a collective resolve in Tamil youth to turn to violent action. By

---

[2] The last real 'free' election in Tamil areas. All subsequent elections were under States of Emergency, held amidst the war, violence and gross malpractice.

the mid 80's, more than 500,000 Tamils had fled abroad, mainly to India, as refugees. The sympathy of Tamil Nadu for Tamils created an opening for interference in Sri Lankan politics. India trained a variety of Tamil militant movements to fight against Sri Lankan forces, while diplomatically pressurizing the Sri Lankan state to find a political solution. The political expectation of the Tamil militant movements was towards independence and separation as had happened in Bangladesh. In the violent struggle that ensued, competition among the different Tamil militants resulted in internecine fratricide from 1985.

Sri Lankan forces were gradually restricted to their camps by Jaffna in 1985. In 1987 Sri Lankan forces captured Vadamarachi and arrested young boys aged from 15 to 35 years. Some of them were shot to death. Others were chained and put in the cargo ship and sent to prison in Boosa. The first LTTE suicidal cadres demolished a military camp in July 1987 by driving a vehicle loaded with explosives. It became a saying in the militants that *"It is better to sacrifice the life to revenge the enemy rather than be captured to be tortured and be killed and burned and buried"*. Later a suicidal squad, the "Black tigers", was established in the LTTE. It became a very terrifying dimension of the war—a powerful live weapon of counter terror.

Under the Indo-Sri Lanka peace accord in 1987, an Indian Peace Keeping Force (IPKF) came to implement the accord. The LTTE resisted the Indian approach. One LTTE cadre in protest, fasted to death even without taking water. Later a group of LTTE cadres committed suicide after having been detained by the Sri Lankan forces despite the cease fire and the IPKF presence. It aroused violent emotions and reaction. IPKF started their military operations against the LTTE from October 1987. Artillery shells rained down in Jaffna day and night. Tanks were also used. Indian troops were unable to differentiate between the LTTE and the public and lashed out indiscriminately. People were totally unprepared. In one telling incident on the traditional Theepavali day, the IPKF entered the Jaffna Hospital and proceeded to massacre over 60 patients and staff despite the absence of militant presence. The Indian Government was never made to answer for the war atrocities against the people. The LTTE gradually frustrated the Indian efforts by continuous guerilla attacks. IPKF left the country in early 1990 following persistent demands from the new President, Premadasa who had developed an understanding with the LTTE. The truce between the Sri Lanka State and the LTTE broke down and another phase of the war, so called Elam war II, commenced.

In June 1990, battle for the old historic Dutch Fort began in earnest at Jaffna. A garrison of more than 200 Sri Lankan police and Army personnel were surrounded by the LTTE. Sri Lankan government used a variety of bombers and helicopters to counter act. Aircrafts began to pound Jaffna city mercilessly and the densely populated urban area was evacuated. General Hospital, Jaffna also moved out of the city to Manipay where it was subsequently bombed.

A fragile peace came with the elections in 1994. But the Elam war (III) re-started in 1995 and is still continuing. There was a massive exodus of people from Jaffna in October 1995. In 1996 people resettled back in their own places except for those areas in the high security zone. The peak of arrests and disappearance, over 600, occurred in the later months of 1996. It is now being brought to light by the mass graveyards at Chemmani. Again, in April–May, 2000, over 100,000 people were displaced from the Thenmarachi area as fresh fighting broke out. The LTTE captured the massive military camp with the old Dutch fort at Elephant Pass, strategically located at the isthmus to the Jaffna peninsula. The fighting became highly technological with massive firepower that used artillery, shells, missiles, multi-barrel rocket launchers, jet fighters, helicopter gunships, fast attack sea crafts etc. The protagonists started trading shells from a distance instead of bullets with greater destruction, death and trauma for the civilians. The experience was mind shattering.

Economic Cost of War. The pre-occupation with an ethnic conflict, the soaring expenditure and ravages of war were to ruin the country's economy. The increasing militarization of the whole country has seen a soaring defense budget expenditure which has now officially reached over 44 billion rupees (US$754 million), more than on health and education combined, accounting for 22 percent of government spending. The total cost of the war has been estimated at Rs. 1443 billion (Marga, 2001). But this may be only the 'official' tip of an iceberg of what is actually spent. Other funds, votes and resources, for example foreign aid and loans for development and rehabilitation, have been increasingly unofficially diverted towards military objectives.[3] The extensive colonization schemes in the North and East have not only been completely state–funded Sinhala settlements, but also created the infrastructure to service them. Rehabilitation funds and material also have found their way into the military effort or have favored an ethnic group. However, at the same time, the ethnic war brought all economic development in the North and East to a complete halt. More, it has led to the utter devastation of the land, buildings, institutions, resources and property; contamination with landmines and large-scale displacements that makes the North and East look today like ancient ruins of some long lost civilization. The contrast with the South, where modern developments have kept pace with the rest of the world, for example in technology, communications, mass media, electronics and consumerism, is striking. The North and East have gone backward to candle light, bicycles and the bullock cart. The war also has given the state the opportunity to push ahead with its colonization schemes with extra vigor and protect it with the army as well. The peace dividend, if and when it comes, will be very

---

[3]Thus the whole Accelerated Mahaveli Programme, especially the "L" scheme—where the once Tamil *Manal aru* was turned into the Sinhalese *Weli Oya* through state sponsored settlements (UTHR-J, 1994), are part of the state's overall military strategy and heavily funded covertly through foreign governments and agencies.

high indeed particularly for the civilians caught up in the conflict areas. But, then the vested interests in the ongoing conflict, political, military, economical as well as psychological (the kind of extreme ethnocentrism that makes ethnic wars possible) will have to be reversed.

SOCIAL-PSYCHOLOGICAL PROCESSES THAT LED TO CIVIL VIOLENCE

Decline of the Welfare State

The early social statistics of Ceylon show that under its expensive (35% of budget) welfare programs, its citizens had attained a high standard of health and enjoyed a good quality of life, education and democratic freedoms. However over the years, the parameters of social ill health have shown a marked increase: poverty, unemployment, suicide rate, homicide rate, and more recently, extra-judicial killings, violence, arrests, detentions, and "disappearances". Thus Sri Lanka, for a low-income country, has one of the highest literacy rates (90%), long expectancy of life (72 years), and one of the lowest infant and maternal mortality rates. But at the same time, a quarter to half (depending on the definition of poverty) of the population is below the poverty line and the poor have become poorer. From the time these figures have been available, Sri Lanka has had a remarkably high suicide and homicide rate (WHO, 1986). For example in 1968, an average year that was uneventful and 'calm', she had the highest reported suicide rate of 17.2 per 100,000 and the fourth highest homicide rate (2.2) in Asia (WHO, 1986). These figures have been steadily increasing to 47 per 100,000, now the highest suicide rate in the world, being most marked in 15 to 24 years age group (Kadiragamar, 1996). Today, the country is second only to Iraq in the number of "disappearances". Thus more than anything else, the high rates of homicide, suicide and poverty, belied the appearance of prosperity and calm of this 'island paradise' and indicated a smoldering and festering socio-economic problem within, which was to be displaced onto a convenient scapegoat, the Tamils.

Religious and Cultural Mechanisms in Violence

Buddhist Paradox. Uyangoda (1988) states the current problem facing Buddhism (as well as the other religions practiced on this island) very succinctly:

> The ethnic war in recent years has indeed produced a deep crisis in the Theravada Buddhist culture in Sri Lanka. To put this crisis in rather crude terms, violence and death, in its most cold blooded form has engulfed a land where the teachings of the compassionate Buddha are supposed to guide the individual as well as social life. Has contemporary Sri Lankan Buddhism seriously addressed itself to this cruel and unfortunate paradox?

Thus there appears to be a fundamental contradiction in what we see happening in Sri Lanka. Though Buddhism preaches non-violence, widespread manifestations of the cruelest violence is in evidence (Palihawadana, 1983). Similar developments were seen in another Theravada Buddhist country, Cambodia but not in Thailand. In Sri Lanka, the Buddhist monks have always played an active if not decisive role in politics, earning the term, *'militant Buddhism'* (Thambiah, 1992). In Vietnam, Buddhist monks used to play an active role but in more non-violent ways. In Tibet, under the Dalai Lama, non-violent methods have held the forefront. When analyzed in this manner, though the 'militant' Buddhist monks in Sri Lanka have played an important role in politics, it cannot be traced to anything inherent in Buddhism itself. Similar violent developments have been manifested in other religions throughout the ages, including the Christian Crusades. In fact, the greatest tragedy that has befallen Sri Lanka is that despite her rich religious heritage was their failure to check the violent deterioration that happened. There was a singular lack of true spiritual men to guide and lead the people through this crisis.

Hindu Tamil Reaction. As for the Tamils, their main religion, Hinduism, also strongly advocates '*Ahimsa*' or non-violence. However considerable violence has been generated by the Tamils during this conflict. It has been standard rhetoric by Tamils that they first tried non-violent 'Gandhian' methods and then turned to violence only when that repeatedly failed. Initially the violence was a form of what Fromm (1973) described as *'defensive aggression'* against a threat to the Tamil community. Devaluation of its language meant a threat to its identity; state sponsored colonisation was perceived as invasion of its territory, political discrimination meant degradation to second class citizenship and socio-economic deprivation threatened its very survival. Recurrent mob violence against persons and property and increasing violent repression by the state provoked the youth to take up arms as a form of reactive aggression.

But with time, violence took a more virulent and malignant form. The malignant transformation was characterized by fanatic intolerance to any forms of opposition or difference of view, internecine fratricide, spate of political and extra-judicial killings, fascist and totalitarian rule. The malignant transformation also appeared in the massacre of men, women and children of the 'enemy'; in torture and killing of fellow Tamils (the infamous 'lamp posting'); and acting as mercenaries in foreign countries (e.g. Maldives). The primacy given to mechanical weapons more than life (such as cadres sacrificing their lives to save a weapon), glorification of the dead cadres (a martyr cult, elaborate public funerals and rituals, sacred burial sites, statues, posters, poems and writings, posthumous military ranks); suicide squads and the cyanide capsule; a preoccupation with death in the conscious, unconscious and dream material of the cadres; while at

Table 2. Malignant Transformation of Aggression

Factors	Description
Decrease of social cohesion	Modernization, westernization, migration, social change, impact of repeated violence and political suppression
Reduction in social control	Abdication of primary role by elders, Breakdown of social institutions (family, village, caste, religious)
Change of norms	Breakdown in ethical values and traditional beliefs
Politics	Marginalization of moderate politics and politicians while grudging, covert admiration for violent action by those in power
Mass media	Popularity of thriller videos and violent heroes, violence on TV and other popular media showing the success of violent methods
Militarization	Military logic, brutalization of the younger generation (through beatings, detention, torture, killings etc.), institutionalization of the violence against them etc.
Traumatophilia as an adverse coping strategy to deal with trauma	Addiction to violence in militants with malignant PTSD (see text)
Anomie	Gradual isolation and separation of the North East from the mainstream of development and modern progress.
Helplessness	A generation pushed into feeling helpless and powerless in the face of repeated mob violence against their ethnic group, brutal treatment by the authorities etc.
Hopelessness leading to suicide and homicide	Frustration of hopes and dreams through closing of avenues for advancement through blatant discrimination in education, employment, scholarships etc.

the same time, desecration of dead bodies of the enemy, and public exhibition of parts of their bodies amounted to almost a 'necrophilia'. The rapid change from defensive aggression to what Fromm (1973) called *'malignant aggression'* seems that one sort of violence rapidly deteriorates in to the other, at least in humans, under certain difficult life conditions and socio-cultural conditions (Staub, 1989). Thus the apparently non-violent Hindu religion too could not inhibit the expression of violence from within the Tamil Society (Table 2).

Caste. In fact, one of the strongly imbedded institutions within the Hindu socio-cultural system, that of caste, has been responsible for considerable covert violence throughout history. There had been some struggle by leftist organizations, trade unions and progressive artists in the 60's against the caste discrimination, for example the temple entry movement. The migration abroad for jobs such as to the Middle East creating a new class of *nouveaus riches*, had also added an economical impetus to the loosening of caste barriers as had modernization in general. But it was the current war that made considerable inroads into the caste system. During the mass displacements people could not observe the usual caste exclusions as people were thrown together in unexpected circumstances and many relationships across caste were stuck up. There were some rare exceptions, where even under the threat of death, people held onto caste distinctions such as refusing to stay in certain refugee camps with lower castes. In the various Tamil militant movements, castes become a non-issue, particularly in the leftist leaning movements. Thus with the progress of the war, caste has lost its tight hold on society, though it lingers on in for example, marriage arrangements. Whether it will come back once the war is over is difficult to say but in all probability it will not have the same stranglehold it once had.

Women. Similarly, Tamil society had always suppressed women into a subservient position. Modern education starting in the colonial period had loosened this to some extent and some women managed to get free. However, it was the war that has had a liberating role for women. Some males left seeking jobs and other opportunities abroad. It was also the males who initially joined the militants, were killed, migrated or left the area out of fear, seeking asylum in foreign countries for obvious reasons. For all these reasons the women were left behind to shoulder the responsibility of family, home and keep the society functioning during this critical period (Sivachandran, 1994). While men left their wives and children behind, women did not leave their children or husband to emigrate or flee the area (with the exceptions in cases of Middle East housemaid jobs).[4] They were left to face the trauma of war all alone. They looked after their families and generally 'kept the home fires burning' during this crisis in the Tamil society. As a result, women were forced to take a more leading role, thus freeing them to a large extent.

Some women have also been induced to join the militants. One factor inducing them to leave society was the tight control, domestic life and bleak future they faced. Joining the militants was a liberating act, promising them more freedom and power (Trawick, 1999). In some cases, the family actively encouraged their daughter(s) to join when their poor socio-economic state did not allow them to put by a good dowry for their daughters. The observed cruelty of the women fighters could be psychologically related to this loosening of social control and emancipation, a form of 'pathological liberation'.

Christianity and Islam. As for Christianity, members from both ethnic communities were Christians. The Christian church divided along ethnic lines. As Christianity straddled both ethnic groups, church leaders and the Christian community could have played a constructive role in bringing the two groups together. This was not to be as language and 'ethnicity' proved stronger

---

[4]This was more of a social problem in the South and East of Sri Lanka.

than religion. In contrast, Muslim religious leaders, and Mosques organizations, have played a more subdued, if not a constructive role, particularly in the East where they have tried to bring the communities together.

However, emotional and charismatic non-orthodox religious movements have been very popular during this time of war and traumatization. Apparently they have filled an important need during this time. Since the island boasts of such a rich resource of religions, it should be possible, as a method of reconciliation, to rekindle religious practices that encourage tolerance, non-violence, understanding and compassion.

Rather than to look to religion, we have to look to the socio-cultural, historical, economic and psychological context for the origins of the violence as discussed below.

Origins of the Conflict

The central factor in the ethnic conflict in Sri Lanka as in many parts of the world (the old USSR and Yugoslavia; India, Cyprus, Rwanda, N. Ireland and Spain) has to do with group identity or ethnic consciousness. When this identity and belonging is threatened, it strikes at the very core of the being, evoking anxiety and a deep sense of insecurity. Thus, it is no surprise that individuals and groups will react with considerable emotion and fight with a survival instinct as if their very group life was at stake. It was the assertion of the Sinhala–Buddhist identity of the majority, using the state machinery at the expense of the minorities, that led to the growing reaction to save the Tamil identity. The driving force behind the confrontation has been the two ethnic identities—Sinhala and Tamil.

Sinhala–Buddhist Identity. The emergence of the Sinhala–Buddhist identity was a gradual historical development, but took its current form only from the end of the last century (Gunawardena, 1990; Kumari Jayawardena, 1986). It started initially as a reaction to the proselytizing Christianity and Westernization which threatened the Buddhist identity of the Sinhalese.[5] Many of the Sinhalese Buddhist elite also became enamored with the European notions of race, believing themselves that Sinhalese were part of the Aryan race. This was owing to the work of some scholars like the well-known German Indiologist, Max Muller, who classified Sinhalese as an Aryan language (Gunawardene, 1994). However, at this time there was no conflict of interests between the Sinhalese and Tamil elite.

The popularization of the Sinhala–Buddhist identity took place through popular meetings, literature, mass media, political demagogue and anti-minority conflicts, against, in chronological development, Christians, Muslims, Indian

---

[5]This developed into a movement led by Anagarika Dharmapala and was later taken up by other aspiring Sinhala leaders.

Tamils, Malayalis and finally Sri Lankan Tamils. The construction of the Sinhala-Buddhist identity based on *'race, religion and language'* which is perceived to be threatened by the 'alien' Tamil 'invaders' from South India has had a profound influence on the Sinhalese people, spurring them to action, politically and violently against those that it was told threatened this historic identity. It was this appeal to the core identity of the Sinhalese by the upcoming parochial leaders that provided the driving force to unseat the English educated national elite in 1956, and made the majority governments undertake affirmative action to correct perceived 'historic' injustices to Sinhala Buddhism. These strong feelings were to grow into virulent Sinhala Buddhist chauvinism from 1956 and culminated in the 1983 race riots. Since that emotional outburst, there has been some realization and rethinking among the Sinhalese, though vestiges of extremist thinking linger in such organizations as the "*Veera Vithana*".

Tamil Identity. The Tamil identity developed mainly as a reaction to the increasing dominance of the Sinhala Buddhist identity (though there had been a short lived Hindu revival in the last century as a response to the Christian Missionaries). As successive Sinhala leaders rose to power by exploiting emotions relating to Sinhala–Buddhism and then proceeded to use the state machinery to enforce Sinhala as the only language (1956 Bill), enshrine Buddhism as the state religion (1972 constitution), discriminate in favor of the majority Sinhalese in education, employment, allocation of resources and land (state sponsored colonization schemes), and encourage periodic mob violence (1958,'77,'81,'83) against the minority Tamils, they in turn began to fear that their very identity, cultural existence as a separate and unique group was threatened.

Thus although the Tamil identity crystallized more in opposition to the threat from the state, yet it was not a *de nova* synthesis. Language was the vital element of the Tamil identity, with territory, a homeland in the North and East of Sri Lanka forming another aspect. The key role of language in the Tamil identity is shown by the fact it crossed religious, caste and territorial differences. Thus it was more important that one was a Tamil than if one was a Hindu, Christian or Muslim. They were treated this way by the Sinhalese and initially felt bonded by the ties to a common language. This was similar to developments in India where identities crystallized along language rather than other loyalties leading to lingual federalism. The Tamil language had an ancient heritage with a rich literature. In the later stages of the struggle, the Hill Country (Indian) Tamils and Muslims were forced to assert their unique cultural differentiation, as were other (territorial) groups, for example, Tamils from Batticaloa and Trincomalee, who resented dominance from Jaffna Tamils.

Identity Crisis in the Youth. It was the elder generation who first gave voice to the increasing insecurity felt by the Tamils, the reaction taking 'moderate' political form. The elders' arousing rhetoric of the principles of self-determination, autonomy, freedom, separation and the virtues of Tamil nationalism, fired up the idealistic youth but failed to achieve any positive results in the face of increasing violent persecution by the State. They were in time debunked from the leadership as too compromising, accommodative and submissive. It was left to the youth to redeem the Tamil identity and honour, to take up the mantle and meet the challenge for group survival with a violent defiance. It was the educated youth that felt most the closing of the doors to higher education and occupational opportunities. When in the 1983 riots Tamils as a group were humiliated, the youth took up arms to prevent a complete eclipse of the group's identity. That they did so in thousands with complete dedication, determination and resourcefulness is a mark of the deep threat that was felt at the core of their beings, a fear for their identity as a group.

The crucial role of the youth in the Tamil 'identity crisis' and the subsequent ethnic war can be understood from a study of the psychology of identity formation (Erikson, 1968). The phenomenal success of the dominant Tamil militant group, the LTTE, to win the continuing support of a segment of the population and attract a large number of dedicated youth into their ranks has been their ability to identity themselves with the Tamil socio-cultural identity and represent Tamil nationalistic fears, suspicion and aspirations at its deepest and fundamental level. Thus the LTTE became the ideal, the alter-ego, acting out the inner longings, wishes and paranoia of the Tamils.

Racial Myth. There is no scientific evidence that Sinhalese and Tamils of Sri Lanka belong to different races (the mythical Aryan/Dravidian split). Historically it would appear that both started from the same stock of autochthonous *Veddas* and after centuries of intermarriage with migrants from India, mainly South India, the Sinhalese and Tamils share the same genetic pool. Indeed some of the elements of identity have a mixed origin. Most Tamils were Buddhist in early history and many of the Sinhalese nobility were Tamils, while Tamil was their court language. Considerable assimilation of South Indian migrant groups into the Sinhalese society, has also taken place over time and still continues (e.g. the fishing community in Negombo).[6]

Territoriality. In *The Territorial Imperative*, Ardrey (1967) attributes most of man's ills to his drive to conquer and maintain a geographical territory. The problem of territoriality is at the center of the Sinhala–Tamil ethnic conflict. The Sinhalese consider the whole of Sri Lanka as their home territory—*Sinhaladipa*, and hence have a right to colonize and settle in any part of it. They strongly feel that the other ethnic groups inhabiting the island are migrants whose home territory is

---

[6]Such as the Cinnamon growers, *Salagamas* and the Karawas.

elsewhere. The '*bhumaputira*' theory holds that they are the legitimate '*sons of the soil*' and have all rights procuring from it. The Tamils on the other hand also regard themselves as heirs to the land, a well demarcated but restricted area—the North and the East of the island and claim to have been living in their homeland from historic times. The separatist demand for a state of Tamil *Eelam* is based on this very concept of home territory. In fact one militant group, the EROS, also include the hill country—*Malainadu*—as part of the Tamil territory as it has been settled and developed by 'Indian' Tamils. There is further disagreement as to whether the North and East is to be merged and whether the Muslims have a right to a territory of their own. Even India's intervention can be seen as a defense of her 'geopolitical' territory—India now expanding her conceptual territory to include the whole of South Asia (Nehru, 1991).

This fundamental dispute over territoriality, evoking as it does the baser instincts and strong emotions of those concerned, is the crux of the ethnic conflict and can be taken to show that man is after all a territorial animal.

State sponsored colonization

A major area of ethnic conflict and one of outstanding grievances of the Tamils is the change in the demographic pattern of the Northeast by state sponsored Sinhalese colonization. The Tamils perceive the influx of Sinhalese as a threat to the integrity of their 'traditional homeland' where they want to retain their voting majority, control over their own affairs and cultural identity, if not at least the name of their villages. The dominant Sinhalese politics on the other hand does not recognize this claim to exclusive territoriality but looks upon the whole island as belonging to the Sinhalese (*Sinhaladipa*). However, it is important to note that almost half of the Tamil population actually lived outside the North and East, which they claim as their homeland. The Hill country Tamils comprises 15% of the population in the central zone. There has been considerable internal migration following periodic anti-Tamil violence from these areas to the North and East. In addition, there has been an exodus of Tamils to India and other countries since 1983, when the civil war broke out. The Tamil Diaspora to every part of the world (which started with the Sinhala-only policies of the state and periodic anti-Tamil violence beginning in 1956), the consequent brain drain on the home community, the adaptation and assimilation of the migrants to the host country and the asylum issues including repatriation are burning current problems.

Economical and Socio-political Factors

Essentially, Ceylon failed to diversify its economy and maintain a sustained balanced growth to keep pace with its rapidly increasing population. The population grew due to a high standard of health and soon outstripped the available natural resources and cultivable land. Consequently there was chronic unemployment (particularly among educated youth), landless disgruntled peasants, galloping inflation and increasing pauperization of the poor. The poor have actually grown poorer and the rich richer (NORAD, 1988). About 40–50% of the population is estimated to be below the absolute poverty line.

Due to the population explosion and the consequent lack of land and opportunities for educated youth, there has been a large scale migration of the population from the villages to the city, seeking employment, creating a politically volatile rootless lumpen proletariat in the city slums and ghettos. Patronage, nepotism, and corruption with *mudalalis*[7] and *goondas*[8] have largely characterized the working of the establishment (Thambiah, 1986). Close ties with the criminal underworld, as well as with sinister extra-judicial units have become routine for politicians holding high office.

The increasing differences between the poor and affluent, exposure to unattainable luxury goods and unrealistic expectations of prosperity, and unemployment, particularly among the educated youth, has generated considerable discontent, anger, hostility and aggression that have manifested in such social pathological indices as high suicide, homicide rates and the continuing youth unrest and violence, specially the JVP insurrection in the South.

Universal free education had been introduced in 1943. By the mid 50's with no corresponding economic development, there was strong competition for limited government jobs. Just as the ideological thrust of Sinhalese chauvinism was first turned against Muslims just before 1920, then against Indian workers occupying laborers' positions in government departments in the 30's, followed by a reaction against Christian influence, it was now increasingly turned against educated Ceylon Tamil white collar aspirants. Although the Sinhalese and Tamils were both led by the small English educated elite and their conflict of interests did not involve the peasant masses. But in order to mobilize electoral support, both found themselves raising communal slogans to get others, at least emotionally, involved.

Since 1956, with the establishment of the Sinhala Buddhist dominance, there has been growing discrimination against the Tamils in a bid at 'assertive action' to redress perceived imbalances. This has led to 'over determination' whereby the Sinhala majority now enjoys a gross advantage in university admissions particularly to the important fields of medicine, engineering and law, employment in the public and private sectors, recruitment into the armed forces and administrative posts. Due to minimal economic expenditure and development in Tamil areas (Committee for National Development, 1984; Manogaran, 1987), Tamils perceive themselves as a besieged minority who are being squeezed economically. This has in turn led to the 'separatist response' where

---

[7]Local bosses.
[8]Muscle-men, criminal elements, underworld.

Tamils demand the right to control or determine their own economic development and destiny.

Recruitment and Indoctrination of Child Soldiers

Sri Lanka has become well known as one of the areas around the world where children are being used for war. This includes the use of children for work by the army for odd jobs around the camp, in the so called home guards but more alarmingly as direct frontline soldiers by the LTTE. The LTTE has increasingly turned to children and females, as the older males are no longer joining. The older youths have matured enough to see through the propaganda to become disillusioned with the whole struggle. To a large extent, under the LTTE, recruitment has remained 'voluntary'. There was the horrendous period during the Indian Army intervention when the EPRLF[9] indulged in forced conscription of youth for their ill fated Tamil National Army. The terror of those days when youth hid in their homes or fled the region has left deep scars in the community as a whole.

Children because of their age, immaturity, curiosity and love for adventure still remain susceptible to 'Pipe Piper' enticement through various psychological methods. From public displays of war paraphernalia, funerals and posters of fallen heroes, speeches and video, particularly in school, cleverly drawing out feelings of patriotism, restrictions on leaving for the target age group by the LTTE and of course the actions of the Sri Lankan forces all have created a milieu where they are psychologically compelled to join. The UN Convention on the Rights of the Child (CRC) does speak of the Right of the child to make decisions however much adults may doubt their capacity to do so. More recently, the LTTE has introduced compulsive military type training for all eligible ages in areas under their control. Obviously this will instill a military thinking and lead to more joining, particularly when faced with the entry of the army. (As they have already been trained, capture by the army would mean detention.) When children are thus cynically manipulated to end up as cannon fodder in hopeless or suicidal missions and when we see the malignant traumatization in the survivors as the case histories presented elsewhere (Somasundaram, 1998) and below under Malignant PTSD show, there can be only strong advocacy for banning all recruitment of children.

However, it may not be enough to merely condemn the recruitment of children. One may have to address the wider socio-political and economical oppression that forces children to fight if we are to prevent their occurrence. Children in the North often have no other alternative. Those with money, influence and connections abroad have taken or sent their children out of the area. The

---

[9]Eelam People's Revolutionary Liberation Front, a leftist, Tamil militant group that has now joined the 'democratic' mainstream.

children who remain are faced with experiencing deaths or injury within the family, destruction of their homes, grinding poverty, deprivation of food, lack of opportunities for schooling or further education, unemployment, displacement, uncertainty about the future, insecurity and fear for their lives. Tamil youth are the ones specifically targeted by the security forces in their routine checking and search operations and detained for interrogation, detention, torture, execution or even rape. During the so called "*Operation Liberation*" in 1987, youth were either summarily shot or shipped off in chains to the Booza camp in the South by the army. Fifteen percent of the 600 disappearances in 1996 within Jaffna were children. In the recent Druaiappa Stadium and Mirusivil evacuations, remains of children were found. Thus it is no surprise that most of the young men tried to escape the 'Herodian' solution adopted by the Sri Lankan army to crush the militancy.[10] So when faced with the possible entry of the army, many youth will rather join than face, in their eyes, certain detention and death.

Many of the children now joining are from the lower socio-economical classes. Economical pressures within the family, lack of opportunities in the wider society drove many youth to join. Many families that are displaced, without incomes, jobs, or food may encourage one of their children to join so that at least they have something to eat. Education and schools have become disorganized in the north. Opportunities for further education, foreign scholarships or jobs have been progressively restricted by successive Sinhalese governments, despite the ethnic ratio rhetoric (Somasundaram, 1998).

The psychosocial rehabilitation of these child soldiers when they are captured or they surrender, when large scale demobilization takes place once peace is restored will need careful planning. Currently, child militants who are captured (a rare event as they are indoctrinated to bite their cyanide capsule to avoid capture) or who surrender are rehabilitated by the army. Their rehabilitation should not be in the hands of the military but come under civilian authority as has been recommended in all such rehabilitation programmes the world over (Jareg, 1999). This should include education, vocational training, psychosocial help (including psychotherapy for example for those with malignant PTSD), expressive creative opportunities, relaxation etc. However, currently they are viewed as 'criminal elements' who need to be re-educated to the right path. It should be understood that many of these youngsters took to militancy out of altruistic motivation to help their community, which was under threat. It is those responsible for the recruitment, training and deployment of child soldiers who should be charged as war criminals. If the process of reconciliation and reintegration back into society is to succeed, the young ex-militants should be given recognition for

---

[10]It may be no coincidence that there were reports that Israaeli Secret Service agents working from the US embassy special interest section played a central role in the planning and execution of the *Operation Liberation* as advisors to the security forces.

their sacrifice and treated with due respect. Any peace settlement should give priority to the process of demobilization. Specific arrangements should be made for the rehabilitation and reintegration of ex-militants and soldiers. Opportunity structures in the form of jobs, positions and function in society commensurate with their previous roles is needed. They should be given the opportunity to put to use for the benefit of society the motivation and ideals that made them join the fighting in the first place.

DISPLACEMENT

External Displacement (Refugees)

The world-wide refugee crisis has reached enormous proportions (see chapter 1). A significant contributor to the international refugee population is the Tamil Diaspora. Starting in the wake of the 1958 race riots, the continuing Tamil exodus from the island is estimated to have removed more than 50% out of a total of 2,400,000 (Department of Census and Statistics, 1995) from their homes. The early migrants were well educated—contributing to the crippling brain drain—and have integrated well into their host country. The present waves of refugees starting from the 1983 ethnic holocaust have suffered a worse fate. About 225,000 were to leave the Island, seeking asylum in Europe, Canada, etc. They have had to face increasing restrictions and barriers and have been detained in camps or even forcefully repatriated. The problems faced by refugees seeking asylum abroad are compounded by having to first face unsympathetic and hostile authorities and later adapt to a new culture and integrate into a different society. Many Tamils abroad developed various types of mental disorders and some were forced to return.

Refuge in India. An estimated 150,000 were to escape to India, many making the risky journey across the Palk Straits in make-shift or fiber glass motor boats. Some never made it to Indian shores, being captured by the Sri Lanka Navy patrols or drowning when the overcrowded boats capsized. With the killing of Rajiv Gandhi, the attitude and the treatment by the Indian authorities became completely negative. Repatriation, with varying degrees of compulsion-*refoulement* (Ruiz, 1994) and resettlement, of the refugees back to Sri Lanka with UNHCR assistance was begun with the Indo-Lanka accord of 1987. A major concern expressed by local workers is the issue of safety for those being resettled. Often they face similar dangers that led to the initial displacement and have been frequently displaced repeatedly even after "official resettlement". At times the direct cause has been the state security forces. Those being sent back by western governments after they have been refused asylum there are usually arrested by the authorities on or shortly after arrival. Many have been released after questioning. However, refugees continue to cross the treacherous Palk Straits upto date. In more recent developments of the new millennium, due to the hostile attitude of the Indian authorities, the refugees are unloaded on sand bars off the Southern Coast of India where they have to wait several days to be picked up by sympathetic Indian fisherman or authorities. Several have died, collapsed or women abducted during this deadly vigil.

The Internally Displaced

There has also been the more tragic problem of the internally displaced (IDP) from one part of Sri Lanka to another, involving all three communities—Sinhala, Tamil and Muslim.

Displacement created deep psychosocial changes in Tamil society. The ties to home (*vidu*) and village (*uur*) are very deep and forms a prominent part of the Tamil identity (Daniel, 1984). When they finally abandoned their home and village, which had been part of their families for generations, they disrupted an organic tie that could not be repaired. Many developed a deep sense of guilt. Even when they returned they could not re-establish that close relationship. Further, many never returned to their homes after the 1995 exodus.

The accumulated stress of leaving their homes and usual habitat was accentuated by a complete disruption of normal life patterns, together with lack of food, rest, medical attention and a continuing atmosphere of fear and terror. The problems faced by the internally displaced refugees have been studied more systematically (Reppesgard, 1993; Somasundaram, 1998), which show considerable traumatization and the debilitating effect of indirect stresses like poverty, unemployment and lack of food. They manifested with somatization, depression (Reppesgard, 1993) and disturbance within the functioning of the family system (Jeyanthy, Loshani, & Sivarajini, 1993).

On the positive side, some adapted well to the stress of displacement and showed hidden strengths and leadership qualities. Particularly encouraging was that individuals, considered as troublemakers or administrative headaches during normal times, acted with heroism and initiative.

These IDP populations have become the forgotten symbols of war—uncared for and rejected by all, and a daunting challenge to post-war rehabilitation and resettlement.

EFFECTS ON SOCIETY

The war has had a tremendous impact. During the current war whole communities or villages have been targeted. One can mention the systemic attacks on all the Tamil villages in the Trincomalee District, which eventually displaced all of them into the city or to other districts. Another example is the Moslems of the

North, who were suddenly forced to leave *en masse* without their belongings. Apart from direct attacks, whole villages of all three communities have been disrupted, displaced and uprooted due to the ongoing conflict. One terrible example is the fishing community, another the farmers. From the beginning, for various security reasons, fishing in the North and East has been restricted. This has included ban on fishing from and in certain areas, restrictions on distance where fishing can be done (usually restricted to short distance offshore). Whole fishing communities have been displaced. Fisherman have also been at increased risk to death, disappearance, detention, and injury due to the nature of their work which takes them into the sea, a highly contested area in the war. As a result the highest number of widows are from this community. This has had a terrible toll on this community. Many have shifted to other occupations, some are still unemployed living off government rations, others have left the area. They have lost their way of life and culture. Many yearn for the days when they were able to fish freely and lead a fisherman life in their village. Before 1983, fishing was a very fruitful occupation, the catch was good off the long North East coast, and a considerable part of the fish was transported to Colombo and other areas in the Island. In the whole island the North East was a leading area for fishing. It has been a similar tale with farmers, many of whom have been displaced from their traditional lands, and have lost all their equipment. Some are unable to cultivate their land, as it is located in contested areas or are mined. Some have abandoned their traditional occupation as it no longer profitable, given unavailability or cost of agricultural inputs like fertilizers, insecticides, fuel or lack of access to markets for their product. Other traditional trades like carpenters, masons and so on have been affected similarly. The Muslims who were a very prosperous business community as well as specialized in other occupations like tailoring, tinkering, leather work and so on have lost their occupations and way of life due to displacement and other disturbances. The Sinhalese were well known bakers in the North and East, but have now all left.

In the various rural communities, the village and its people, way of life and environment provided organic roots, a sustaining support system, nourishing environment and network of relationships. The village traditions, structures and institutions were the foundations and framework for the their daily life. In the Tamil tradition, a person's identity was defined to a large extent by their village or *uur* of origin (Daniel, 1984). Their *uur* more or less placed the person in a particular matrix. All this has been destroyed by the war. Some villages have ceased to exist. Due to displacement people have been separated so that the network of relationships, structures and institutions have been lost. Kai Erikson (1976) described it as a "loss of communality". Even when people have returned to their villages, as it has happened in Jaffna in 1996, the village was not the same. Many were complete newcomers. The old structures and institutions were no longer functioning. Thus the protective environment provided by the *uur* is no longer there.

Collective Trauma

Another phenomena, given the widespread nature of the traumatization due to war, has been that psychosocial reactions have come to be accepted as a normal part of life. Indeed, it would be more appropriate to talk of collective trauma (Somasundaram, 1996) or cultural bereavement (Eisenbruch, 1991). This normalization can be seen in the prevailing cultural coping strategies. Some coping strategies that may have had survival value during intense conflict may become maladaptive during reconstruction and peace. For example the Tamil community had learned to be silent, non involved and stay in the background. They have developed a deep suspicion and mistrust. People learned to simply attend to their immediate needs and survive to the next day. Any involvement or participation carried considerable risk, particularly at the frequent changes of those in power. At these shifts in power, recriminations, false accusations and revenge were very common. For example, as happened in 1987, 1990, 1996 and is feared will happen again if the LTTE takes over. Those with leadership qualities, those willing to challenge and argue, the intellectuals, the dissenters and those with social motivation have been weeded out. They have either been intimidated into leaving, killed or made to fall silent. Gradually people have been made very passive and submissive. The repeated displacement, disruption of livelihood have made people dependent on handouts. People have lost their motivation for advancement, progress or betterment. They have developed dependence on help from outside sources, on relief, losing their old self-reliance. Further they have lost their trust in their fellow human beings as well as the world order. The signs of collective trauma can be seen in all social institutions, structures and organizations in present day Jaffna. There is a general *ennui*. Most have left their houses and property in disrepair, not taking the effort to start repairs. In offices and organization the work output had declined considerably. Once the work ethic had dominated this hard working society. Most are now not inclined to work, merely sign their names in the work register and take the day off at a slightest excuse. More effort and interest is spent on obtaining relief items, rations, incentive payments, risk allowances and such like. There is a crisis of leadership. No one comes forward to take leadership positions like chairmanship, presidency and director. Most positions go by default. There is a complete lack of quality in all aspects of society, partly due to crippling brain drain, but also the devastating effect of the war. There is a marked deterioration in social values as shown by sexual mores (for example in the refugee camps in Vavuniya and in general society, medical personnel report increased unwanted pregnancies, teenage abortions and child sexual abuse) and social ethics (robberies of the houses and property of those displaced is now claimed as a right).

Some new community organizations have emerged in some areas for widows, the disappeared and so on. Particularly noteworthy is leadership of women in many of these grass-root organizations. Several NGO's have worked to create such community organizations. Some new religious movements, particularly the charismatic, emotive ones, have proven popular. Evidently there is a need felt in the community for them at this time. They are able to provide emotional support, fellowship, leadership and meaning to events.

The impact of the war on the macro, meso and micro levels of society can be studied. Wealth status ranking of the community was done by the Participant Rural Appraisal (PRA) technique (Goodhand, Lewer, & Hume, 1999). People gave the top wealth status ranking to those who obtain income from abroad, mainly from relations. The lowest rank was given to those who lost their earning members due to the war. The recruits for the war on both sides have come from the rural poor. Apparently joining has improved the socio-economic status of their families (Marga, 2001).

Effects on Civilians

War can have devastating effects not only on individuals (Somasundaram, 1998), but also on their family, extended family, group, community, village and wider society. The following section will summarize data from a series of studies on the psychosocial and medical effects on the traumatized populations. As a way of understanding the characteristics of help seeking behaviour who may need special attention, the results from the community survey (Somasundaram & Sivayokan, 1994) are compared to finding in those seeking treatment at Out Patient Departments (OPD) (Somasundaram, 2001).

While Table 3 shows the exposure of the population to a wide variety of stresses, Figure 1 shows the psychosocial effects.

Figure 1 shows that among the general population and OPD attendees, somatization ranks as the most common manifestation in both groups (88% and 42% respectively) and PTSD, anxiety and depression also rank high.

Somatization was defined as more than five somatic complaints without organic cause due to war stress while other problems included functional disability, social withdrawal, and change in religious beliefs. The above mentioned studies found a strong relationship between the stress score and the somatization score. Thus the somatic complaints of the patients are directly proportional to the impact of the stress they have been exposed to. Similarly the correlation between the stress score and psychosocial sequelae was significant.

General Hospital Attendees (OPD)

As can be expected, those affected don't seek help for their psychological traumatization per se but were going to general hospital Out Patient Departments (OPD's), GP's and the traditional healers with somatic complaints

Table 3. Distribution of War Stress in the Community

Stress factors	Community (%) (n = 98)	OPD (%) (n = 65)
Direct stress		
Death of friend/relation	50	46
Loss to property	46	55
Injury to friend/relation	39	48
Experience of bombing/shelling/gunfire	37	29
Witness violence	26	36
Detention	15	26
Injury to body	10	9
Assault	10	23
Torture	1	8
Indirect stress		
Economic difficulties	78	85
Displacement[a]	70	69
Lack of food	56	68
Unemployment	45	55
Ill health[b]	14	29

[a] Before the 1995 mass displacement when the figure would have reached almost 100%.
[b] Ill health due to war related injuries including amputations due to landmine blasts, epidemics like malaria, reduced resistance to infections (due to stress and malnutrition), septicemia due to lack of drugs etc. had debilitating mental effect.

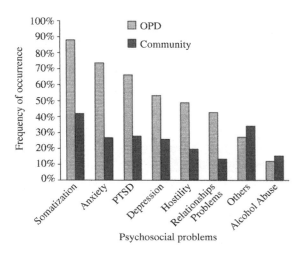

Figure 1. Psychosocial and psychiatric problems in the OPD compared to the community.

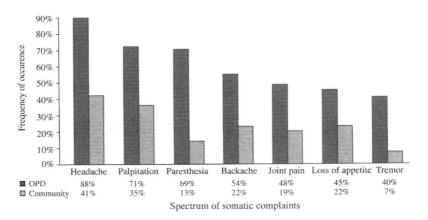

Figure 2. Common somatic complaints without organic cause in OPD patients, compared to the community.

(Somasundaram, 2001). For example, in the Out-Patients Departments (OPD) of a general and district hospital in Jaffna we found a high prevalence of psychological problems presenting as somatization as shown in Figure 2.

The level of traumatization (as shown in Table 3) and symptom formation was higher among OPD patients than in the general population (Figures 1 and 2). This has several explanations. First, patients with psychological problems tend to attend the OPD on their own initiative or they are referred to the OPD by primary care workers. A second explanation is that they may seek help for their psychological problems in the health sector. The mean stress score for the OPD attendees (41.4) was significantly higher than in the general population (36.2).

Figure 2 also shows that the spectrum of somatic complaints among the OPD patients reflects the spectrum of somatic complaints in the community, but the OPD patients suffer from it more often. As such they are seeking relief at the OPD. However, due to the predominant physical complaints they often receive inappropriate physical treatment in the form of somatic drugs. Their real underlying psychosocial problems, in this case the war traumatization, manifesting as somatic complaints, thus go undetected and untreated. More awareness and training of the medical staff at the OPD's and other health outlets in recognizing somatization, looking for the underlying causes, and then treating them appropriately with simple mental health measures will go a long way in offering relief to this large number of help seekers.

Effects on Women

In Northern Sri Lanka the male to female ratio for admission remained close to 1:1 from before the war upto 1986. In low-income countries of Asia and

Africa a preponderance of males in the ratio of 1:2 (female to male) is usual (Ihezue, 1986) while the reverse is true of developed countries (Shepard, Brown, Cooper, & Kalton, 1966). The higher number of females may reflect the sex ratio of the resident population due to the absence of young males in the age group where mental illness is common (70% of the mentally ill are form the 20–44 year group). Some in this age group left seeking jobs and other opportunities abroad. It was also this age group that joined the militants, were killed, or left the area out of fear, seeking asylum in foreign countries. It is also noteworthy that it was the same age group that swelled the ranks of the militants; a vicious cycle where the increasing repressive policies aimed at this age group forced them to join the militants or flee abroad.

For all these reasons the women were left behind to shoulder the responsibility of family, home, filling in for the absent male in what had been up to then, traditional male roles. They rode bicycles in greater numbers, went to the shops, met and argued with authorities, took their children to schools and temples, and generally kept the homes functioning during this crisis in the Tamil society. They were thus under considerable stress and more vulnerable to breakdown. The sex ratio of admission tilted even further towards female preponderance as the war continued, due to accentuation of this process (for example by 1991 the ratio of female to male was 1.2:1). In the final analysis this may have been the price women had to pay to save the Tamil society from collapse.

Effects on Children

The trauma of war appears to have caused considerable problems in the children of the north and by the 90's we found an increasing number coming for treatment. For example, children (up to 18 years) formed 12.6% of 1st visits at the outpatient psychiatric clinic at the G.H Jaffna and 8% of admissions at D.H Tellipallai in 1994. Studies of the student population shows that this is just the tip of the iceberg and psychological problems are widely prevalent in the schools up to and including the University (Somasundaram, 1998). It is significant that the Health Reach Program at McMaster University (Perera, 1996) did a detailed study of children in the Eastern Province of Sri Lanka, in addition to their studies in Yugoslavia, Palestine and Iraq, and found considerable more war trauma and psychological problems in Tamil (including Muslim) children compared to Sinhalese children.

Two small studies were carried out on 3–6 year olds in the Jaffna Peninsula. One was an in-depth one year observational study of 76 children in the Kokuvil and Kondavil area (just north of Jaffna town) identified as having been exposed to war trauma, out of whom 18 were 3–6 years old (Lakshman & Sivashankar, 1994). In the second, randomly selected 50 pre-school children studying in Montessories in the Vaddukoddai cluster area were studied (Rasiah & Nadarajah, 1994). Common disturbances reported by parents and teachers are shown in Table 4.

Table 4. Common Symptoms in Pre-school Children (n = 68)

Symptoms	Percentages
Refusal to sleep alone	71
Irritability	63
Sleep disturbances	48
Crying	39
Temper tantrum	35
Withdrawal from play	34
Disturbed at sounds resembling gunshots	30
Hyperalertness	30
Listlessness	29
Phobia for army or uniformed personnel	22
Aggression	21
Sadness	20
Symptoms of PTSD	11

Table 5. Common Symptoms in School Children (n = 305)

Symptoms	Percentages
Sleep disturbance	77
Irritability	73
War vocabulary	64
Decline in school performance	60
War games	54
Hyperalertness	50
Aggressiveness	46
Clinging	45
Anti-social behaviour	44
Sadness	43
Separation anxiety	40
Cruelty	30
Withdrawal	25

An extensive study of the Vaddukoddai cluster schools in conjunction with the Department of Education showed wide prevalence of traumatization among students (43%) and a wide variety of behavioral disturbances reported by parents and teachers (Arunakirinathan, Sasikanthan, Sivashankar & Somasundaram, 1993). A salient finding was the pervasiveness of indirect stresses such as poverty and displacement. A more detailed description is given elsewhere (Somasundaram, 1993). A summary of the commoner symptoms is given in Table 5.

The symptoms of hostility such as anger, aggressiveness, cruelty, antisocial behavior, pervasiveness of war vocabulary and games indicative of brutalization in the war milieu are very disturbing recent developments. Thus school aged children who were born and grow up in a war milieu show the pervasive effects in their emotions, cognition and behavior.

Adolescence

Adolescence is a critical period of transition to adulthood when childhood developmental stages and identity formation comes to a climax. We have now several studies of youth in Jaffna (Geevathasan, Somasundaram & Parameswaran, 1993; Arunakirnathan et al., 1993) and Killinochchi Districts (Somasundaram, 1998), while a study of the new entrants to the Jaffna University has been completed in the faculty of agriculture (Somasundaram, 1998). Common types of war stresses experienced by youth are shown in Table 6.

The great majority of students had experienced multiple stressors. Many stressors were chronic. The psychosocial sequelae found in adolescent students assessed with the help of the Stress Impact Questionnaire (SIQ) is given in Figure 3.

DESNOS

The psychological consequences for children and youth who had become militants were severe. In those that came for treatment, we found that they had joined the movement when very young and been exposed to massive trauma where they have witnessed gruesome deaths and mutilating injuries to many of

Table 6. War Stress in Adolescents in Rank Order (n = 613)

	Frequency
Direct war stress	
War death of relation	195 (32%)
Witnessing violence	156 (25%)
Threat to life	154 (25%)
Injury	45 (7%)
Detention	39 (6%)
Torture	23 (4%)
Indirect stress	
Displacement	241 (39%)
Economic problems	208 (33%)
Lack of food	92 (15%)

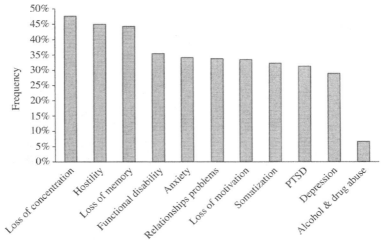

Figure 3. Psychosocial problems in adolescents (n = 625).

their comrades or had themselves been badly injured. They had frequently been involved in atrocities, having been responsible for many cruel deaths and torture. They present with very disturbed, aggressive outbursts when they re-experience traumatic events. Death scenes and battles repeatedly overwhelm them in the form of flashbacks and vivid hallucinations. During these periods they completely lose control over themselves becoming very violent and destructive.

The condition of addiction to violence or *Malignant PTSD* was first described by Rosenbeck (1985), where the US Vietnam war veterans come to feel most alive when they are in a situation of intense conflict or potential danger, and feel bored or depressed in the absence of such a situation. Many were anxious or paranoid in crowds or public places and could get irritated or argumentative in such situations. More recently, something similar was considered for inclusion in the DSM IV as Disorders of Extreme Stress not Otherwise Specified (DESNOS), characterized by alterations in regulating affective arousal with difficulty in modulating anger, self-destructive and suicidal behaviour and impulsive and risk-taking behaviour. In addition, chronic characterological changes with alterations in self-perception: chronic guilt and shame; feelings of self-blame, or ineffectiveness, and of being permanently damaged, a tendency to victimize others and alterations in systems of meaning such as despair and hopelessness or loss of previously sustaining beliefs has been described (de Jong, 1997). The ICD-10 of WHO (1992) also includes permanent hostility and distrust. Whether these are similar conditions manifesting differently in different cultures will need more research.

We observe that children, specifically adolescents, are particularly vulnerable during their impressionable formative period, causing permanent scarring of their developing personality. Military leaders have expressed their preference for younger child recruits as "they are less likely to question orders from adults and are more likely to be fearless, as they do not appreciate the dangers they face" (AI, 1998). Their size and agility makes them ideal for hazardous assignments. Their immaturity makes them more open to manipulation and indoctrination. However this is the pathodynamics, their personality being plastic is easily formed in a malignant direction that is difficult or impossible to reverse.

Case History 1. A youth was admitted with aggressive behaviour and suicidal ideas to District Hospital, Tellipallai. He had a depressive mood and talked to himself. His sleep was disturbed. He was irritable, with hostility, aggressiveness and given to outbursts of violence.

He had joined a militant group when he was 14 years old. While in action a shell had fallen and exploded close to him. A friend of his was injured in the posterior aspect of neck and bled. His friend cried "Iyo" and had fallen down. He was unconscious with deep breathing. He was taken to Teaching Hospital Jaffna. Two days later his friend died. He never went to see his friend. It was a terrifying experience for him.

He left for the Vanni and there he had loved a girl. Later he traveled to Vavuniya where he was arrested by the Army and assaulted and handed over to the Police. He had been tortured in the "Joseph Camp" after being blindfolded. Then he was sent to Bandarawala Rehabilitation Camp, later he was transferred to Tellipalai Rehabilitation camp. He used to smoke 'Beedi'.... The camp supervisors, also ex-militants, did not like this habit. They complained to the military officer. They had punished him by assaulting him and forced him to chew the Beedi and swallow it. After that he had become aggressive and violent.

He used to sleep after lunch, but the supervisors poured water over him. He had an affair with a girl close to the camp, and later was punished by the officer. Then his self care deteriorated. So the supervisors forced him to bath and remove the dirt by rubbing coconut coir until he got abrasions. He developed attacks of aggressive behavior and tried to assault others often. So they brought him to the hospital.

After admission he developed a good rapport with the counsellor who showed a good empathy. With the "sandbag technique" (where the client is asked to take out his anger by hitting a sandbag that is hung from the ceiling) he named two officers, A&B, who had assaulted and beaten him with a broomstick while using vituperative language. He shouted, "Hai A you see, son of bloody bitch.... I will destroy you". He cried and beat the sand bag. Then he said that all was finished. Then he turned to B. Then he said take them to Hospital by Ambulance. "Later we will see him". He had later beaten the sandbag with a broomstick until it broke. Later he was very thirsty and drank a lot of water. Then he said not to tell anybody this story.

At the same time he was treated with anti-depressant medication, relaxation exercises, art therapy and occupational therapy. He made a dramatic recovery from the state he was in when he came and was eventually sent home from the camp.

Case History 2. A 36 year old average built man was admitted to District Hospital, Tellipallai with complaints of loss of sleep and loss of appetite of one year duration. He had been conversing with the goddess Amman for the past 2 days. He was afraid of army personnel and got terrified when dogs start barking. He also complained of heaviness of the head. He was anxious to build a temple for Lord Kannan.

He was from a Sinhala Buddhist family from Kandy. Later, his father, a navy officer at Trincomalee, married another Tamil girl. He was taken by his father to Trincomalee. He studied upto grade 7 at the local Sinhala Maha Vidyalaya. As he was made to work hard at home he gradually developed an aversion for his family. He left the home and stayed with a Christian family as a domestic servant. Later he left them also and stayed with another family where he built a small shrine for worship. At the age of 11 he went to Batticaloa. He met and lived with a Hindu Guru who had trained him in the art of charming, sorcery etc. like locking the jaw of dogs leading to its death, give life to a still born foetus and directing it to cause the death of others, exorcism, and telling the past, present and future events. He then used this skill to earn his livelihood. He arrived in Jaffna when he was 22 years of age. He promptly used his skills with a still born foetus to kill others.

He joined the LTTE in 1991 and fought in the epic Elephant pass battle. He was buried in a bunker after an air raid and had to be dug out. He had an injury in his head and had lost consciousness. Many of his colleagues had been killed or injured in a gruesome way on the days before and during this incident. After recovery from the head injury, he had developed behavioural disturbances such as sleep disturbances, aggressive outbursts and suicidal ideas. He was admitted to the Psychiatric unit and was found to have frequent re-experiencing of the incident where he was injured and the events that preceded it where his colleagues had died. He experienced frequent intrusive memories of the event. At times he could hear his colleagues crying out in agony. At other times he heard the army talking. He was very aggressive and given to violent outbursts where he assaulted anyone around, including the ward staff. He would drive his fist through the window pane. It was difficult to control him at these times. Only other militants were able to hold him down. None of the strong tranquillizers like Chlorpromazine or haloperidol in high doses had any effect on him. Carbamazepine too was tried with no benefit. He was given psychotherapy but was inaccessible during these outbursts. Art therapy, relaxation exercises, anti-depressants and the "sandbag" technique was tried on him. He gradually settled down.

He left during the 1995 exodus and later returned to Allaveddy where he settled down by marrying a hospital attendant and has a child. After his marriage he has continued his practice of regular puja to God Kannan, Anuman, Muthumar and Sudalaikuli. Before the puja he builds an imaginary barrier around himself. He says by this action he ties the God during the day time and unties him during the nights. In the process of worship he goes into a trance and performs "Karaagam" where he places a pot on his head and dances. He had danced on the edge of a sharp knife without injury. Sometimes he cuts his forearm and offered the blood to God. By these actions he is able to foretell the future, tell where something that is stolen is hidden, or create attraction between a male and female for marriage. He is very popular and sought after for his skills. One year back he had been arrested by the army and beaten. His face had been covered with a petrol drenched polythene bag. He was released after two weeks.

OBJECTIVES OF THE PUBLIC MENTAL HEALTH PROGRAMME

As outlined above, the psychosocial sequealae to the ongoing war have been immense (Somasundaram, 1998) and a program to start systematically addressing the increasing trauma was needed. The catchment area for this mental health programme is the Jaffna Peninsula. The number of Internally Displaced who have now returned to the Jaffna Peninsula total around 500,000. The number of clients who have come for psychosocial treatment to the psychiatric units at District Hospital Tellipallai and General (Teaching) Hospital, Jaffna are shown in Table 7.

A multidisciplinary team with Canadian support consisting of psychiatrist, medical officers, psychiatric nurses, counsellors, psychiatric social workers, occupational therapists, relaxation therapists, child therapists, family counsellors, alcohol counsellors, drama therapists and masseuse collaborate with the psychiatric unit to render treatment and support.

The mental health programme uses a public mental health approach in combination with psychosocial intervention strategies. Local community workers

Table 7. Treatment at the Psychiatric Unit, General Hospital, Jaffna and District Hospital, Tellipallai (1996–2000)

Mental Health services	1996	1997	1998	1999	2000
Total Clients	13,800	14,800	15,600	16,500	17,300
New Clients	800	1000	800	800	700
No of groups got treatments	15	23	40	70	88
No of family	20	25	28	50	110
The Needs					
Mental health problems	–	–	40%	42%	43%
Psychological problems	–	–	55%	56%	53%
Medical problems	–	–	5%	2%	4%

receive a basic theoretical and practical training regarding psychosocial issues. The mental health programme trains a target group of people such as teachers, health-workers, healers and welfare workers to be able to help people in local communities to identify their emotional and social difficulties and to feel empowered to find their own solutions to these problems. Towards this end a manual, *Mental Health in the Tamil Community*, has been adapted from the TPO-Cambodia, *Community mental health in Cambodia*, which in turn was an adaptation of the WHO/UNHCR manual *"Mental Health of Refugees"*.

A community-based approach to address psychosocial problems was used, and the interventions were aimed to include:

- Training community health workers in identification and intervention for psychosocial problems, thereby
- Develop their knowledge and skills to use a variety of psychosocial interventions
- Develop practical structures in the community for promotion of psychosocial well-being, and
- Develop referral and treatment possibilities for those suffering from severe mental illness at the local hospital
- Identify and help the most vulnerable such as women, widows, children, the displaced and the poor.

Selection, Training and Supervision

Training of Specialized Staff and Trainers (TOT). Although initially, there was no formal training in trauma therapy for the few medical doctors and clinical psychologist working in the field, through sheer practical experience (and later updated by reading the relevant literature and additional training) they have become skilled trainers. Thus they have become quite capable trainers of the variety of trainees mentioned below.

The senior counselors who initially underwent training at Shantiam,[11] have now become trainers themselves. They were given theoretical lectures, demonstration and role plays exercises for 6 months. Then they practiced counselling under supervision and met for case supervision and discussion. At the end of one year they underwent an examination and were then certified as counsellors. This process is repeated each year for new batches of trainees.

---

[11] The Association for Health and Counselling (Shantiam) was started in Jaffna in 1988 by locally concerned individuals, particularly from the medical sector with the help of the Quaker Peace and Service to help those traumatized by the war. Shantiam has been training a batch of counsellors each year and running counselling services. There are outreach counselling through the hospitals and other centres.

Counselling supervision is done through weekly case conferences at General Hospital, Jaffna and Shantiam.

Training of Different Sectors. At the Primary Health Level all Medical Students, Nurses and Public Health Midwives (FHW or the Primary Health Worker) in Jaffna undergo teaching and training in basic mental health as shown in Table 8.

Two texts have been written in Tamil (Damian, 1994; Somasundaram, 1993). A module based on the UNICEF manual, *'Helping Children in Situations of Armed Conflict'* (Nikapota & Samarasinghe, 1995) has been used to train FHW's and other staff. The WHO has supported the adaptation and publication of the WHO/UNHCR book, *Mental Health of Refugees* (De Jong & Clarke, 1996), for the Tamil culture: *Mental Health in the Tamil Community* (Somasundaram & Sivayokan, 2001). This manual is being used to train Trainers (TOT) who will then train community mental health workers and others working at the grass-root level with UNICEF support.

As for the general community, a 45 hour 'Introduction to Counselling' weekend course at the Extra Mural Studies Unit at the University of Jaffna was run. Following the recognition of the seriousness of traumatization in students shown by several studies already mentioned, a detailed long-term programme has been instituted by the Department of Education, Shantiam and Jaffna University Department of Psychiatry. Initially all the schools in the Jaffna peninsula and some outside were given a general awareness programme. The stress faced by students in a war situation and traumatization were discussed, while means of coping were explained. Then more intensive training was given for selected teachers starting with the Chankanai Division. This is to be extended to other areas after feedback evaluation and modification. A group of selected teachers (1 per 300 students) will undergo training as 'skilled helpers' (and in the future as teacher counsellors) to function as health promoters in schools. Programmes for pre-school teachers have also been held in the Jaffna Municipality and Moolai Nursery Institute.

Table 8. People Trained in Mental Health

Trainees	
Medical student	500
Counsellors	150
Public health midwife	200
Nurses	300
Extramural students, University of Jaffna	300
Relaxation therapist	25
Multidisciplinary team	20
Grama Sevaka	100

Management

As described above, the wide spread problem of collective traumatization is best approached through community level interventions. Further, community based approaches will enable one to reach a larger target population as well as undertake preventive and promotional public mental health activities at the same time (Somasundaram, 1998). In these circumstances it may be more meaningful to look at how the community as a whole has responded, how the community coped, and what we can do at the collective level (Somasundaram, 1996). For example, it may be more beneficial to consider strengthening and rebuilding the family and village structures as well use the traditional resources widely available in the community, a natural source of help to which people turn when in distress. Recourse to traditional or western medical and psychological methods to treat individual traumatization will be needed in special cases.

Help-seeking Behavior. Help seeking behavior of the people depends on their educational and socio-economic status, availability of help givers and social stigma of looking for mental help. Most people appear to, in time, seek some form of help for their problems when faced with intolerable stress. They will seek help with the expectation of relief related to their beloved ones, property, job, marriage, travel abroad or business.

People with psychosocial problems would go to different healers, including traditional and modern, seeking help. The traditional healer may divine the cause of the problem in terms of cultural beliefs and then set right the harmonious relationships between people, their deities and the environment. In doing this they would involve the family and society in the ritual practice and in the solution. The western biomedical practitioner would treat the physical complaint (somatization) with drugs. Sometimes, the person seeking help may have to go to several healers till some remedy for his or her misfortune is found.

Traditional Healing Methods. The traditional healing methods have evolved from the local and Indian culture, particularly from the Ayurvedic and Siddha systems of medicine as well as folk beliefs and practices. They can be a source of strength, support and meaning. Cultures and villages have their own rituals and traditional functions to deal with trauma. Funeral rites, the 31st day and subsequent anniversary observance are powerful social mechanisms to deal with grief and loss. Particularly, funeral ceremonies can be very effective ways to find comfort. The gathering together of relations, friends and the community is an important social process to share, work through and release deep emotions, define and come to terms with what has happened and finally integrate the traumatic experience into social reality. In addition to funerals, religious and temple rites, cultural festivals, dramas, musical fares, exhibitions and other programs, meetings and social gatherings provide the opportunity for people to discuss, construct meaning, share and assimilate traumatic events. In war, when due to the disturbed situation these rituals are not possible or improperly performed, the trauma is never fully accepted or put to rest, as in the cases of "disappearances" where there is no finality about death. Ideally the social processes should work to promote feelings of belonging and participation, where the group is able to give meaning to what has happened, adapt to the new situation, and determine their future. Communities should be encouraged to hold traditional rituals and arrangements made for this.

Patricia Lawrence (1998) has brought out the psychosocial value of the traditional oracle practice of *"vakuu choluthal"* in Batticaloa, particularly in cases of disappearances, where the families are told what has happened to the disappeared person in a socially supportive environment. When a member of the family is detained, the relation will make a vow (*nerthi*) to the God or temple asking for his/her release and fulfill it (*nerthi kadan*) if they are released. Religious festivals, folk singing and dancing can be ways of meeting, finding support and expressing emotions. Other local practices would include *bajan* (devotional singing), temple festivals, repetition of mantras, religious sermons and explanations of the Hindu concept of Karma (there is now a popular explanation that the Tamil community must have done something 'bad' to have had to experience the effects of this war), bad time or evil influence of planets etc.

The help given could be categorized as rituals of misfortune (Helman, 1994)

> The aim of these public rituals is visibly to restore the harmonious relationships between man and man, man and his deities, and man and the natural world. Rituals of misfortune usually have two consecutive phases: the phase of diagnoses or divination of the cause of the misfortune, and the treatment of the effects of the misfortune and removal of the cause.

Some of the methods that are in use in Northern Sri Lanka could be broadly categorized as those establishing the cause and those providing a remedy (Somasundaram & Sivayokan, 2001), though often both are involved in the same method. During the helping session the practitioner often will take the opportunity to give prescriptions of do's and don'ts; for example, to avoid a calamity or undo a "bad" deed. Religious beliefs, cultural practices, rituals, explanatory expositions, philosophy, counseling, theories of karma, advice on right living, relationships, marriage and so on will be imparted during these sessions. When diviners/healers go into a trance and speak in an oracular language often being possessed by a God or deity, they will show certain cultural stereotyped actions, sometimes in the form of a dance (*Kalai or Uru eduthu adal*) and speak in the voice of the particular god or deity. These performances are social actions in front of a large audience, usually in a sacred place such as a temple. Thus what is done has considerable social legitimacy, authority and power which can heal relationships between family members or in society. People can be asked to do things, set right relationships, give importance to a neglected person (for example an overworked housewife) that they would not normally do but will now follow.

Case History 3. A 30 yr old gentleman working in Palmyrah Coconut Developmental Society at Chunnakam, was arrested in mid August, 1996 at Chemmany while he was cycling to his office in the morning. His parents and three sisters searched for him and learnt he had been arrested by the military forces. They had complained to the Army 512 Brigade, Government Agent, ICRC and Human Right Commission. But nothing was fruitful.

They went to hear the horoscope from the Sasthirakarran. He told them that he had the "bad period". Three months later they went to hear the Vaku (Oracle) at the Sivahamy Amman Kovil, at Mirusuvil. After performing a ritual, She said that he is living in the South. Six months later, they went to Kokuvil, where the Oracle worshipped Kannan (Lord Krishnan), and said that he was living, pray to Lord Kannan. (To date they have continued to pray to Lord Kannan). Later, they went to another oracle at Alaveddy where also they were told that he was living.

Meanwhile, the mother got sick, lost her appetite, found it difficult to speak and died one year later. Father also became depressed and started to neglect his self-care. Sister also has poor concentration in her normal work. But they said with tears that they are praying that one day their beloved one might come back.

Case History 4. A 18 yr old girl had been suffering from severe headache, loss of appetite, poor concentration in studies of 3 month duration. Her parents took her to see several doctors and finally they went to Teaching Hospital Jaffna. As the physical examination and investigation were normal, no medication was given except placebo and paracetamol. But the symptoms did not subside.

Later she went to the traditional healer in Chulipuram. The lady who is the traditional healer worshiped in the prayer hall of the small house. Around 10–15 people gather there every Tuesday, Friday and Sunday. She worships Nagamma (Snake god) and then does the Vaku cholluthal (oracle) to relate what the help seeker needs. There was a cobra also in the room. (Actually it is dwelling there.)

She asked this girl about the problem. The girl related that her parents wanted her to marry her cousin who is abroad. But she hates going abroad. She said, "If I go abroad I will have to stay in a small room and I have to depend on others. There is no freedom, very soon I will become obese." She wishes to stay with her parents and wants to study the Advanced Level so that she can enter the university. She never tells the problem to any others.

After the ritual, the lady performed movements like a cobra and told her that "This time is not good for traveling abroad. So study. I (Goddess) will help you. Go and worship me at Nainatheevu (Temple of Nagamma) donating a copper cobra as a merit. The parents too accepted this and the girl is now studying without any symptoms.

In our experience we have found that the traditional sector is quite effective in managing minor mental health disorders, including the after-effects of the war. However, they are not able to treat the major mental disorders like schizophrenia, and indeed many of their actions like exorcism through whipping and other injurious procedures can be quite detrimental (Somasundaram & Sivayokan, 2001).[12] The majority of the experienced traditional practitioners are able to make the distinction between minor and major mental disorders, readily referring the later for western medical treatment.[13] We in turn encourage many of our patients suffering from minor mental health problems like somatization and hysteria to use the traditional sector. In fact we have been trying to include a traditional practitioner in our multidisciplinary team. At present we have a yoga instructor, traditional masseuse, Brahmin, and Catholic priest in our team.

The Psychosocial and Mental Health Interventions

Despite all the shortcomings of a war situation, the Mental Health Services have continued to function as the overall statistics for the period show (see Table 7). The type of problems encountered and the interventions used are shown in Table 9.

The following box shows the different types of interventions.

Box 1. Therapeutic Interventions for Trauma

1. Psycho-education
2. Crisis Intervention
3. Psychotherapy
4. Behavioural-Cognitive methods
5. Relaxation Techniques
6. Pharmacotherapy
7. Group therapy
8. Family therapy
9. Expressive methods
10. Rehabilitation
11. Community approaches (see box-3)

---

[12]It is interesting that a herbal preparation of rauworlfia alkaloids made from the local medicinal plant, rauwolfia serpentica, used for centuries in the treatment of psychosis has an action similar to the western anti-psychotics.

[13]Particularly after an elderly and respected traditional practitioner, Ambalavanar, specializing in mental disorders was murdered by a psychotic patient who he had been treating for months. The patient who had been restrained by a wooden block used for this purpose, took an axe lying close by and killed the practitioner when the later released him for his meals.

Table 9. Common Psychosocial Problems and Interventions

Specific group	Problems	Intervention
1. Children	Learning disorder	Play therapy, art therapy
	Conduct disorder	Family therapy
	Trauma	Referred for child therapy
	Child soldier	Rehabilitation
	Child abuse	
2. Women	Somatization	Find out the social cause
	Anxiety neurosis	Counseling, relaxation
	Depression	Social case work
3. Alcoholics	Chronic alcoholism	AA, Medical therapy
	Acute alcoholism	De-toxification, aversion therapy
4. War victims	PTSD	Medication, rehabilitation, relaxation exercises, counseling
5. Drug Abuse	Addiction	Withdrawal, behaviour therapy & counselling
Neuropsychiatric problems		
1. Children	Epilepsy	Antiepileptic drugs + play therapy Advice to go to school, counselling for "social stigma".
	Mental retardation	Play therapy, music therapy, family counselling, referral to ARK
2. Schizophrenia	1. Acute emotional problems	Psychotropic medication & ECT
	2. Chronic illness	Maintenance medication, observe for side-effects, dose titration, compliance, reduce Expressed emotions at home
	3. Social problems	Social case work
	a. Economic	Occupational therapy, employment
	b. Marriage	Martial counselling
	c. Security	Yellow ID card
	d. Social stigma	Mass media propaganda

Psycho-education. Basic information about trauma and normal responses to stress can be very reassuring. Suggestions on what to do and coping techniques can be helpful. Several informative pamphlets and media publications for the public on trauma and related issues were undertaken. The World Mental Health Day on October 10, is observed each year by a cooperative effort of all the mental health organizations working in the area with a view of increasing public awareness on mental health issues.

Psychotherapy. From the initial contact an atmosphere of mutual trust and therapeutic alliance was sought to be established. Basic counselling was sufficient and appropriate in a large number of cases. An opportunity to "tell their story" in a non-threatening and accepting atmosphere, express their repressed emotions, and receive the support and the warmth of the therapist was all that was needed. Brief psychotherapy, testimony method of therapy, bereavement counselling, crisis intervention, problem solving, relaxation techniques and other short term therapies were carried out where necessary. Counseling sections attached to the University Psychiatric Unit and the Association for Health and Counselling is carrying out such therapeutic work. Similar centres will be needed in other districts. The staff for these centres are trained at Shantiam.

Spiritual beliefs. Spiritual beliefs and strengths have been found to make people more resilient. Thus a much more ambitious aim, termed logotherapy (Frankl, 1959) is to find meaning in what happened. For once meaning is found most clients appear to recover quickly. Again the cultural and religious beliefs, for example the doctrines concerning Karma and suffering, central to Hindu system, were important. Attempts were made to co-opt sympathetic traditional resources such as priests, monks and healers as co-therapists or in the traditional nosology, as allies, in the therapeutic endeavour (see Box 2).

Box 2. Collaboration with the traditional sector

We refer patients to the experienced Yoga Asana Specialist, Swami Sithananda Yogi at the Divine Life Society, Nallur. Several of our members have been or will be going to Vivekananda Khendra school in Bangalore for extensive training, supported by the MADAM trust under Dr. Ponna Wanigaraja. In northern Sri Lanka, there was considerable resistance to referral of 'psychiatric patients' to a well known yoga centre. The board at first refused to accept such referral, voicing fear that the negative stigma of mental illness will be passed onto their centre as well. It was only after the swami in charge, with whom we had already built a strong relationship, stood firm that the practice of referral was begun. In time, the board and other members as well as the public realized that only people with minor mental health disorders (people very much like themselves) were being referred and were able to see the benefit that individuals referred there were receiving. This led to several programmes where mental health education was given to the public through the centre and the swami and other adepts were able to give talks and demonstration of yoga to a wider audience through the medical and academic systems.

Group therapy. Group therapy has been found useful. The formation of ex-detainee groups, widow groups, ex-alcoholic (A.A.) groups and other groupings of affected individuals have happened out of need in some cases and was encouraged wherever possible.

Family therapy. Family therapy is an important therapeutic tool. In the Tamil culture where the family bonds are very strong, the family is an essential resource that can be used in therapy. The principles of family dynamics were used to facilitate supportive and healing relationships while counteracting damaging and maladaptive interactions. Communication of individual problems leading to an awareness of each other, one's role and encouragement towards mutually interdependent functioning was used to build up family unity.

Relaxation techniques. Based on Jacobson's Progressive Muscular Relaxation, culturally acceptable methods of Yoga practice were used for several of the consequences of traumatization, namely states of arousal, anxiety and somatization. Tensed muscles are the cause of much of the somatic pains in traumatized, particularly torture victims. Relaxation will counteract this. Similarly Hyperventilation is a common problem and the basis for many of the psychosomatic complaints. Slow, deep, relaxed breathing can be taught to rectify this tendency. Four basic methods adapted to the culture and religion of the client have been developed by us:

- *Breathing exercises.* For Hindus, the yogic method of *Pranayama*, was taught. A mantra or word (*OM*) can be said such as *O* while breathing in and *M* while breathing out. For others, regular abdominal breathing was explained.
- *Progressive muscular relaxation.* For most clients, Jacobson's technique can be taught. Hindu clients can be taught the technically similar Yogic exercise, *Shanti* or *Sava Asana*.
- *Repetition of words.* In this method of *Japa*, a meaningful word, phrase or verse is repeated over and over to oneself. For Hindus the Mantra given to them during initiation by their Guru or the *Pranava mantra*, '*OM*', was selected. For Catholic Christians, the Jesus prayer (*Jesus Christ have mercy on me*) or prayer beads was used.
- *Meditation.* Various meditation practices were used.
- *Massage* has been found useful in treating victims of torture, particularly the common complaints of musculo-skeletal pains. In addition to directly focusing on painful areas like the sole of the feet, head, neck, back, joints and other areas that may have been injured, leaving scar tissue, the massaging induces a state of relaxation, warmth and trust that is useful in therapy. Massage using traditional methods like *Ayurvedic* or *Siddha* oil massage are both culturally familiar and effective. It was our practice to involve traditional practitioners and others in therapeutic programmes, for, in addition to mobilising available resources, it will help to spread awareness and knowledge about trauma in the community. Further, it can tap into hidden talents and skills. For example the traditional practitioner giving oil massage in our unit was found to be very good at communicating with her clients, many, particularly young combatants recovered from their problems by just talking to her.

Calling these cultural techniques as relaxation exercises may be a misnomer leading to an underestimation of their value. When methods are culturally familiar, they tap into past childhood, community and religious roots and thus release a rich source of associations that can be helpful in therapy and the healing process. Further, mindfulness and meditation draw upon hidden resources within the individual and open into dimensions that can create spiritual healing and give meaning to what has happened. Although these techniques do no formal psychotherapy, they may accomplish what psychotherapy attempts to do by releasing cultural and spiritual processes.

At the community level, considerable effort was put into the training of personnel in the aforementioned Yoga techniques, teaching it to the public, and specifically in the treatment of traumatized individuals, particularly torture victims. It was felt that with sufficient trained personnel and motivation, Yoga could be introduced into the regular school curricula and thereby benefit a large number of students. When Yoga is practiced regularly in the correct way, it helps the child to express pent-up energy and emotions in a healthy way and thus is a promotive, preventive and curative method of health that can be used at a community level.

Pharmacotherapy. In PTSD too, there was positive improvement with antidepressants, particularly in the intrusive phenomena and nightmares. Low doses of imipramine (25–50 mg) worked in the majority of cases.

Expressive therapy. Artistic expression of emotions and trauma can be cathartic for individuals and the community as a whole. Art, drama, story telling, writing poetry or novels (testimony), singing, dancing, clay modeling, and sculpturing are very useful emotive methods in trauma therapy. The Multidisciplinary team in the University Psychiatric clinics were trained to use these methods, particularly in children.

A socio-drama on the psychological effects of war was produced.[14] The drama went a long way in creating awareness about trauma among the public and helped traumatized individuals to ventilate their emotions or seek treatment. Local drama groups have used drama, including street drama (*theru kuthu*), to work with affected populations in the community and refugee camps. It has been found a powerful method to increase awareness, promote catharsis and encourage discussion about pressing problems.

Children in particular, who usually are unable to express their thoughts or emotions verbally, benefited from the above mentioned expressive methods and play therapy. Structured play activity was introduced in many of the refugee camps in the North and East. They proved to be very popular with children and adults alike. The children's time could then be usefully structured and physical energy channeled in a healthy manner. More important, it helped in organizing camp activity, building friendships and peer relationships and giving an opportunity for

---

[14]Psychological dramas called "*Annai Ida Thee*" and "*Vellvi Thee*", were produced by Kulanthai Shanmugalingam and Sithambaranathan of the Jaffna University Fine Arts Department. The roles were played by medical students.

the child to bring out his or her creative impulses. One example of story telling used in Sri Lanka was the use of the "Little Elephant" book to build family unity and encourage positive interactions in traumatized families (Baron, 1994). Many were able to identify with the little elephant who had lost his father in the conflict. The story was also staged several times.

A very innovative approach to encourage the child's imagination, creative potential and playing impulse by linking it with the nurturing, supporting and healing power of mother earth has been started in Batticaloa.[15]

Occupational therapy. Individuals can benefit from being taught basic social skills and specific crafts to help them re-find employment and integrate themselves back into society. In addition, occupational training, by structuring time and channeling physical activity into satisfying goals helps the individual regain his or her sense of control and mastery, his or her worthiness and usefulness and thus establish their self-respect and self-esteem. In the long-term, occupational skills are empowering and produce self-sufficiency. The Occupational Therapy department with a group of volunteers at the Tellipallai District provided such therapy and training.

Rehabilitation. The rehabilitation of the individual back into his community forms an essential if not the most important part of the overall treatment. Unfortunately in the North and East such opportunities for trauma victims have been completely lacking. A network for helping victims was established through the NGO Forum together with such active NGO's as TRRO and the Centre for Women and Development.

Community approaches. Given the widespread nature of the traumatization due to war, a Community based approach will enable one to reach a larger target population and undertake preventive and promotional public mental health activities as well.

Box 3. Community approaches

- Awareness
- Training of community workers
- Public mental health promotive activities
- Encourage indigenous coping strategies
- Cultural rituals and ceremonies
- Community interventions
  1. Family
  2. Groups
  3. Expressive methods
  4. Rehabilitation
- Prevention

---

[15]Started by the Canadian MacMaster University Health Reach artist, Paul Hogan, as the Butterfly Garden project, it was based on his work with the Spiral Garden project in Toronto, Canada.

As already mentioned, training of grass root community level workers in basic mental health knowledge and skills is the easiest way of reaching a large population. They in turn would increase general awareness and disseminate the knowledge as well as do preventive and promotional work. The majority of minor mental health problems could be managed by them and others referred to the appropriate level.

Indigenous coping strategies such as the traditional practices for death—funeral rites, disappearance—*vaccu cholluthal* (oracles) and detention—*nerthi* (vows) that have helped the local population to survive should be encouraged.

PROBLEMS PRESENTED TO THE MENTAL HEALTH PROGRAMME

Despite all our very well meant efforts, it is very difficult to heal a traumatized patient in a war milieu. Further, the ongoing war will continue to produce more and more traumatized individuals.

When working in community settings, for example refugee camps or with children, unconscious values like non-violence and peace guide our agenda. These basic assumptions that are being promoted can go against the values those involved in fighting are trying to encourage, particularly in motivating for recruitment or support for the war. Thus the community work can create a conflict of interests, even become risky under some circumstances. And at times, the heroic fighting spirit, anger and resistance may have survival value—those who remain may get killed while those who join the militants may escape the periodic rampages of the state military.

A serious problem for mental health workers has been burn out. Several of the long-term workers have over the years developed personal problems, lost their motivation and some have left. Considerable in-fighting, jealousies and conflicts have developed. One reason could have been lack of adequate support groups and rest. The few involved in this mentally strenuous type of work have overworked themselves, without recourse to rest, holidays or support from others. This was particularly noticeable after the mass exodus when everyone was affected, including the mental health workers themselves and a kind of "collective trauma" set in affecting the whole community.

Prevention

After working in a war devastated area and seeing the untold misery it causes, one begins to realize the enormous physical, psychological, social and spiritual cost. There can truly be no neutral position in war. It is obvious that one way to prevent the trauma is to stop the war. Health workers in areas of conflict have started emphasizing that as health professionals we can't remain silent, we need to consider the ethics and take principled stand for victims and society (Armenian, 1989; Zwi & Ugalde, 1989).

Another area of intervention, both for prevention and reconciliation is at the national level by influencing policy making, rehabilitation and international aid programmes. Such a role has become possible through membership in national bodies such as the Presidential Task Force on Disaster Management, Child Protection Authority and Framework process. For example the Framework process being directed by the World Bank is: "an effort to develop a framework for relief, reconciliation and rehabilitation. This effort will be supported technically by international donor agencies and will address present bottlenecks and constraints as well as look to new opportunities. The Framework will provide common direction and basis for effective assistance to war-affected communities in Sri Lanka, through formulation of policies, strategies, mechanisms and guidelines". Workshops with the theme of Healing of memories with guidance from experts from South Africa, have been organized by the Presidential Task Force on Disaster Management. WHO has developed the concept of using *Health as a Bridge for Peace* (HBP) and have already carried out two training course for Health staff in Sri Lanka. The overall objectives of the HBP (Pagani, 1999) is

- the development of an understanding of the dynamics of conflict situations and of the role that health personnel may play as a bridge for peace
- The raising of the capacity of considering conflict scenario in the planning and implementation of health programs, and
- The development of a specific sensibility that the planning and implementation of any health program must be compatible with the framework of international human rights principles and of international humanitarian law.

The training courses were found to be extremely useful and well appreciated by local health staff from all ethnic groups. The UNICEF Education for Conflict Resolution will be a very effective programme for introduction into schools (Wijeyasekara, 1996). More recently UNICEF (1999) has developed

> peace education as the process of promoting the knowledge, skills, attitudes and values needed to bring about behavior changes that will enable children, youth and adults to prevent conflict and violence, both overt and structural; to resolve conflict peacefully; and to create the conditions conducive to peace, whether at an intrapersonal, interpersonal, intergroup, national or international level.

Their more recent publication edited by Bush and Saltarelli (2000), "The Two Faces of Education in Ethnic Conflict" is a powerful critique of the way education can be an aggravating factor in ethnic conflict and how it can be used more positively for solving such problems. Similarly the distorted histories that have been written for the school curricula will have to re-written in a more neutral, factual and towards the aim of producing national harmony (Siriwardene, 1984). Learning both the national languages, with English too, should be implemented in the schools.

It would be possible to influence policy by making use of some of the conclusions mentioned in the above analysis under such headings as the origins of the conflict, context, assessment and background.

COLLABORATION

There has been close collaboration between the Department of Psychiatry, Faculty of Medicine, University of Jaffna and the Association for Health and Counselling (Shantiam) on many of the mental health programmes. Similarly with the Ministry of Health Provincial Health Service, Teaching Hospital Jaffna and Jaffna Municipal Health Office in training for the health staff and running of the psychiatric clinics. The Department of Education extended its support for the training of teachers. The Mental Health Society based at the Tellilpallai District Hospital has worked closely on mental health programmes (see Figure 4).

Several NGO's, notably the TRRO, gave considerable assistance. The NGO Forum, Jaffna helped to form a functioning network for mutual referral. The UNICEF, SCF, FORUT, Centre for Women and Development collaborated and supported many programmes. UNICEF has provided several ongoing training for various categories of staff. Diplomatic Missions from Canada and NORAD have given considerable financial assistance. Canada has funded the Multidisciplinary team while the WHO is supporting the development of the manual for training community level workers. The main ongoing service work is done through the Health Ministry of the Government of Sri Lanka and the training through the Psychiatric Department of the University of Jaffna.

CONCLUSION

Due to sustained work over the years disseminating the knowledge and skills of basic mental health, particularly in regard to the trauma of the ongoing war, there has been a growing awareness in the public in general and among community workers in particular about the problem. Thus more are willing to come for help, while others are able to recognize problems in themselves or others and take appropriate action. This has included several simple self-help

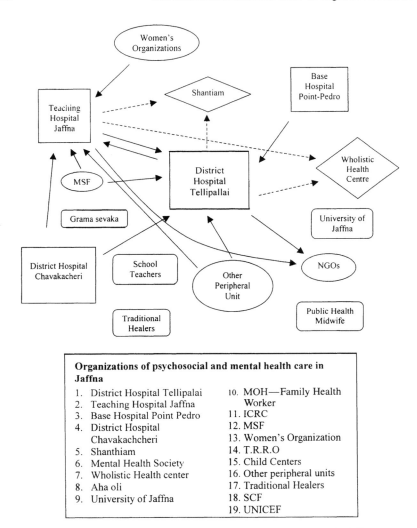

Figure 4. Organizations of psychosocial and mental health care in Jaffna.

measures such as the traditional relaxation methods. Various levels of health staff, such as doctors, nurses, Primary Health Workers (FHW's and PHI's), health volunteers; Educational staff such as teachers, principals, pre-school teachers and directors; Governmental staff such as Grama Sevakas (Village Headman) and others; NGO staff, Camp workers, Volunteers and others have been trained. Thus under times of crises there are many in the community who are able to respond to psychosocial needs of others. This was brought out during the massive 1995 exodus, when psychosocial issues were dealt with as one of the five priorities in the different areas. The Tamil militant organization is now more willing to acknowledge the problem (and seek help) among their own cadres and in the community. The NGO sector as well Governmental organizations are also now including psychosocial aspects as part of their programmes. Some health staff, teachers and counsellors have been given extensive training so that they are able to offer more specialized help as well as act as trainers.

One serious problem among this group has been burn out. Due to the ongoing war without respite many have had to face repeated personal and family hardships. No proper mechanism has been evolved to provide ongoing support for this group. There are no programs for them to go on relief, take holidays, and receive support from others. As a result of burn out many of those who were trained have left the area or stopped working in this field. Interpersonal problems among the workers have also cropped up. Due to ongoing stress, some of these problems have not been sorted out satisfactorily. Sustaining long-term counselling and other programmes due to lack of funding from donors is another problem. Of course the stigma attached to this kind of work has not been completely erased within the community. As such it is still difficult for some one with psychosocial problem to acknowledge it or seek help.

Considerable research, publications, and pamphlets on psychosocial issues have come out over the years. Experience and expertise in working in this difficult field has been slowly built up. Innovations, such as the use of traditional yoga methods, adaptation to local forms of drama, evolution of Tamil terms for psychosocial words and concepts have also been achieved.

REFERENCES

Amnesty International. (1998). *Child soldiers*. London.
Ardrey, R. (1967). *The territorial imperative*. New York: Atheneum.
Armenian, H. K. (1989). Perceptions from epidemiological research in an endemic war. *Social Science & Medicine, 28*, 643–647.
Arunakirinathan, T., Sasikanthan, A., Sivashankar, R., & Somasundaram, D. J. (1993). *A study of psychological consequences of traumatic stress in school children under 12 years*. Paper presented at the Ninth Annual Scientific Sessions, Jaffna Medical Association, Jaffna, Sri Lanka.
Bandura, A. (1973). *Aggression: A social learning analysis*. Englewood Cliffs, NJ: Prentice Hall.
Baron, N. (1994). *A little elephant finds his courage*. (Trans. into Tamil Sivathamby, K., Kamalanathan, M., & Shanmugam, M.) Colombo, Sri Lanka.
Bush, K. D., & Saltarelli D., (2000). *The two faces of education in ethnic conflict*. Florence, Italy: UNICEF.
Committee for National Development. (1984) *Sri Lanka: Ethnic conflict (Report)*. New Delhi, India: Navrang.
Damian, S. (1994). *Ula Vallathrurai* [Counselling]. Jaffna, Sri Lanka:
Daniel, E. V. (1984). *Fluid signs—being a person the Tamil way*. Berkeley, CA: University of California Press.

de Jong, J. T. V. M. (1997). *TPO program for the identification, management and prevention of psychosocial and mental health problems of refugees and victims of organized violence within primary care of adults and children.* Amsterdam: Transcultural Psychosocial Organization. Internal document.

de Jong, J. T. V. M., & Clarke, L. (Eds.). (1996). *Mental health of refugees.* Geneva: World Health Organization.

Department of Census and Statistics. (1995). *Statistical Abstracts (Annuals).* Colombo, Sri Lanka.

de Silva, K. M. (1981). *A History of Sri Lanka.* New Delhi, India: Oxford University Press.

Eisenbruch, M. (1991). From post-traumatic stress disorder to cultural bereavement: Diagnosis of Southeast Asian refugees. *Social Science & Medicine, 33*(6), 673–680.

Erikson, E. H. (1968). *Identity, youth and crisis.* London: Faber & Faber.

Erikson, K. T. (1976). Loss of communality at Buffalo Creek. *American Journal of Psychiatry, 135*(3), 330–335.

Frankl, V. E. (1959). *Man 's search for meaning: An introduction to logotherapy.* Boston: Beacon Press.

Fromm, E. (1973). *The anatomy of human destructiveness.* Middlesex, England: Penguin Books.

Geevathasan, M. G., Somasundaram, D. J., & Parameshwaran, S. V. (1993). *Psychological consequence of war on adolescents.* Paper presented at the Ninth Annual Scientific Sessions, Jaffna Medical Association, Jaffna, Sri Lanka.

Goodhand, J., Lewer, N., & Hume, D. (2000). *NGOs and peace building: Sri Lanka study.* Institute for Development Policy and Management, University of Manchester, INTRAC and the Department of Peace Studies, University of Bradford.

Greiger, W. (trans.) (1964). *The Mahavamsa.* London: Pali Text Society, Luzac and Company.

Gunawardena, R. A. L. H. (1990). The People of the Lion: the Sinhala identity and ideology in history and historiography. In J. Spencer (Ed.), *Sri Lanka: History and the roots of conflict.* London: Routledge.

Helman, C. G. (1994). *Culture, health and illness* (3rd ed.). Oxford, England: Butterworth-Heineman.

Hirsch, H. (1995). *Genocide and the politics of memory.* Chapel Hill, NC: The University of North Carolina Press.

Ihezue, U. H. (1983). Psychiatric in-patients in Anambra state, Nigeria. *Acta Psychiatrica Scandinavica, 68*, 277–286.

Jareg, E. (1999). *Rehabilitation of child soldiers.* Workshop on "Taking up the Challenge of Child Soldiers" arranged by the Save the Children Alliance and UNICEF, in Colombo, Sri Lanka.

Jayawardena, K. (1986). *Ethnic and class conflicts in Sri Lanka.* Dehiwala, Sri Lanka: Centre for Social Analysis.

Jeyanthy, K., Loshani, N. A., & Sivarajini, G. (1993). *A study of psychological consequences of displacement on family members* (III MBBS Research project University of Jaffna, Departement of Community Medicine, Jaffna, Sri Lanka).

Kadiragamar, L. (1996). *Mental health in Sri Lanka.* Keynote address for the National Council for Mental Health, Colombo, Sri Lanka.

Lakshmman, N., & Sivashankar, R. (1994). *War stress in children.* Paper presented at a seminar on Child Mental Health, Shantiam, Jaffna, Sri Lanka.

Lawrence, P. (1998). Grief in the body: The work of oracles in eastern Sri Lanka. In M. Roberts (Ed.), *Sri Lank: Collective identities revisited* (Vol. 2, pp. 271–294). Colombo, Sri Lanka: Marga Institute.

Manogaran, C. (1987). *Ethics of conflict and reconstruction in Sri Lanka.* Honolulu, HI: University of Hawaii Press.

Marga Institute. (2001). *The Cost of the War.* Colombo, Sri Lanka.

Nehru, J. (1991). *The discovery of India.* New Delhi, India: Oxford University Press.

Nikapota, A., & Samarisinghe, D. (1995). *Training manual for helping children in situation of armed conflict.* Colombo, Sri Lanka: UNICEF.

NORAD (1988). Growth strategy and Sri Lanka's poor. *Lanka Guardian, II*(3).

Obeyesekere, G. (1984). *The cult of the goddess Pattini.* Chicago: University of Chicago Press.

Obeyesekere, G. (1988). *A meditation on conscience*. Colombo, Sri Lanka: Social Scientists' Association of Sri Lanka.
Pagani, F. (1999). *Objectives*. Presentation at the WHO workshop "Health as a Bridge for Peace", Colombo, Sri Lanka.
Palihawadana, M. (1983). *Violence in a Buddhist society*. Weekend, Sept. 11, 1983, Colombo, Sri Lanka.
Perera, J. (Ed.) (1996). *The health of children in conflict zones of Sri Lanka*. Hamilton, Canada: McMaster University, Centre for International Health and the Centre for Peace Studies.
Piyadasa, L. (1984). *Sri Lanka: The Holocaust and after*. London: Marram Books.
Rasiah, S., & Nadarajah, K. (1994). *A study of psychological consequences of environmental stress on pre-school children*. Paper presented at the Seminar on Child Mental Health, Shantiam, Jaffna, Sri Lanka.
Reppesgard, H. O. (1993). *Studies on psychosocial problems among displaced people in Sri Lanka: How to counsel and to set up a counselling organization*. Colombo, Sri Lanka: FORUT.
Rosenbeck, R. (1985). The malignant Post-Vietnam Stress Syndrome. *American Journal of Orthopsychiatry, 55*(2), 319–332.
Ruiz, H. A. (1994). *People want peace*. Washington, DC: US Committee of Refugees.
Shepard, M., Brown, A. M., Cooper, B., & Kalton, G. W. (1966). *Psychiatric illness in general practice*. Oxford, England: Oxford University Press.
Siriwardene, R. (1984). National identity in Sri Lanka: Problems in communication and education. In Committee for National Development (Ed.), *Sri Lanka: The ethnic conflict*. New Delhi, India: Navrang.
Sivachandran, S. (1994). Health of women and the elderly. In S. Arulanantham, S. Raatneswaran, & N. Streeharan (Eds.), *Victims of war in Sri Lanka*. London: Medical Institute of Tamils.
Social Science Association. (1985). *Ethnicity and social change in Sri Lanka*. Colombo, Sri Lanka:
Somasundaram, D. J. (1993a). *Child Trauma*. Dr. A. Sivapathasundaram Third Memorial Lecture, University of Jaffna, Jaffna, Sri Lanka.
Somasundaram, D. J. (1993b). *Mana vadu* [Psychological trauma]. Jaffna, Sri Lanka: University of Jaffna.
Somasundaram, D. J. (1996). Post traumatic responses to aerial bombing. *Social Science & Medicine, 42*, 1465–1471.
Somasundaram, D. J. (1998). *Scarred mind*. New Delhi, India: Sage Publications.
Somasundaram, D. J. (2001). War trauma and psychosocial problems in patient attenders at Jaffna. *International Medical Journal, 8*(3), 193–197.
Somasundaram, D. J., & Sivayokan, S. (1994). War trauma in a civilian population. *British Journal of Psychiatry, 165*, 524–527.
Somasundaram, D. J., & Sivayokan, S. (Eds.). (2001). *Mental health in the Tamil community*. Jaffna, Sri Lanka: Shantiam.
Spencer, J. (Ed.). (1990). *Sri Lanka: History and the roots of conflict*. London: Routledge.
Staub, E. (1989). *The roots of evil*. Cambridge, England: Cambridge University Press.
Thambiah, S. J. (1986). *Ethnic fratricide and the dismantling of democracy*. Chicago: University of Chicago Press.
Thambiah, S. J. (1992). *Buddhism betrayed?: Religion, politics, and violence in Sri Lanka*, Chicago: University of Chicago Press.
Trawick, M. (1999). Reasons for violence: A preliminary ethnographic account of the LTTE. In S. Gamage & I. B. Watson (Eds.), *Conflict and community in contemporary Sri Lanka: 'Pearl of the East' or the 'Island of Tears'* (pp. 139–163). New Delhi, India: Sage Publications.
United Nations Children's Fund (1999). *Peace education in UNICEF*. New York.
University Teachers for Human Rights, Jaffna (1994). *From Manal Aru to Weli Oya*. Jaffna, Sri Lanka.
Uyangoda, J. (1988). Dharamasiri Bandaranayake's 'Echoes of war': Peace, please. *Lanka Guardian, 10*(23).
Vittachi, T. (1958). *Emergency '58*. London: Andre Deutch.

Wijeyasekera, A. (1996). *Education for Conflict Resolution*. Presentation at the Asia-Pacific Expert Group Consultation on the UN Study on the Impact of Armed Conflict on Children, Manila, Philippines.

World Health Organization. (1965–1986). *World Health Statistics, 1965–1986* (Annual reports). Geneva.

World Health Organization. (1992). *The ICD-10 Classification of Mental and Behavioural Disorders*. Geneva.

Zwi, A., & Ugalde, A. (1989). Towards an epidemiology of political violence in the Third World. *Social Science & Medicine, 14*, 633–646.

5

Addressing Human Rights Violations
A Public Mental Health Perspective on Helping Torture Survivors in Nepal

MARK VAN OMMEREN, BHOGENDRA SHARMA, DINESH PRASAIN, and BHAVA N. POUDYAL

BACKGROUND

In 1990, the Centre for Victims of Torture Nepal (CVICT) was established to provide medical services to native Nepalese who were tortured during or before Nepal's 1990 people's movement that led to multi-party democracy. The initial assumption was that that there would be no more torture in a democratic Nepal, but this assumption proved to be naïve. Torture resurfaced after the 1991 parliamentarian election as a means of controlling activists from opposition parties. Non-political torture—i.e., torture of suspected criminals during police investigation—never stopped. Thus, since 1991, CVICT has worked against continuing torture in Nepal. CVICT defines torture as:

> Intentional infliction of severe physical or mental suffering by the state's law enforcing institutions or armed opposition on a person under the physical control of the perpetrator, for any reason (Van Ommeren, Sharma, & Prasain, 2000).

In 1991, when large numbers of Nepali-speaking tortured Bhutanese refugees entered Nepal, CVICT organized services. Between 1994 and 1997, CVICT ran a community-based rehabilitation program providing medical and psychosocial care for tortured Bhutanese refugees. These Nepali-speaking Bhutanese refugees were forced to leave southern Bhutan to escape persecution from the Bhutanese authorities, who appear to have feared a pro-democracy movement led by the Nepali-speaking population (Hutt, 1996).

Since 1996, Nepal's human rights situation has worsened, because of a spreading armed Maoist movement, which has resulted in an indiscriminate, hard-line government reaction. Between February 1996 and December 2000, 1396 people have died because of this insurgency (Informal Sector Service Centre, 2001). Most of the 909 people killed by the police were innocent villagers branded by the government to be Maoists. These villagers were murdered during alleged Maoist attacks. The Maoists themselves are estimated to have killed 234 policemen and 253 civilians (Informal Sector Service Centre). Maoists are also torturing political opponents within and outside their party, applying similar techniques as those used by the police. CVICT, an independent non-governmental organization (NGO), treats people who have been tortured by the police, army, forest guards, or armed Maoist opposition.

The aim of this paper is to analyze the activities of CVICT from a public mental health perspective. We will cover four areas: (a) population-based studies on torture survivors living in Nepal, (b) clinic data on help-seeking native Nepalese torture survivors, (c) care of Bhutanese refugee torture survivors and training of Bhutanese refugee counselors, and (d) care of native Nepalese torture survivors and training of native Nepalese counselors. For the purpose of this paper, we use the term *native Nepalese* to refer to a person who is born in Nepal and has Nepalese citizenship.

POPULATION STUDIES ON TORTURE SURVIVORS LIVING IN NEPAL

Torture: How Common?

A public health perspective on torture calls for data on the percentage of torture survivors for a given population. Reliable estimates of the number of native Nepalese torture survivors have not been available. However, evidence exists that torture has occurred in Nepal throughout history (Guragain, 1994). State-sponsored torture was widespread during Nepal's autocratic Panchayat regime (1962–1990). The Nepal Medical Association has estimated that more than 5000 people were tortured during the people's movement for democracy in the spring of 1990 (Forum for Protection of Human Rights, 1991). On the basis of contacts with survivors and policemen, CVICT believes that routine torture occurs in every police station in Nepal. Our national survey conducted between 1994 and 1997, covering all prisons and an estimated 95% of all prisoners in Nepal, indicates that 70% of prisoners reported a history of physical torture that had occurred most often in police custody. Recently, in the context of the Maoist insurgency, the police have severely beaten and threatened the majority of people in specific villages accused of supporting Maoists.

CVICT has been able to estimate the percentage of people with a history of physical torture among the Bhutanese refugees in camps in Nepal. In 1994, CVICT in cooperation with Bhutanese political parties and human rights organizations, collaborating agencies, and ex-patients, identified and registered 2331 survivors of physical torture in the camps. The identification process involved a hut-to-hut survey. By the end of 1994, there were 85,078 refugees in the camps, implying a history of self-reported physical torture among 2.7% of the refugees (Shrestha et al., 1998).

Population Mental Health Data

When discussing a social problem such as torture from a public health perspective, it is important to look at population data of health consequences—which requires representative samples. Globally, most data sets on health consequences of torture are not representative, because the data have been collected from the select group of mostly Asian and African refugees who managed to escape to the West. However, the vast majority of the world's torture survivors live in low-income countries. Until recently, representative data from populations of torture survivors have not been available.

CVICT—in collaboration with the Amsterdam-based Transcultural Psychosocial Organization—has conducted two population-based mental health surveys among torture survivors in the Bhutanese refugee camps in Nepal. Because of the existence of a register of torture survivors in the camps, random sampling was possible. The first of the two surveys occurred in 1995 and focused on symptomatology. The results indicated that tortured Bhutanese refugees, compared with nontortured Bhutanese refugees, are, as a group, at increased risk of physical complaints and symptoms of anxiety, depression, and posttraumatic stress disorder (PTSD) (Shrestha et al., 1998).

The second survey was conducted in 1997 and focused on diagnosed *ICD-10* psychiatric disorders (Van Ommeren et al., 2001). The survey compared a representative sample of 418 tortured Bhutanese refugees with 392 nontortured Bhutanese refugees using face-to-face structured diagnostic interviews. The tortured Bhutanese refugees were more likely to report recent (within the previous 12 months) *ICD-10* PTSD, dissociative (amnesia and conversion) disorders, and persistent somatoform pain disorder. In addition, the tortured refugees were more likely to report having had one of the following disorders at one point in their life: PTSD, dissociative (amnesia and conversion) disorders, persistent somatoform pain disorder, affective disorder, and generalized anxiety disorder. The data indicate that the differences between tortured and nontortured refugees in terms of rates of affective and generalized anxiety disorder disappear over time—implying that affective and generalized anxiety disorders are not chronic for most refugees with these disorders. However, lifetime rates of dissociative (amnesia and conversion) disorders and persistent somatoform pain disorder were similar to 12-month rates, indicating that these reported disorders have a chronic course in this population. Furthermore, even though men were more likely to report torture, tortured women (compared to tortured men) were at higher risk for most disorders (Van Ommeren et al., 2001).

Both surveys are limited because concurrent validity (agreement with another criterion) has not been established. Nevertheless, the research has strengths in terms of content validity (relevant content), semantic validity (adequate translation), and technical validity (concern for response set issues) (Van Ommeren, 2000).

Generalizability of Mental Health Findings

The generalizability of our research findings to other populations of torture survivors is unknown. Research reviews indicate that results of psychiatric epidemiological surveys among refugees vary enormously (Boehlein & Kinzie 1995; Marsella, Friedman, Gerrity, & Scurfield, 1996). We ourselves have also been confronted with different findings of different studies on the same population. Psychiatric epidemiological data are extremely sensitive to variations in methods used to collect data. Moreover, because of cultural and language differences, responses to questions cannot be assumed to be comparable across cultures (Malpass & Poortinga, 1986; Van Ommeren et al., 1999). For these reasons and the aforementioned difficulty of obtaining random samples, the state of knowledge about the exact prevalence rates of disorders among populations of torture survivors is still very much limited. For example, we do not know to what extent the results of the studies among Nepali-speaking Bhutanese refugees generalize to native Nepalese torture survivors. Nevertheless, to the extent that our data are generalizable, our population-based research suggests a need to pay attention to PTSD, (medically unexplained) persistent pain, and (somatoform) dissociative disorders among torture survivors. Even in the West, treatment outcome researchers still have not identified empirically-supported effective treatment for the latter two disorders (Chambless et al., 1996). Treatment outcome research for complaints related to these disorders is needed.

A limitation of assessing disorders in terms of international classification systems, such as the *ICD-10*, is the possibility of missing local categories of distress (Kleinman, 1977). In 1997, among the Bhutanese refugees, an epidemic of medically unexplained illness ("mass hysteria") occurred, involving fainting and dizziness. Our research shows that history of trauma was one of the predicting factors that placed people at risk during this epidemic (Van Ommeren et al., in press). Thus the finding that trauma is a risk factor for mental health may generalize beyond *ICD* or *DSM* disorders into local illness categories.

CLINIC DATA ON HELP-SEEKING NATIVE NEPALESE TORTURE SURVIVORS

Demographic Information

In 1999, 680 torture survivors were treated at CVICT clinics. Out of 680, 407 (60%) were native Nepalese torture survivors who sought help from CVICT for the first time. Of 407 new clients, more men (n = 324; 80%) than women (n = 83; 20%) sought help from our services. Eighteen (4%) were younger than 15 years and 21 (5%) were older than 60 years. The vast majority (n = 368; 90%) were between 15 and 60.

CVICT has three clinics. The main clinic is in Kathmandu and the two subcenters are in Biratnagar and Nepalgunj, respectively in East and West Nepal (see Figure 1). Each of the three clinics received between 130 and 140 clients in 1999. The clinics did not vary much in terms of age and gender distribution of clients. However, the 3 clinics differed in terms of ethnicity of its clientele. While the clinic in Kathmandu treated mostly high caste Hindus living in the hills (n=109; 79%), the clinic in Nepalgunj treated mostly people belonging to the ethnic groups living in southern Nepal (n = 100; 75%). The client population at the clinic in Biratnagar was more evenly distributed in terms of ethnicity.

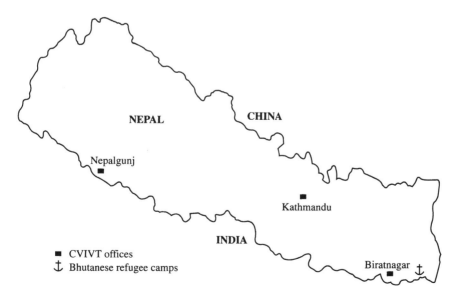

Figure 1. Map of Nepal with locations of the Centre for Victims of Torture Nepal (CVICT) clinics and the Bhutanese refugee camps.

Torture Experience and Presenting Complaints

Almost all of the torture was reported to have been perpetrated by Nepal's police and army. However, in Nepalgunj, 32 people (24%) and, in Kathmandu, 12 people (9%) reported having been tortured by Maoists. The three most common forms of torture reported by the 407 survivors are beatings on various body parts, verbal torture (e.g., threats), and deprivation (e.g., insufficient food). The torture inflicted by police on accused Maoist-leaders has been particularly brutal in terms of number and types of techniques.

Most of the complaints reported by help-seeking Nepalese native torture survivors involve somatic pain. If we define a prevalent complaint as one that is presented by more than 10% of the clients, then more than half (n=7) of the 13 prevalent complaints in 1999 concerned somatic pain (Center for Victims of Torture Nepal, 2000). Many somatic pain complaints among our clients remain medically unexplained after examinations and investigations. The frequent presentation of medically unexplained (psychosomatic, functional) complaints may be because of a variety of reasons: Limited knowledge about the body's functioning and belief that the body has been damaged leads Nepalese survivors to attribute any pain to torture (Sharma & Van Ommeren, 1998). Also, many local people are not aware that help can be offered for mental distress. Common beliefs are that mental distress, in contrast to bodily distress, is not serious unless you're mad (i.e., display psychotic behavior) and that one should be strong enough to deal with mental distress.

In addition to pain, survivors often present affective symptoms and vegetative symptoms (such as sleep disturbance, loss of appetite, and weakness) (Center for Victims of Torture Nepal, 2000). Interestingly, in contrast to what one would expect from our population-based research findings, simultaneous presentation of PTSD re-experiencing, avoidance, and hyperarousal symptomatology is not often identified in the clinic. As we will argue next, this may be because CVICT does not systematically check for PTSD symptomatology for every client who seeks help. Rather, so far, emphasis has been given to the symptoms that are most meaningful to the client—which tend to be somatic symptomatology.

The absence of help-seeking through presentation of PTSD symptomatology may be interpreted as meaning that the PTSD concept has little relevance (i.e., low content validity) to the mental health of Nepalese torture survivors. However, our interpretation is as follows: Help-seeking behavior is likely influenced by expectations of help available, and help-seekers who do not expect treatment to be available for a certain symptom (e.g., anxiety) are unlikely to present that symptom. Moreover, as mentioned above, if people focus on the somatic aspects (such as body pain) of a psychosocial problem (such as traumatization), they are less likely to present psychological aspects (such as anxiety) even though they may experience much psychological distress. Considering that substantial PTSD rates have been identified in various cultures (Marsella et al., 1996) and not withstanding cultural variations (Marsella et al.), we believe that PTSD is a relevant concept for transcultural research and practice. Nevertheless, so far, in our clinic, our focus has been on presenting complaints, which typically are somatic complaints by survivors who focus on and expect treatment for somatic complaints. We are currently planning to conduct a study to identify the prevalence of PTSD symptoms among help-seekers who present somatic complaints only.

STRUCTURING SERVICES FOR TORTURE SURVIVORS

In this section, we will describe (a) the structure of CVICT's previous community-based health service for tortured Bhutanese refugees, (b) the training and supervision of Bhutanese refugee counselors, (c) the structure of CVICT's current health services for native Nepalese torture survivors, and (d) the training and supervision of native Nepalese counselors.

Structure of Community-Based Project in The Bhutanese Refugee Camps

Background. CVICT became initially involved with the Bhutanese refugees in 1991, when most of the refugees arrived from Bhutan. At that time, CVICT organized and provided emergency medical care for refugees settling haphazardly at the banks of two large rivers in eastern Nepal. Because of observations made during medical missions, CVICT felt the need for specialized treatment for torture survivors, including women raped by Bhutanese soldiers or police.

In 1992, CVICT launched a program to support female torture survivors and selected female volunteer helpers from among the refugees. These volunteers were trained in basic communication and counseling skills and in maintaining confidentiality. The women worked through informal channels, going from hut-to-hut to identify and befriend the torture survivors. These volunteers were supported by counseling supervisors, social workers and medical personnel from CVICT. The volunteers' main task in the initial stage was to serve as a link between existing facilities and persons in pain. One advantage of this approach was that the volunteers, being Bhutanese, shared a similar background and could, therefore, better relate to clients than would be possible for native Nepalese helpers. Furthermore, these Bhutanese refugee volunteers were readily available in the camps.

As of January 1994, an integrated community based program for both male and female torture survivors was initiated. Male and female community health workers (CHWs) were hired and trained in listening and problem-solving skills, relaxation exercises, and yoga. A monthly medical clinic, which included a female doctor for female torture survivors, was organized with the help of the volunteers and some Bhutanese human rights organizations. The cases that were too difficult to manage at the camp level were referred to CVICT's clinic in Kathmandu, which is a 1-day bus trip from the camps. The monthly medical clinic program, however, posed two drawbacks: (a) they served only a few people at a time, and (b) the expense was high.

Community-Based Rehabilitation Program. In March 1994, on the basis of repeated requests by refugee organizations, CVICT signed an agreement with the United Nation High Commission of Refugees (UNHCR), the agency responsible for the Bhutanese refugee camps, to become an implementing partner and start a community-based rehabilitation program for torture survivors. Within the UNHCR-coordinated aid structure, CVICT was given the responsibility for the care of all torture survivors in the camps. The program consisted of 1 doctor (who also served as local project director), 2 counseling field supervisors (1 nurse-counselor and 1 psychologist [B. N. P.]), a health assistant (i.e., a paramedical worker) for each of the 6 camps, and 30 CHWs. Except the doctor and psychologist, all CVICT field staff were Bhutanese refugees.

CVICT used the following case management procedure in the camps: Help-seeking torture survivors were either referred to CVICT by community leaders or were identified by a CHW. A trained staff member, either a CHW or a supervisor, then completed a screening format that included identification of the patient, history, and presenting problems. After screening and documentation, the case was presented to the team, including community health workers, a health assistant, a counseling field supervisor, and the doctor. The team jointly assessed the case. On the basis of this assessment, the case was subsequently managed in the camps. The CHWs would usually provide counseling. The doctor visited each of the camps approximately one day a week and was responsible for general medical care and prescription of medication. The health assistants treated minor medical problems and monitored medication. Professional assistance from a consultant psychiatrist was sought every month for the treatment of cases with complex or severe psychiatric disorder. As before, difficult cases were referred to the CVICT clinic in Kathmandu or to hospitals for investigation, management, or both. On the basis of need and availability, some torture survivors were sent for participation in skills development and income generation programs, organized by two NGOs, namely, Oxfam UK and Bhutanese Refugee Aid for Victims of Violence (BRAVVE).

By April 1997, CVICT had provided treatment to approximately half of the 2,520 Bhutanese refugees torture survivors. The other half never sought help. By 1997, the caseload had decreased to about 200 clients seeking CVICT services. The UNHCR asked CVICT to hand-over the 200 service seekers to be cared for through the existing basic medical facilities provided by Save The Children Fund United Kingdom (SCF-UK; also an implementing partner NGO of the UNHCR). To facilitate the hand-over, CVICT provided a ten-day counseling training to the SCF-UK health staff. As we shall argue later, in hindsight, we believe that the impact of our training was limited, because of the lack of proper follow-up supervision.

Training and Supervising Bhutanese Refugee Paraprofessionals

Training of paraprofessionals is becoming one of the main components of psychosocial programming for traumatized people in low-income countries. Teaching basic psychosocial counseling skills is challenging, because these basic skills are, for a large part interpersonal skills (e.g., active listening, attending, responding with empathy, probing, encouraging, self-disclosure, brainstorming, focusing, challenging) (Egan, 1994). Even though it is easy to explain the basic counseling process, instilling good long-term counseling habits is much more difficult. As is well-known among counseling and psychotherapy educators in the West, regular and thorough supervision is necessary to ensure lasting effects of training. However, when counseling training takes place outside the West, the supervision component is typically neglected. In this section, we will discuss CVICT's efforts to train Bhutanese refugee professionals. A recurring theme is the observation that counseling skills are only gained after field supervision.

CVICT provided a combined six weeks of training in 1994 and 1995 to the CHWs and health assistants. The training for CHWs primarily focused on counseling skills, mental health, first-aid, relaxation, and case discussions. The training for health assistants focused on mental health as well as general and forensic medicine. All staff underwent an orientation on human rights and local law. The six weeks of training was not enough to instill basic counseling skills in the paraprofessionals, because most trainees had difficulties refraining from advising, lecturing, suggestive questioning, and communicating their own explanations for clients' problems. However, after the training, it was easier for the field supervisors to show and teach paraprofessionals how to counsel.

As part of its ongoing collaboration with the Transcultural Psychosocial Organization, CVICT conducted another training program for the same group of CHWs and health assistants in 1996. This training was based on the WHO/UNHCR manual *Mental Health of Refugees* (De Jong & Clarke, 1994). A core group of CVICT staff consisting of doctors, counselors, social workers, and psychologists studied the manual. Irrelevant parts of the manual were adapted or deleted. Subsequently, the manual was translated into Nepali by CVICT's consulting psychiatrist, Dr. N. M. Shrestha. On the whole, the manual was perceived by the core group as a very useful resource for community workers, because the manual is simply written and covers core content. Adapting the training to the paraprofessionals' level and using multiple role plays, however, appeared essential to ensure learning of core content.

The ten-day training program for CHWs covered the content of the manual: basic listening skills, problem solving, stress management, progressive relaxation, managing functional complaints, understanding and treating mental illness and alcoholism, collaborating with traditional healers, problems of refugee children, and helping torture and rape survivors. The training was conducted for groups of 20 to 25 people at one time. Though the total program covered 10 days, it was split into two 5-day sessions with two weeks in between sessions. This split enabled the participants to use what they had learned during the first five days and then come back for the second part with that experience. During the training, it became clear that the use of technical words confused participants. Explaining the terms using local idioms, metaphors and local situations increased understanding. Most classes focused on group activity and sharing in order to make learning interesting and help the facilitators understand what the participants were learning. After the training, the facilitators felt that classes of 25 people had been too large. Moreover, although ten days was sufficient to cover all information, it was not sufficient to instill the counseling skills necessary to implement the new knowledge. As mentioned earlier, field supervision after training is the essential ingredient to develop such skills.

The two counseling field supervisors, the nurse-counselor and the psychologist, visited each of the camps at least once a week and supervised the health assistants and CHWs. The supervisors checked all the individual records of clients. The supervisors also observed counseling sessions and provided the CHWs with suggestions to enhance skills. During these supervision visits, the CHWs were also encouraged to present cases and to debrief. This mode of supervision provided an environment in which the CHWs could learn from colleagues and, as far as we could tell, it was quite successful in increasing the skills of motivated CHWs. Nevertheless, not all CHWs were motivated or dared to show their weaker sides. It was a continuous challenge for supervisors to instill comfort about being supervised.

The CHWs' educational background ranged from three to ten years of formal education. The more educated CHWs were easier to train but had a tendency to seek and find better paying jobs outside the project. It was found that although previous education was important for the training of more abstract concepts, the most important factors were sensitivity and motivation. Indeed, one of the best-performing CHWs only had a Grade three education.

As mentioned above, in the context of handing-over the project to SCF-UK, the aforementioned training of the manual *Mental Health of Refugees* was also provided to the 117 primary health care refugee paraprofessional staff of SCF-UK. However, in hindsight we are less satisfied with the results of this effort. After the training, supervision was very difficult to arrange, because the trainees were not staff of our organization, and SCF did not have the capacity to provide necessary supervision. Although we did have several large follow-up/supervision meetings after the training, CVICT was not able to give individual field supervision. Without follow-up supervision, counseling training can waste time and resources.

Structure of Current Health Services for Native Nepalese Torture Survivors

Barriers to Access to Services. Most of Nepal's injured or distressed native torture survivors do not seek help for a combination of reasons. First, those torture survivors who are threatened by the police do not feel safe enough to talk about what happened. Second, as mentioned above, since there is no custom to seek help for mental distress other than from traditional healers, survivors are likely to seek help only if they experience physical distress. Third, Nepalese police usually release survivors only after obvious wounds have healed. Fourth, due to mountains and poverty, the country has an extremely poor infrastructure, which inhibits access to health care services. (A Nepalese who lives in the remote mountainous regions may take five days by foot and a day by bus to reach an urban area with modern health care facilities. Moreover, during the monsoon, landslides hinder movement.) Fifth, modern health care services are considered expensive, and the existence of free treatment at CVICT is not known to most torture survivors. Sixth, many Nepalese torture survivors experience stigma about having been in contact with police (Besch et al., 2001) and therefore may feel inhibited to seek help.

The Clinics. As mentioned in the introduction, CVICT has been providing medical and psychosocial services to torture survivors and their families since 1990. The main CVICT clinic is situated in Kathmandu. CVICT has currently two regional clinics in eastern and western Nepal, respectively (see Figure). These sub-centers provide general medical care and counseling for local survivors. As with the Bhutanese refugees, complex cases are referred to the Kathmandu clinic.

The Kathmandu clinic has simple medical diagnostic facilities, counseling rooms, physiotherapy, and a separate room for relaxation exercises. There is no shelter for the survivors. Torture survivors get information about the clinic through human rights activists and organizations, political parties, human rights fact-finding teams, people who participated in training organized by CVICT, CVICT mobile clinics, CVICT's nation-wide bulletins, and, especially, through previous clients. The majority of clients come from outlying districts, reaching the clinic after a very long journey, involving a lengthy bus journey, sometimes a few days of walking, or occasionally both.

CVICT aims to create a warm and safe environment at its clinics. Display of medical devices is minimized in the doctor's room to avoid possible reminders of torture. Also, there are no pictures or drawings of torture in the clinic. The counseling rooms are comfortable with glass to allow clients to see outside the room. To build trusting relationships and to avoid unnecessarily reminders of the torture, no uniforms are allowed, i.e., none of the doctors wear white coats. (Although torture by doctors is uncommon in Nepal, doctors have been accomplices in terms of manufacturing records.) Staff are trained to respect all clients. Considering the torture and Nepal's enormous class and caste distinctions, providing respect is very important.

Although survivors can refer themselves to CVICT, CVICT has recently started to ask for supporting documents or referrals from known persons to prevent misappropriation of services. However, enough flexibility exists so that services are not denied to apparent genuine survivors who lack supporting documents.

Case Management in the Clinics. As with the Bhutanese refugees, CVICT uses a casework model to help native torture survivors. On arrival, a patient is assigned to one counselor (i.e., a psychologist, a social worker, or a nurse or health assistant trained in counseling) who takes responsibility for the case. An initial interview is then held during which the client is told about CVICT and what it offers. The counselor subsequently documents demographic information and the history of imprisonment and torture. To reduce potential stress for the client, the information is sometimes documented over various sessions. At intake, clients are not pressured to tell all the details of the torture. The counselors inquire about accommodation and food and check whether the client feels physically safe in Kathmandu. Financial support for meals is provided to those who need it, and contact is made with concerned organizations to house those in need.

Each client undergoes extensive physical examinations. A counselor is usually present during the doctor's investigations and plays an active role in planning and implementing treatment. When necessary, clients are referred for more tests to nearby hospitals. For those with medical and psychosocial problems, counseling is carried out alongside the medical treatment, with the client coming in for various sessions. Occasionally, when clients need to be hospitalized, counselors and volunteers regularly visit and hold consultations with doctors and nurses. At CVICT, physiotherapy is offered when deemed useful. Short-wave diathermy has been found useful in terms of treating joint and muscle problems of clients.

As with the treatment of Bhutanese refugees, CVICT's consultant psychiatrist provides care for clients with severe mental disorder. Most of such clients want and receive medication. Moreover, CVICT gives emotional support and information to their families. In the future, CVICT hopes to organize training and supervision in brief family therapy for its counselors. Currently most of the counseling service provided at CVICT is individual counseling.

Counseling. Long term psychotherapy is typically impossible because most clients are farmers from afar and cannot stay for treatment for a long time. Hence, counselors see clients with psychosocial problems as often as possible during the limited time that they are in Kathmandu, with an estimated average of two to three sessions during a 1-week stay. When the problem is more or less satisfactorily managed, clients often do not want to endure strenuous travel for a follow-up visit. Nevertheless, most clients do return when follow-up appointments are scheduled. Because of the clients' short stay, the range of interventions that can be implemented is limited. Counseling at CVICT may be described as follows:

Gaining Understanding of Illness Experience Before a decision can be made on how to help, the client needs to be understood from his or her perspective. Western textbooks often focus on the importance of assessment of psychopathology, presenting problems, the client's current life setting, personal history, and family history. Even though all of these areas are important, at CVICT, the counselors are being encouraged to pay special attention to understand what medical anthropologists call *illness experience* (Kleinman, Eisenberg, & Good, 1978). Illness experience includes: (a) clients' and community perceptions of the causes, nature, severity, and consequences of the illness (e.g., *"Because of last year's torture my blood vessels are broken, causing my leg to hurt. I will probably die because of my broken blood vessels. I am weak, I cannot work, and I am therefore useless. People in my village look down on me, because I am weak, and because I do not work."*) and (b) reasons for seeking help and expected outcomes (e.g., *"I traveled here to get pills for my broken vessels. The pills will heal my vessels but I will remain weak."*). Counselors are encouraged to use variations of questions phrased by Kleinman et al. to elicit illness experience, such as *"What do you think has caused your problem? ... What do you think your sickness does to you? How does it work? ... What do you fear most about your sickness?"* (p. 256). In addition, counselors use questions of our local adaptation of the Explanatory Model Interview Catalogue (EMIC; Weiss 1997), which was used during a recent study into illness experience among Nepalese help-seeking torture survivors (Besch et al., 2001). In short, the counselors are taught to use a basic medical anthropological approach to understand clients' illness experience before proceeding to focus on problems and symptoms.

Problem-Management Influenced by Lazarus and Folkman's (1984) work, we distinguish between problem-focused coping (i.e., problem-solving) and problem-impact-focused coping (i.e., the problem situation cannot be reduced or resolved,

Table 1. Resolving Medically Unexplained Somatic Pain: Flexibly Implementing Tasks[a]

Task	Description of task
1. Understanding	Establishing working relationship. Obtain description of pain and a typical pain day. Identify disability. Identify client's attributions (explanations) for the pain, worst fears, and expected treatment. Use empathy. Ensure that client feels understood. Is pain client's personal or sociocultural idiom of expressing distress? Interview relatives if possible.
2. Examination	Refer for medical examination and investigation.
3. Examination results	Collaborate with medical examiner while giving results. Inform client of good news that there is no serious disease. Never say: "*nothing is wrong.*" Acknowledge presence of symptom and suffering. Avoid unnecessary further tests, even if client insists.
4. Client reaction to examination	Elicit client's reaction to news that medical examination showed no serious disease.
5. Understand details of client's explanation for pain	Explore client's explanation for suffering and the client's detailed perception of damage in the body. If the client says "*you are the doctor, you should know*", be persistent and explain that to help best you need to understand the client's view of the "damaged" body. Identify client's understanding of anatomy, physiology, and traditional-folk conceptualizations of the body and suffering in general.
6. Correcting incorrect medical explanations	Educate client if the client has incorrect understanding of anatomy or physiology. Does the client have questions? Do not argue with client.
7. Reattribution	Assess if client has significant anxiety, grief, or sadness. If so, explain in simple words how bodily sensations can be related to such feelings. For example, discuss—as appropriate—relations between: (a) worry—stomach ache, (b) demoralized and believing that body is damaged—body pain, (c) minor chest wall pain—fear of heart attacks, and (d) worry—muscle tension, body ache, and headache. Does the client have questions? Do not argue with client. Avoid using psychiatric terminology.
8. Avoid medication	Tell the person firmly that medicine will not help. Unless the client is also clearly depressed, or has severe tension headaches, do not give psychotropic medication. Do not reinforce the view that something is wrong with the body through placebo treatment.
9. Bridging	Try to bridge discussion to psychosocial aspects of life. For example, (a) *"When does it hurt most?" "What are you thinking or doing at that time?"*, (b) Ask when problem started, and explore if it may relate to any stressors, (c) Ask about successes and failures trying to self-manage pain, (d) Ask about impact of pain on person's life, and explore, (e) Ask what family and community think of this pain, and explore reinforcing beliefs and social stigma, (f) Ask if the person knows other people with similar problem. What is their story? Is the client identifying with somebody else? (g) Explore worst fears relating to problem not being treated the way client had hoped, (h) Assess current

	problems in client's life spheres [family, children, work, community]. Are these problems likely related to the pain experience? (j) Start discussing emotions. (e.g., *"you look sad"*). Be empathic.
10. Problem-management counseling	If any significant personal or social problems are present, counsel to solve (or cope better) with these problem situations. Counseling may involve family or may lead to the decision to see a traditional healer when the problem situation is in the spiritual sphere.
11. Relaxation training	Consider training client in relaxation (e.g., progressive muscle relaxation, guided imagery).
12. Trauma	If symptom appears to be trauma-related (e.g., pain as a trauma reexperiencing symptom, a body memory), help client cope better with trauma, as appropriate.
13. Anxiety, depression, grief	The body pain may be bodily sensations associated with anxiety, depression, or grief. Counsel for anxiety, depression, or grief, as appropriate.
14. Ways of coping	Brainstorm together on ways to better manage pain. If the person has become inactive, encourage the person to gradually become more active.

[a]This list of tasks integrates experiences at CVICT with approaches advocated by: Gask, De Jong, and Sell (1994), De Jong (personal communications, August 22, 1999), Kleinman, Eisenberg, and Good (1978), Sharpe, Peveler, and Mayou (1992), Goldberg et al. (1989), and Creed and Guthrie (1993).

but strategies can be devised to reduce the impact of the problem). We use the term *problem-management* for the process of working together with the client to identify and implement strategies for either (a) resolving or reducing the problem situation or (b) managing the impact of the problem situation.

Torture survivors, once they are released from prison, often face many serious personal and social problems, such as unemployment, lack of income, social isolation, realistic fear of persecution, stigma of having been in jail, conflict within the survivor's political party, changed relationships with family and community. These problems often lead to emotional and associated bodily distress. The Nepalese torture survivor will then present their medically unexplained somatic distress in the clinic, expecting medical intervention, such as medication, X-rays, or injections. Once the doctor considers the somatic distress to be without organic cause, the helper's task is to see whether the somatic distress is accompanied by emotional distress that is caused by a problem situation in the client's life. If a problem situation appears to be a contributing factor to the emotional and somatic distress, then counselors use a problem-management approach.

Various problem-management approaches are available in the literature (D'Zurilla, 1986; Egan, 1994; Gath & Mynors-Wallis, 1997)—some of which have been shown to be effective in rigorous research in the West (e.g., Gath & Mynors-Wallis, 1997). CVICT counselors have been trained in Egan's (1994) problem-management approach, a framework that emphasizes the flexible implementation of the following overlapping and interacting tasks: (a) helping clients identify, explore, and clarify their problem situations and unused opportunities, (b) helping clients identify what they want in terms of realistic goals that are based on an understanding of problem situations and opportunities within the sociocultural context, (c) helping clients develop strategies for accomplishing realistic goals, and (d) helping clients act on what they learn throughout the helping process through goal-accomplishing action. Attending, empathic listening, probing, challenging, and brainstorming are the core communication skills needed for successful implementation of this framework.

This type of pragmatic framework has a distinct North-American flavor, especially when implemented in a linear manner (Ivey, Ivey, & Simek-Morgan, 1993). The framework is based on two assumptions that are widespread in modern western psychotherapy, namely, (a) systematic approaches to helping (e.g. therapy protocols) are beneficial, and (b) helping is most efficient if the helper aids the client in identifying and implementing ways of coping. Even though these assumptions are non-native, both Nepalese counselors and clients appear comfortable with this approach. Nevertheless, problem-management counseling can be enhanced through understanding of local ways of successful problem-management.

Symptom Management To manage symptoms, the following four specific types of interventions are used at CVICT: (a) emotional support, (b) relaxation, (c) reattribution through education, and (d) exposure therapy.

Emotional Support Emotional support involves mostly listening, empathy, encouragement, and communicating understanding of the clients' feelings and point of view. Variations of aforementioned Kleinman et al.'s (1978) and Weiss' (1997) medical anthropology questions are very useful to enhance understanding. During the earlier years of CVICT, emotional support was the main psychosocial intervention. Emotional support may lead to remoralization, resulting in reduced symptoms and relief of distress (Frank & Frank, 1991).

Relaxation CVICT uses both western and traditional relaxation methods. Frequently used Western relaxation methods include progressive muscle relaxation, deep breathing, and guided imagery. Certain yoga *asanas* (postures) are used for low mood, while other asanas are used for back and pelvic problems reported by rape survivors. Of note, even though yoga is a Hindu construct, for many Hindu villagers, yoga is as foreign as progressive muscle relaxation.

Reattribution through Education Reattribution through education (cf. Goldberg, Gask, & O'Dowd, 1989) has been useful when helping Nepalese torture survivors cope with medically unexplained pain. As mentioned before, the vast majority of medically unexplained pain is interpreted by clients as physical disease or injury (cf. Van Ommeren, Sharma, Makaju, Thapa, & de Jong, 2000). These interpretations are frequently the result of clients' unsuccessful attempts to understand their body in terms of biomedicine. Once the CVICT counselors fully understand the details of their clients' inaccurate medical explanations, the counselors rectify the clients' misperceptions of biomedicine.

Counselors do not use such reattribution approach for those clients who use spirituality to explain their body pain. In such instances, counselors try to discuss matters within the clients' worldview (cf. Frank & Frank, 1991), providing emotional support and encouraging culture-sanctioned interventions, such as traditional healing and *puja* (worship). However, most clients report medical explanations rather than spiritual explanations, because most clients tend to consider CVICT as a health clinic where one is expected to present medical rather than spiritual problems. Second, client have access to traditional healers all over Nepal, and are likely to have already sought help from traditional healers if they have perceived a spiritual cause.

It is not uncommon for clients to give multiple explanations for suffering, involving spiritual, sociopolitical, and inaccurate biomedical explanations. For example, a somewhat anxious male client may misattribute his stomach aches to broken nerves and cancer. Furthermore, he attributes the broken nerves to police torture, for which he blames a local politician who has left the area. He attributes his overall misfortune to having angered a God. Treatment may include: (a) a medical examination and relevant investigations followed by the good news that there is no serious disease or injury, (b) education that his nerves are not broken, (c) reattribution, i.e., explaining why many people experience stomach pain when feeling anxious, (d) emotional support for his feelings towards the local politician. Moreover, (e) the client's perception of having angered a God is approached as a problem situation to be managed. After brainstorming for solutions, the client may decide to appease the God by visiting Pachupatinath, Nepal's most holy Hindu temple in Kathmandu. Table 1 shows our guidelines for managing medically unexplained pain.

Exposure-Based Interventions Treatments involving exposure are most likely to reduce trauma-related symptoms according to western treatment-outcome literature (Van Etten & Taylor, 1998). Counselors have been taught in the basics of Direct Therapeutic Exposure (De Jong, 1994) but seldom implement this approach because clients come from afar and stay too short to start this involved treatment. Moreover, as we will discuss later, few clients are willing to engage in this therapy. For this reason, CVICT has interest in alternative approaches, which also include an exposure component.

Alternative Approaches The counselors occasionally use two alternative interventions, particularly (a) Eye Movement Desensitization and Reprocessing (EMDR; Shapiro, 1995), which is a new approach involving a variety of procedures, including therapist-directed alternating sensory stimulation coupled with brief exposure of trauma memories and related associations, and (b) techniques based on energy psychology, which are highly alternative techniques based on the assumption that, by tapping on various body parts while focusing on the traumatic memory, one can undo emotional distress, which is assumed to be caused by an imbalance in hypothesized energy meridians in the body (e.g., Craig & Fowlie, 1997).

Several CVICT helpers have been keen to apply these new techniques. These new approaches are interesting for work outside the West for various reasons. First, these approaches appear to deliver rapid relief. Rapid relief is expected by clients who often can only attend few sessions and who have been conditioned to expect rapid relief after treatment by shamans. Although CVICT has no long-term data on the efficacy of its use of these new techniques, they appear to facilitate therapeutic relationship building, rapid subjective relief of distress, improved sense of well-being, remoralization, and symptom reduction. Second, these alternative approaches involve physical actions (eye movements, hand tapping) that may be experienced as ritual. Local people have been conditioned to experience healing through combinations of animistic, Hindu, or Buddhist rituals (and through herbal and western medications), but they typically do not know or believe that healing may potentially occur through talking. Talking is not considered treatment by most people in Nepal: psychotherapy is for many an unknown construct. Third, the manuals of these approaches provide clear guidelines to counselors who often communicate discomfort with the ambiguity of conventional western counseling guidelines. Fourth, unlike many cognitive-behavioral therapies, these alternative approaches do not involve homework assignments. In our experience, most Nepalese clients are not interested in therapy-related homework (cf. De Jong, 1999). Fifth, unlike cognitive therapy, these alternative approaches do not involve the difficult task of eliciting and challenging clients' distorted thinking. Sixth, unlike exposure therapy, the client is not required to tell the details of the torture or to repeatedly relive the details of the worst moment of it. In our experience, clients are not easily convinced to talk about the details of their trauma because they neither understand nor agree that such conversation will give long-term relief. The strong cultural belief is that it is best not to try to think about painful memories. Seventh, paraprofessionals can learn these approaches easier than more complex conventional therapy. (Nevertheless, before learning these approaches, counselors *need* to have solid basic skills and substantial experience in helping trauma survivors.)

Several CVICT counselors have been able to selectively apply these alternative techniques within a supportive and problem-management approach to helping. However, the techniques are applied very conservatively. So far, EMDR has almost only been used when the following three conditions apply: the client clearly wants treatment for PTSD re-experiencing symptoms, the client is emotionally stable, and the client is not leaving town within a day after treatment. Although such conservative approach leads to only occasional use, results appear consistent with EMDR's overall very positive treatment outcome literature

(Van Etten & Taylor, 1998). An EMDR protocol for pain management exists (Grant, 1998), and, CVICT will field test it in the near future.

Training and Supervising Native Nepalese Counselors

The original native Nepalese counselors at CVICT include two nurses, a health assistant, and a social worker. After an initial training at the International Rehabilitation Counsel for Torture Victims in Denmark in 1992, they received a 1-week training by an Australian psychologist and a 2-week training by two American psychologists. As a result of these training occasions, the counselors adapted a person-centered approach to helping, emphasizing problem-management, relaxation, and, especially, emotional support. After this training, the counselors occasionally received additional training by a range of foreign mental health professionals who often used part of their holiday time in Nepal to train CVICT staff. In addition, counselors were able to attend a few short training programs abroad. Overall, the collective impact of this diverse training was very positive. By 1996, the CVICT counselors had developed into confident helpers with strong basic skills.

Between 1996 and 1998, the Amsterdam-based Transcultural Psychosocial Organization stationed an expatriate mental health professional (M. V. O.) in Nepal to uplift the care and conduct research at CVICT, focusing mainly on the Bhutanese refugees. As part of this community-based project, the native Nepalese CVICT counselors studied and adapted the WHO/UNHCR *Mental Health of Refugees* manual (De Jong & Clarke, 1994; see the *Training and Supervising Bhutanese Refugee Paraprofessionals* section of this paper). As a result, the helpers became highly familiar with the important content of this manual. During this time, the expatriate professional was a resource person for questions, and he introduced interventions (see the *Counseling* section of this paper).

In 2000, the same expatriate professional returned to CVICT to focus on training and supervising native Nepalese counselors. This led to the development and implementation of a 4-month internship program to thoroughly train six native Nepalese counselors, who subsequently gained employment at CVICT. Five out of six counselors had been part-time Master of Arts-level clinical psychology lecturers at the local university but had not previously worked with clients.

The 4-month internship consisted of four parts: (a) a 2-week psychosocial counseling pre-practice training at CVICT in Kathmandu, (b) six 2-week rotations at the three CVICT clinics and at two local NGOs, (c) daily 1.5 hour supervision at CVICT in Kathmandu for those stationed in Kathmandu during rotations, and (d) in between rotations, regular two-to-five-day meetings at CVICT in Kathmandu for supervision, feedback, and further training.

Interns were trained in communication skills, problem-management counseling, resolving medically unexplained pain, helping children and adolescents, eliciting explanatory models and other illness experience, stress and coping, relaxation, and prioritizing problems. Moreover, the interns were trained in major mental disorders, suicide, trauma reactions, systematic desensitization for phobias, exposure therapy for trauma reactions, energy therapy techniques, and conducting focus groups. Focused lectures, minimal reading, numerous role plays, and extensive practice with clients involving daily supervision appear to have been a good combination to convert motivated, yet inexperienced Nepalese psychologists into competent helpers who can make a difference.

Since September 2000, CVICT has held a routine of 1-hour clinic-supervision meeting at the end of each day. The daily meeting is an opportunity to discuss cases, including counselor's emotional reactions to cases. During each meeting, a different staff member acts as the facilitator-supervisor. Guidelines for supervision have been drafted on the basis of our experience and on the literature (Shanfield, Matthews, & Hetherly, 1993). These guidelines are available upon request.

The work of the counselors is difficult, because many of the problems have no resolution. The CVICT counselors' ability to accept their limitations and cope with the challenges of their work appears strong. Currently, regular supervision and support seems to help them to remain focused and pragmatic. Nevertheless, during the last ten years, temporary burn-out has occasionally occurred, which may be related to factors that were present at those occasional times: (a) heavy case loads, (b) less than perfect relations among staff, and (c) counselors' realistic fear of police. Although the counselors are certainly influenced by their work, thus far, we have not observed long-term vicarious traumatization among the staff.

PREVENTION

From a public health perspective, the obvious way to prevent the health sequelae of torture is to prevent torture itself through sociopolitical action. CVICT has a strong human rights agenda and has been involved in a variety of activities to stop torture in Nepal: CVICT has written the draft of the Torture Compensation Act, which has been accepted by Nepal's parliament in diluted form. CVICT is currently lobbying for a stronger Torture Compensation Act. CVICT provides legal aid to torture survivors, which mostly focuses on obtaining compensation from the government for torture survivors. CVICT has been involved in successful public interest litigation, which has resulted in a Supreme Court order to the government to form a Human Rights Commission. Because of this and other pressures, the government formed a Human Rights Commission in 2000. Through numerous workshops and bulletins and through various media, CVICT has been involved in raising human rights awareness among the general public and among professionals from the fields of health, law, and education. CVICT currently chairs the Alliance of Human Rights and Social Justice Nepal, an alliance of major Nepali human rights organizations, and is thus involved in coordinating human rights activities. CVICT has been very active in facilitating penal reform, including training more than 90% of Nepal's prison wardens in prison management with concern for prisoners' rights. CVICT has been studying community mediation from a sociological perspective (Prasain, in preparation), and, on the basis of this research, a pilot project will start on facilitating community mediation in Eastern Nepal. CVICT organizes fact-finding missions to document torture and organizes international appeals for political prisoners and disappeared persons in collaboration with Amnesty International and the World Organization Against Torture (OMCT/SOS Torture). Finally, because violence is learned behavior and is common in Nepali schools, CVICT has developed a training program for teachers on non-violent forms of discipline. Thus, a focus on description and treatment of health sequelae of torture does not hinder meaningful action against torture and related social suffering.

Providing health services to torture survivors is sociopolitical action in itself. Through providing services, CVICT communicates to the Nepalese government that their torture is noticed, and that people are working to undo its effects.

REFERENCES

Besch, K., Van Ommeren, M., Poudyal, B. N., Jha, R., KC, R., Loksham, C., Pradhan, H., Regmi, S., Shrestha, S., & Sharma, B. (2000). *Impact of torture: A pilot study of stigma and illness experience in Nepal.* Manuscript in preparation.

Boehlein, J. K., & Kinzie, J. D. (1995). Refugee trauma. *Transcultural Psychiatric Research Review, 32*, 223–251.

Centre for Victims of Torture Nepal (2000). *Annual report 1999.* Kathmandu, Nepal.

Chambless, D. L., Sanderson, W. C., Shoham, V., Bennett-Johnson, S., Pope, K. S., Crits-Christoph, P., Baker, M., Johnson, B., Woody, S. R., Sue, S., Beutler, L., Williams, D. A., & McCurry, S. (1996). An update on empirically validated therapies. *The Clinical Psychologist, 49*, 5–18.

Craig, G., & Fowlie, A. (1997). *Emotional freedom techniques: The manual.* Novato, CA.

Creed, F., & Guthrie, E. (1993). Techniques for interviewing the somatising patient. *British Journal of Psychiatry, 162*, 467–471.

De Jong, J. T. V. M. (1994). Helping victims of torture and other violence. In J. T. V. M. De Jong, & L. Clarke (Eds.), *Mental health of refugees* (prepublication version) (pp. 147–159). Geneva: World Health Organization.

De Jong, J. T. V. M. (1999). Psychotherapie met immigranten en vluchtelingen [Psychotherapy with immigrants and refugees.] In T. J. Heeren, R. C. Van der Mast, P. Schnabel, R. W. Trijsburg, W. Vandereycken, K. Van der Velden & F. C. Verhulst (Eds.), *Jaarboek voor psychiatrie en psychotherapie 1997–2000* (pp. 220–237). Houten, the Netherlands: Bohn Stafleu Van Loghum.

De Jong, J. T. V. M. & Clarke, L. (1994). *Mental health of refugees* (prepublication version). Geneva: World Health Organization.

D'Zurilla, T. (1986). *Problem-solving therapy: A social competence approach to clinical intervention.* New York: Springer.

Egan, G. (1994). *The skilled helper: A problem-management approach to helping* (5th ed.). Pacific Grove, CA: Brooks/Cole.
Forum for Protection of Human Rights. (1991). *Dawn of democracy: People's power in Nepal.* Kathmandu, Nepal.
Frank, J. D., & Frank, J. B. (1991). *Persuasion and healing: A comparative study of psychotherapy* (3rd ed.). London: John Hopkins Press.
Gask, L., De Jong, J. T. V. M., & Sell, H. (1994). Functional complaints. In J. T. V. M. De Jong & L. Clarke (Eds.), *Mental health of refugees* (prepublication version) (pp. 41–48). Geneva: World Health Organization.
Gath, D., & Mynors-Wallis, L. (1997). Problem-solving treatment in primary care. In D. M. Clark, & C. G. Fairburn (Eds.), *Science and practice of cognitive behaviour therapy* (pp. 415–431). Oxford, England: Oxford University Press.
Goldberg, D., Gask, L., & O'Dowd, T. (1989). The treatment of somatization: Teaching techniques of reattribution. *Journal of Psychosomatic Research, 33*, 689–695.
Grant, M. (1997). *Pain control with Eye Movement and Desensitization and Reprocessing: An information processing approach.* Sydney, NSW.
Guragain, G. (1994). *Indelible scars: A study of torture in Nepal.* Kathmandu, Nepal: Centre for the Victims of Torture.
Hutt, M. (1996). Ethnic nationalism, refugees, and Bhutan. *Journal of Refugee Studies, 9*, 397–420.
Informal Sector Service Centre (2001). *Human Rights Year Book 2000.* Kathmandu, Nepal.
Ivey, A. E., Ivey, M., & Simek-Morgan, L. (1993). *Counseling and psychotherapy: A multicultural perspective* (3rd ed.). Needham Heights, MA: Allyn & Bacon.
Kleinman, A. (1977). Depression, somatization and the new cross-cultural psychiatry. *Social Science and Medicine, 11*, 3–10.
Kleinman, A., Eisenberg, L., & Good, B. (1978). Culture, illness, and care: Clinical lessons from anthropologic and cross-cultural research. *Annals of Internal Medicine, 88*, 251–258.
Lazarus, A., & Folkman, S. (1984). *Stress, appraisal, and coping.* New York: Springer.
Malpass, R. S., & Poortinga, Y. H. (1986). Strategies for design and analyses. In W. J. Lonner & J. W. Berry (Eds.), *Field methods in cross-cultural research* (pp. 47–84). Beverly Hills, CA: Sage.
Marsella, A. J., Friedman, M. J., Gerrity, E. T., & Scurfield, R. M. (Eds.) (1996). *Ethnocultural aspects of posttraumatic stress disorder: Issues, research, and clinical applications.* Washington, DC: American Psychological Association.
Prasain, D. (2001). *Community level dispute resolution in eastern rural Nepal.* Manuscript in preparation.
Shanfield, S. B., Matthews K. L., & Hetherly, V. (1993). What do excellent psychotherapy supervisors do? *American Journal of Psychiatry, 150*, 1081–1084.
Shapiro, F. (1995). *Eye movement desensitization and reprocessing: Basic principles, protocols, and procedures.* New York: Guildford.
Sharma, B., & Van Ommeren, M. (1998). Preventing torture and rehabilitating survivors in Nepal. *Transcultural Psychiatry, 35*, 85–97.
Sharpe, M., Peveler, R., & Mayou, R. (1992). The psychological treatment of patients with functional somatic symptoms: A practical guide. *Journal of Psychosomatic Research, 36*, 515–529.
Shrestha, N. M., Sharma, B., Van Ommeren, M., Regmi, S., Makaju, R., Komproe, I., Shrestha, G. B., & De Jong, J. T. V. M. (1998). Impact of torture on refugees displaced within the developing world: Symptomatology among Bhutanese refugees in Nepal. *JAMA, 280*, 443–448.
Van Etten, M., & Taylor, S. (1998). Comparative efficacy of treatments for post-traumatic stress disorder: A meta-analysis. *Clinical Psychology and Psychotherapy, 5*, 126–144.
Van Ommeren, M. (2000). *Impact of torture: Psychiatric epidemiology among Bhutanese refugees in Nepal.* Doctoral dissertation, Vrije Universiteit, Amsterdam, The Netherlands.
Van Ommeren, M., de Jong, J. T. V. M., Sharma, B., Komproe, I., Thapa, S. B., & Cardeña, E. (2001). Psychiatric disorders among Bhutanese refugees in Nepal. *Archives of General Psychiatry, 58*, 475–482.

Van Ommeren, M., Prasain, D., & Sharma, B. (2000). *Defining torture.* Manuscript submitted for publication.
Van Ommeren, M., Sharma, B., Komproe, I., Poudyal, B., Sharma, G. K., Cardeña, E., de Jong, J. T. V. M. (in press). *Trauma and loss as determinants of medically unexplained epidemic illness in a Bhutanese refugee camp.* Psychological Medicine.
Van Ommeren, M., Sharma, B., Makaju, R., Thapa, S., & De Jong, J. T. V. M. (2000). Limited cultural validity of the Composite International Diagnostic Interview's probe flow chart. *Transcultural Psychiatry, 67,* 123–134.
Van Ommeren, M., Sharma, B., Thapa, S., Makaju, R., Prasain, D., Bhattarai, R., & De Jong, J. T. V. M. (1999). Preparing instruments for transcultural research: Use of a translation monitoring form with Nepali-speaking Bhutanese refugees. *Transcultural Psychiatry, 36,* 285–301.
Weiss, M. (1997). Explanatory Model Interview Catalogue (EMIC): Framework for comparative study of illness. *Transcultural Psychiatry, 34,* 235–263.

6

Addressing the Psychosocial and Mental Health Needs of Tibetan Refugees in India

EVA KETZER and ANTONELLA CRESCENZI

> As long as human rights are violated, there can be no foundation for peace. How can peace exist in a society where some members oppress their brothers and sisters and knowingly violate their fundamental human rights? How can peace grow where truth is not allowed to surface and speaking the truth is a crime? (His Holiness the XIV Dalai Lama)

BACKGROUND

TPO-Tibet is based in McLeod Ganj/Dharamsala, which is the seat of Tibet's Government-in-exile and the temporary home and headquarters of H.H. the Dalai Lama. Approximately 7000 Tibetan refugees have settled in and around Dharamsala since their escape from Tibet.

Tibet is located along the Himalayan Mountains in the south-western part of today's China. After the Chinese invasion Tibet was divided into six parts of which five were incorporated into neighbouring Chinese provinces. What China refers to as Tibet nowadays is only a part of the original Tibet. It is called the Tibet Autonomous Region (TAR) and covers an area of about 122,200 sq. km. Lhasa is the capital and largest city. Most people live at elevations ranging from 1200 to 5100 m.

Throughout its long history, Tibet has at times governed itself as an independent state and at other times has had various levels of association with China. Regardless of China's involvement in Tibetan affairs, Tibet's internal government was for centuries a theocracy, under the leadership of Buddhist monks. Buddhism was originally introduced from India into Tibet in the 7th century. In the course of time, the Tibetan form of Buddhism evolved into four sects. The head of the largest one was named the Dalai Lama (monk with an ocean of wisdom). He was granted political power in the 1640s.

Historically religion permeated every aspect of Tibetan life. The clergy was at the top of Tibet's feudal society forming about 10% of Tibet's population. The lay population consisted of the aristocracy, land-owning farmers, nomads and landless labourers. Monasteries were the only educational institutions, thus playing a dominant role in political, religious and cultural life.

A turning point in Tibet's history came in 1949 when China invaded and occupied Tibet. Ten years later, during an uprising in Lhasa, H.H. the Dalai Lama escaped to India. Approximately 85,000 Tibetans followed him into exile in 1959. In Tibet the imposition of Chinese rule and the introduction of a communist administration marked the decades that followed. The Chinese Cultural Revolution from 1966 to 1976 was a particularly harsh time during which religious practise in Tibet was completely curtailed, temples and monasteries were destroyed and monks and nuns persecuted. The role of monastic institutions was eliminated and formal Chinese State schooling was introduced. Apart from administrative and political control, China gained economic control of Tibet. The socialist transformation of Tibet caused starvation as food shortages developed with the influx of Chinese settlers while harvests were shipped off to China. Impoverishment through land reforms affected in the first place landowners and farmers. Landowners were not only dispossessed but were also deprived of access to education. Strict Chinese control had a traumatising effect on subsequent generations.

All forms of Tibetan customs and worship, public and private were banned. Arbitrary arrests, detention, torture and executions took place in this period. Large numbers of Tibetans died in labour camps and prisons due to ill treatment and torture. They were imprisoned for participating in demonstrations against the Chinese government or simply for fighting for their basic human rights. Torture against political prisoners has been used as a method of repression since 1949 and continues to be the main form of human rights violation in Tibet to this day. Over the years Chinese torture methods have been modified and physical injuring has been shifted to psychological injuring with the aim of preventing obvious external markings.

It is estimated that 1.2 million Tibetans, about one-sixth of the total population, have died in Tibet since 1949 due to persecution, imprisonment, torture and famine and that over 6000 of Tibet's religious and cultural monuments have been destroyed (Planning Council, Central Tibetan Administration [CTA], 1994).

A change in Chinese policy began in 1979, when Beijing opened a dialogue with the Tibetan government-in-exile. During this period of liberalisation monasteries were reopened and restored but the percentage of monasteries that are active nowadays is still small and the quota of monks is fixed by the Chinese Religious Bureau. This state-run agency oversees all spiritual activity in Tibet, allocates funds for the reconstruction or renovation of monasteries, and screens aspiring monks of whom many are rejected in order to keep the quota low. Recent religious policies have focused on re-educating monks and nuns with the objective of turning Tibet into an atheist country. Atheism is believed to be necessary to promote economic development and to strengthen the anti-Dalai Lama campaign.

From 1979 onwards resistance against Chinese control which culminated in violent demonstrations and Chinese crackdowns on Tibetan monasteries and lay activists triggered new waves of refugees escaping from Tibet to India. The Tibetan exodus continues with 3000–4000 refugees escaping each year (Information from the Tibetan Reception Centre, McLeod Ganj). The main reasons for Tibetans to leave are to meet H.H. the Dalai Lama and to admit their children in a Tibetan school in exile. Political activists escape Tibet to save their lives and to be able to do more for the cause of Tibet from outside. Monks and nuns of whom many are politically active come to India to practise and study Buddhism freely. Poverty and unemployment as a result of continuing sinocisation are other reasons for Tibetans to leave their homeland.

The flight out of Tibet is a dangerous journey across the Himalayan Mountains. The most common way of escaping is to walk over the 5000–6000 m high mountain passes into Nepal. Most refugees escape during the winter months when the escape route is less guarded. At the same time it is more dangerous and strenuous because of the cold which results in many of them contracting frostbite. Almost all of the new refugees visit Dharamsala to receive the blessings of H.H. the Dalai Lama (Figure 1).

With the increasing number of new refugees, the Office of the Reception Centres was established in 1990 as a department of the Central Tibetan Administration (CTA). Its headquarters are in Dharamsala but there are branch offices in Kathmandu and Delhi. Apart from giving relief aid such as food, medical care and accommodation, the Reception Centre also assists in the admission procedure into the various refugee institutions established by the CTA. Tibetans who come to India for pilgrimage are usually well off. Yet many others arrive with hardly anything but the clothes they are wearing and their spiritual devotion to sustain them. Often they do not only suffer from the strains of a long and arduous journey and from the changes in climate and diet, but also from physical and mental health problems due to oppressive living conditions in Tibet. Some also suffer from physical and mental impairment due to torture and imprisonment. Those new refugees who are not in danger of imprisonment are encouraged to go back to Tibet after they have had an audience with H.H. the Dalai Lama or after completing a course in one of the transit schools. As they are not entitled to an RC (registration card) they have no legal status in India.

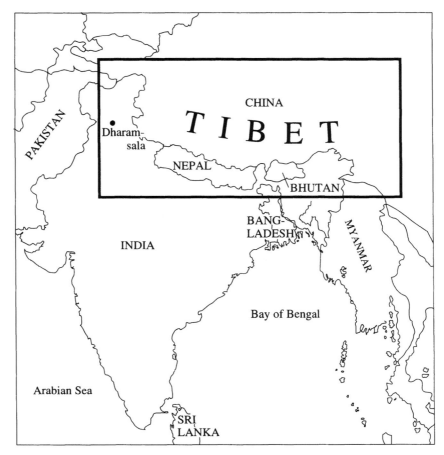

Figure 1. Map of Tibet.

Many of the first group of refugees who arrived in the early sixties landed either in transit camps or in camps building roads for the Indian government. The mortality rate was very high due to the harsh living conditions during this first stage of the refugee situation. Only about 60% of these early refugees had a chance to build a new life in exile. However, it was H.H.'s main concern to organise the refugee groups in such a way that the Tibetan identity could be preserved. The majority of the early refugees were resettled in agricultural-based areas. 54 refugee settlements have been established in India, Nepal and Bhutan since 1959 of which 26 are agricultural, 17 agro-industrial and 11 handicraft based (Planning Council, CTA, 1994). The agricultural settlements are mostly located in south India. All of the settlements set up health centres (for both allopathic and traditional Tibetan medicine), schools, temples, monasteries and co-operatives to market agricultural products as well as the products from handicraft and carpet-weaving centres. Due to the strains of population growth, insufficient agricultural yields and lack of employment opportunities, an increasing number of settlers had to resort to sweater-selling. This has resulted in many of the settlements seasonally being left with only old people and children. Today some 130,000 Tibetan refugees are living in large and small settlements in India and Nepal.

When H.H. the Dalai Lama arrived in India he pronounced the formation of the Tibetan Government-in-exile and established the Central Tibetan Administration (CTA). The CTA functions as the Tibetan Government-in-exile and is responsible for wide-ranging programs. Since 1963 the Tibetan Administration has been developing a democratic system of government. This government has not officially been recognised by the governments of the world, especially the government of India, which granted the Tibetans asylum.

Of all the departments of the Central Tibetan Administration, it is the Department of Home, which is responsible for the rehabilitation of Tibetan refugees. Other departments of the CTA involved in looking after the refugees include the Department of Security which is responsible for the identification and registration of torture survivors, and the Department of Health which is in charge of looking after the health needs of the Tibetan refugee community in India, Nepal and Bhutan. This also includes the rehabilitation of torture victims. In collaboration with the Tibetan Medical and Astrological Institute, the Department of Health is seeking to integrate modern allopathic medicine with the traditional system of Tibetan medicine. Besides a variety of health care projects such as the introduction of primary health care in all the settlements, it has set up a program to provide medical and psychological treatment as well as social support for survivors of torture. The Tibetan TPO Mental Health Care Program is a joint project of the Department of Health and TPO.

As the destruction of religious and cultural institutions in Tibet threatened to wipe out the Tibetan religious and cultural heritage, the importance of the re-establishment of monasteries in exile was realised. Many of the great monasteries in Tibet have been re-built in exile along with most of the big monastic universities in south India. Many newcomer monks have been admitted to acquire religious education, which is not available in Tibet nowadays. For Tibetan nuns it is especially in exile that religious and educational opportunities have been instituted. Tibetan society both in Tibet and in exile depends on the monastic institutions as a source of advice and consolation. Lay people go to the monasteries to have rituals performed by monks in times of crises or they consult Lamas in decision making which is still done by divination. By providing spiritual guidance and by preserving and handing down spiritual culture, monasteries and nunneries function as cultural centres.

While those Tibetans who fled Tibet after the Chinese occupation have been struggling to rebuild their lives in exile, those who stayed in Tibet have been suffering under the Chinese rule of their country. Despite the suppression of religious

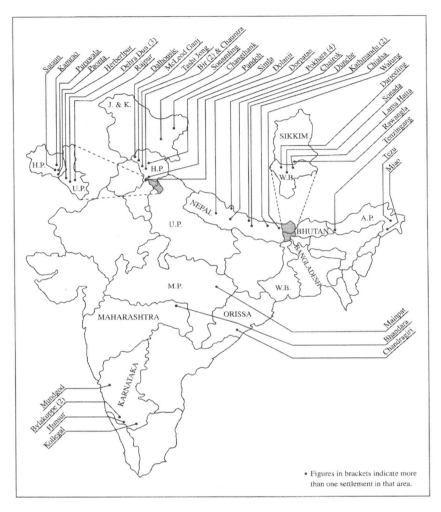

Figure 2. Map of Tibetan settlements in India and Nepal.
Courtesy: Department of Home, CTA.

practice and a lack of formally educated religious teachers, spirituality and devotion for H.H. the Dalai Lama has been kept alive in occupied Tibet (Figure 2).

After decades of living apart under very different conditions Tibetan refugees come together in exile. For all of them religion continues to be the dominant element in every day life as it has been throughout history. Their shared faith in Buddhism and H.H. the Dalai Lama sustains the common identity of all Tibetans. With this religious devotion and unfailing respect for H.H. the

Dalai Lama, the Tibetans have been coping remarkably well as a refuge community despite the ordeals they have been living through. But although the physical hardships of the 1960s and 1970s are gone, the situation is still difficult for new arrivals, many of whom suffer from mental anguish. It is the aim of TPO-Tibet to make a contribution to the wellbeing and rehabilitation of those Tibetans who suffer mentally due to the refugee situation.

DEVELOPMENT OF THE PROJECT

Introduction of Mental Health Issues to the Central Tibetan Administration (CTA)

In 1991 the first contact was made with the Department of Health. It was approached with the question whether the Tibetan Community provided any special service for survivors of torture and people with mental health problems apart from the traditional religious and medical system. After raising the issue we were told that the Tibetan traditional medical system together with Buddhist lamas had been successfully looking after people with mental problems throughout Tibet's long history and that mental health care other than in the traditional way was therefore not considered necessary. However, since 1990 many new refugees have been arriving from Tibet and settling in India, of whom some experienced torture in Chinese prisons. It became indeed a question whether the traditional medical and religious system was providing adequate care to deal with a different range of problems due to the new circumstances. The community was not only faced with the traumatic experiences of torture survivors but also with problems due to the confrontation between old and newcomer refugees. By dealing with the new refugees in every day life, we experienced that tensions had been arising from the contact between them and those who arrived many years earlier or who were born in India. Although the Tibetan government and the institutions have been putting effort into integrating the new refugees smoothly by providing them with basic facilities such as accommodation, education and work, most of these new refugees are uneducated and destitute, which leaves them confused and anxious in the daily context. Their irritable behaviour patterns, especially concerning expectations, requesting help or demanding support, are often perceived as being aggressive by the old comer refugees. Both groups agreed, however, that life in exile as well as in occupied Tibet involved much more stress than they had ever experienced. Since the newly arrived refugees were intended to integrate into the community while reducing stressful situations, it was decided to tackle the issue. With the awareness that stress had increased for both groups of refugees there was also a readiness to expand the traditional way of looking at mental health by focussing on the new situation.

Consequently there was a willingness to consider new concepts and methods on an experimental level.

In order to assess the current opinion on mental health and on the necessity of mental health care we carried out a small survey within the community during which representatives of three levels of the society were asked open questions on mental health problems. The interviewed participants involved five directors of different departments and institutions such as the Department of Health, the Tibetan Childrens' Village, the Tibetan Women Association and the Suja School. Furthermore there were four staff nurses and matrons from the Delek Hospital, the Suja School, the Tibetan Childrens' Village, one health worker, one teacher and eleven newly arrived refugees. The eleven newcomers, all of whom had experienced imprisonment and torture, were asked open questions relating to their life stories and experiences in prison as well as to their present symptoms. Their symptoms were assessed with the help of the Harvard Trauma Questionnaire, which was directly translated during the interviews. The result of the interviews showed that there five of the refugees suffered from PTSD (using a cut-off score >2.5) and the remaining six were presenting mild to moderate symptoms of PTSD.

During this first stage of assessing psychosocial and mental health concerns, the nurses were the first ones to show interest. While looking after patients, they became aware of the fact that some of the patients had mental problems associated with traumatic events, as well as problems related to the adaptation process. And they often felt unqualified to appropriately treat these patients. The members of the upper level of society, who also represent the moral standards of the Tibetan community, expressed more reservation towards the introduction of western style mental health care such as psychotherapy. The prevailing opinion was that the concept of western psychology should be combined with Tibetan philosophy in accordance with the wish of H.H. Dalai Lama and that it should only gradually be introduced into the community. Their main concern was that the community had no knowledge about psychosocial interventions and therefore not in a position to judge whether its introduction would be beneficial or even harmful. "Maybe psychotherapy will cause Tibetans to become as neurotic as some of the westerners", turned out to be a common opinion. This reluctance of the Tibetans to introduce an unknown concept of understanding and dealing with the mind was definitely justified because of their highly developed knowledge and practice of the mind established over hundreds of years. At that time we were only superfically familiar with Tibetan traditional concepts and methods. Our lack of knowledge of the healing impact of traditions became one of the challenging issues in the process of developing the project. We understood that research had to be the first step if we were going to develop and integrate a culturally adapted form of psychotherapy and psychosocial interventions, which would not replace the traditional way of coping but strengthen and complement it.

The results of our survey were presented to the Secretary of the Department of Health who subsequently decided to set up a project in co-operation with the Tibet Support Group of Copenhagen, which was going to focus on the social and mental rehabilitation of survivors of torture. In the meantime the administrator (Dr. Tsetan Sadutshang) and a resident doctor (Dr. L. McDougall) of the Tibetan Delek Hospital conducted a study with a small group of torture survivors with the aim of collecting information about torture types and sequelae, of giving proper treatment for torture survivors and giving guidelines for future treatment approaches. During this study twelve survivors of torture were interviewed and medically examined. The result showed that the physical and mental morbidity among them correlated well with the histories of imprisonment, ill treatment and torture. Based on the result of this study, TPO-Tibet was requested to do an epidemiological study among the group of newly arrived refugees in order to qualify and quantify the mental impact of torture. The government employed one person from the Department of Health to work with us as a counterpart. This research was meant to serve as a base for any implementation and further commitments towards projects of the Department of Health.

Epidemiology

For our research among newly arrived refugees we kept to the definition of the Tibetan Government concerning trauma and torture, according to which 'torture' implies having been imprisoned. Thus everybody who has been imprisoned is considered having been exposed to torture, whereas those who have been involved in political activities and managed to escape before getting imprisoned as well as those who were traumatised under Chinese rule or during their escape, are not considered having been tortured. Although we focussed on the trauma of torture in our study, we were also interested to assess how newcomer refugees were coping with their traumatic experiences and distress during the adaptation process. As research instruments we decided to use the Harvard Trauma Questionnaire and the Hopkins Symptom CheckList 25. The participants included in our research were selected according to the following criteria: (a) arrival in India between 1991 and 1995, with an equal number of participants in each year, (b) age 18 or older at the time of escape, (c) an equal number of imprisoned and never imprisoned participants, and (d) an equal number of men and women in the imprisoned and non-imprisoned groups. We compared 76 previously imprisoned with 74 matched refugees that were never imprisoned. Previously imprisoned refugees reported more anxiety than controls (76% $v.$ 50%). The groups were similar in terms of depression (58% $v.$ 54%) and total number of somatic complaints. Previously imprisoned refugees reported more traumatic events, especially torture and deprivation. Across the two samples, multivariate analyses showed that the total number of experienced traumatic events predicted both anxiety and depression. Ability to read Tibetan acted as a buffer against anxiety. Female sex and escaping by oneself were risk factors for depression (Crescenzi et al., 2001).

Adaptation of the Questionnaire to Tibetan Culture. Before we could start the research the questionnaires had to be translated, a task which took almost eight months. While producing a Tibetan version of the questionnaire, a main problem turned out to be the fact that written Tibetan is very different from spoken Tibetan and that written language is only understood by literate Tibetans. Our research population, however, consisted in the majority of illiterate Tibetans. Furthermore the Tibetan language has three main dialects which are basically three very different spoken languages. Also there were no commonly used terms in Tibetan to express emotional details. To overcome these obstacles we decided to create a questionnaire using only spoken language. Four resident Tibetan nurses were requested to translate the English question into the kind of Tibetan language they would use to ask an illiterate person in an emphatic way. Each of the four translated versions was taped and transcribed. As a next step all the versions were discussed in a focus group with the nurses until one version was agreed upon to come closest to the meaning of the original question in English. This version was presented to the members of the target group of newly arrived refugees in focus groups consisting of 6–10 people who had been selected at random. They discussed the questions and then provided examples to explain the meaning. When the group agreed on an example to reproduce the meaning of the question most appropriately, the translation of this question was accepted. If the example did not properly reflect the meaning, the question was explained and the group was requested to find alternative ways of expressing it in Tibetan. The new versions of the translated question became the subject of discussion for the next focus group. After this process of testing the translation in the focus groups, the final versions were translated back into English by four bilingual Tibetans. In this way a new Tibetan questionnaire was developed in which all rules of proper written Tibetan were broken and which was to be applied only orally. Besides overcoming the problem of illiteracy and of the different dialects in the target group we succeeded in creating a research instrument, which could equally be applied by all interviewers in the sense that the same words and examples were used for asking and explaining questions. In this way we tried to minimise inter-rater bias caused by improvised interviews, which was a concern at this stage when nobody was yet familiar with psychological concepts and terminology. As an example we provide the translation of the fourth question of the Hopkins Symptom Check List—25: "Nervousness or shaking inside".

> *sems 'tshab pa'm gzugs po nang la 'dar bsil rgyag gyi 'dug gas (final Tibetan version)*
>
> 'Nervousness' was translated as *sems 'tshab 'tshab byes*.
> *Sems* is the most colloquial word for 'mind' and was chosen instead of *blo* which is the written form; *'tshab 'tshab* means 'restless, being agitated'.

For 'shaking inside' the nurses' group agreed on the following version: 'Inside' was translated as *snying nang la*. *Snying* means 'heart'; *nang* means 'inside'. In the Tibetan concept mind is located in the area of the heart. To express the shaking sensation *grang bsil bsil* was chosen, *grang* meaning 'cold' and *bsil* meaning 'cool'. The combination of the two words means 'cool coldness in the heart'.

Focus Group 1 and the Department of Health did not understand the meaning of this expression. The translation for shaking suggested by the Department of Health was '*dar bsil rgyag* which means 'physical shivering, shaking and trembling'. *Gzugs po nang la* means 'in the body'. The literal translation of the final version, which the Department of Health proposed, was the one approved by Focus Group 3: "Is your mind restless and do you shake in the body".

The process of developing the Tibetan Questionnaire was an intense learning process for our local staff and for us. By translating they acquired a basic understanding of applying psychological concepts while we learned how 'idioms of distress' were perceived, expressed and dealt with in the traditional way. During this procedure we experienced that in a transcultural setting language becomes a central issue, especially while dealing with intricate concepts such as counselling methods. The prime focus is on the language because it is through language that mental problems are communicated. The local trainees do not only have to understand psychological processes, they also have to be able to convey them via the language and they have to be able to communicate with patients and colleagues in the health care system.

Relations with the Tibetan Department of Health

In the course of the research some of the participants proved to be in need of treatment for their symptoms and the Department of Health requested us to provide it. At that time the Department of Health was starting to offer social support to those victims of torture who had to find ways of rebuilding their socio-economic life in exile. While developing the social support structure, induction of dependency behaviour of the clients had to be prevented. In order to define an appropriate policy we had regular meetings with the staff of the Department of Health, the resident medical staff and the TPO staff. Until then the Department of Health had requested us to treat only torture victims because it was assumed that too much attention to non-ex-prisoners would imply more financial requests to the government. Another concern of the Department of Health was the stigmatising effect, which attending our clinic would have on patients in the sense that it could induce illness behaviour and secondary benefits. Because these were relevant and realistic concerns, it was difficult for us to make the administration see that for patients with psycho-social problems counselling was sufficient to help them find their own solutions. Moreover the experience proved that these patients did not demand extra social support.

We experienced that chronic psychiatric patients who frequented our clinic, although well looked after by their families, often did not receive continuous medical treatment with the result that many developed chronicity and social dysfunctioning. Yet by providing continuous psychiatric treatment their mental condition and social functioning could be helped, thus reducing the strain on their families and the community. Based on the experience that survivors of torture and psychiatric patients improved through clinical interventions, the Department of Health agreed to increase knowledge and skills in mental health care and it was decided to provide training to all health workers. At this stage TPO-Tibet had only two Tibetan employees. The Department of Health requested us not to employ any new staff because the sustainability of a long-term commitment could not be guaranteed and developing of the project was still taking place on an experimental level.

Clinic

The first outpatient clinic, which we set up, consisted of two modest and quiet rooms where people could enter anonymously. The first patients to frequent our clinic were people who had participated in the research. They included survivors of imprisonment and torture as well as non-tortured patients. After a few months the Reception Centres in Kathmandu and Mcleod Ganj started to refer torture survivors and other Tibetans suffering from mental or psychiatric problems to our clinic. Furthermore, resident Tibetans suffering from chronic psychiatric diseases, epilepsy and problems related to alcohol and drug abuse started to attend our clinic and everybody received treatment. Survivors of imprisonment and torture were presented to the Department of Health for social support in order to provide them with basic needs. Other patients with social problems were helped to find support in the existing social network. Before addressing psychological issues during the counselling, the basic needs of the patient should be provided.

In order to meet the needs of the different patients we have been applying a variety of methods. Patients who have undergone torture often present physical symptoms, which receive medical attention and further treatment if necessary. But the physical symptoms often express mental distress and usually the focus quickly shifts from physical symptoms to thoughts and feelings when these physical symptoms appear. To create a link between the physical and mental symptoms we ask our patients to keep a diary and to write down or to keep in mind what they had been doing, thinking and feeling at the time when the symptoms appeared. The patients' realisation that they are not suffering from a physical disease but that the symptoms are the result of their emotional state makes them willing to speak of their life story in more detail. This also gives a chance to gain insight into their personality structure as well as into the traumatic experiences. The patients talk about their traumatic experiences several times during counselling sessions while focussing on associated feelings, thoughts and coping behaviour. That way patients learn to be aware of their feelings and to gain control of their physical symptoms. One way of achieving this is by applying relaxation exercises, which we teach patients during their treatment. Conflicts in relationships with other people, news from Tibet or difficulties to concentrate often trigger the recurrence of symptoms. The current experiences are linked with the traumatic experiences in the counselling sessions. Thus patients get to know their patterns of reaction in such a way that they learn to interpret conflicts and to define alternative solutions. The treatment of torture victims lasts between six month to two years (Box 1).

Box 1. Tenzin Sonam

I was born in 1962 into a farmer's family. My schooling was limited to 3 months of primary education due to my family's economic situation. I helped at home until I was about 16 years old. Then I became a member of the Chinese Youth Congress and later joined the Communist Party of China. This is how I became aware of Chinese policies and of the dangers they were causing to Tibetan culture and religion. I developed the urge to do something for the protection of my own people. So I joined a group of Tibetans who were working for the freedom of Tibet. One of their activities was to put up posters which were demanding human rights, independence, the end of Chinese occupation, stating that H.H. the Dalai Lama is the political and religious leader of Tibet and criticising re-education.

During one such activity I myself put up a Tibetan flag and a poster near the public hall in my home town demanding Tibet for the Tibetans, the end of re-education and the withdrawal of the security police. I was arrested by security policemen, handcuffed and blindfolded in their van, thrown into a dark and cold room and not given a single drop of water for 24 hours. I don't remember how many times I was interrogated and each time I was beaten, sometimes with the belts of the prison authorities; I was tortured with electric batons normally used for cattle, my face and hands were burned with cigarettes, the chains around my feet and hands were pulled tight until my ankles started to bleed, I was hung from the ceiling by rope upside down, I was beaten on my head with a stick until blood was pouring into my eyes and I often fell unconscious. They wanted to know which association the poster and the flag had come from and the names of members of the association. They offered to release me immediately in return for this information but I remained silent. After 6 months of interrogation and maltreatment I was sentenced to 5 years imprisonment for counter-revolutionary activities and transferred to Drapchi prison, which is Prison No. 1 of the Tibetan Autonomous Region. I was a political prisoner, doing forced labour, with never enough food to fill my stomach and not enough warm clothes even in summer. When I was released from prison in 1995 my father had already died. I was very sad that I had not had a chance to talk to him before his death. Also it was impossible for me to find any job as an ex-political prisoner. When an anonymous letter was posted to the People's government stating 'Tibet is an independent country' and demanding human rights and freedom of speech, I was immediately suspected. I had no choice but to leave Tibet. I reached Dharamsala in 1996.

When I was admitted in the Reception Centre in McLeod Ganj my health was in a very bad state. I had constant pain in my knees due to the work I had been forced to do in prison. My vision was disturbed because I had been suffering from snowblindness on my way over the mountains although I had been using plastic bags to protect my eyes from the strong sunlight at such a high

> altitude and I had frostbite and couldn't move my fingers. I was so unhappy that I couldn't eat. I suffered from depression, sleeplessness and from something, which was diagnosed as agoraphobia.
>
> However, I was very happy to get an audience with His Holiness. The Department of Security organised my medical treatment for which I had to go as far as Chandigarh and Delhi. Many problems got better but there were still some associated with the torture I had gone through that continued to trouble me. I still couldn't hear nor see well, I was suffering from backpains and had a heart problem. I used to wake up at night with nightmares from prison and even thought about ending my life. Then I came to the TPO clinic but with a lot of resistance. I had no trust in the doctors and counsellors because the consultations reminded me of the Chinese interrogation. I think I came only because I was so desperate and wanted to try a last resource. It took weeks to build up some confidence and because my memory was so bad I used to forget my appointments. Also I didn't feel like speaking to people and remained very suspicious but I accepted the medication. I received counselling twice every week for one year.
>
> When I eventually got better I started to look for a job. There was a lot of waiting but I was lucky to get social support from the Security and Health Department. Generally my health and my whole situation had improved a lot but there were still things that I found difficult to cope with such as hearing the whistle at the bus station or seeing Indian policemen in their uniforms as this brought back memories of prison. I finally received training and soon found some work. Nowadays I am very happy.

This case demonstrates how difficult it often is for torture victims to trust anybody. Most of these patients consult traditional medical doctors and lamas for their problems while receiving counselling from us at the same time. At present victims of torture patients tend to visit our clinic when they hear of us through other patients who have been successfully treated.

Help-Seeking Patterns. For mental illness Tibetans generally first seek the advice of lamas. These mostly recommend prayers to be performed by monks in the house of the patient. The Tibetans' faith in the capacity of religious people and the effectiveness of religious practises is very strong. Rituals prove to be successful as they involve the whole family or the immediate social environment, which contributes to the nurturing of the patient. Symptoms often disappear by applying traditional practises, and rituals are usually continued over a long period of time. Lamas may also advise to seek treatment with a traditional Tibetan doctor. In cases of recurrent crises Tibetan traditional doctors recommend allopathic treatment or the family themselves seek consultation with a psychiatrist. Medication is usually given only for a short time. If religious and traditional Tibetan medical treatment or psychiatric medication is not successful, families tend to accept the mental disease or retardation of a member as their karma and bear the distressing and sometimes even violent behaviour of the patient. Mentally disturbed family members are treated like any sick people in the house, which implies that they do not have duties in the household and often sit or roam around doing nothing. Retarded children stop going to school after being diagnosed and do not get exposed to any stimulation (Box 2).

> **Box 2. Rinzin Tashi**
>
> Rinzin, 20 years old, is the first of two sons. When he was 14 his mother committed suicide. His father, who has been an alcoholic ever since he retired from the army, used to spend only 2 months a year with his family. After his mother's death Rinzin was admitted into the boarding school of his settlement and had a normal life as a student until he was 17. Then he dropped out of school because he failed his examination. Subsequently he started to develop psychotic behaviour, which became very disturbing for his community in the settlement. He was given Tibetan traditional medicine and various religious rituals were performed which were effective for a short time only. When the girl he liked refused him he developed an acute psychosis with violent behaviour. At that point the Tibetan traditional doctors recommended allopathic treatment. The settlement representative sent him to the Indian mental hospital together with his father and brother, where he was admitted for 6 weeks. With the medical treatment he soon functioned normally but the medication was discontinued when he returned to the settlement. The TPO-team who happened to be on field trip in the settlement put him back on medication and involved his father and the health worker in the responsibility for his treatment. He improved after some time and started helping in the household of his family. Six months later the family decided to send him to the army and stopped the medication, as his behaviour was consistently normal. But shortly after joining the army he developed another episode of acute psychosis and was brought to our clinic. The traditional Tibetan doctor who was also consulted for a joint assessment of his problem stated that Tibetan medicine had no cure for his disease. Then he was admitted to the Tibetan Delek Hospital where his medical treatment was resumed. Within a month he recovered from his acute symptoms and remained stable on a low dosage of neuroleptics. The family, the health worker and the representative of his settlement were informed about his disease and of the necessity to continue medication for the coming years. The health worker was instructed to check the medicine intake regularly as well as to monitor changes in his mental state. Furthermore we suggested that the patient should have a stable every day life routine, doing a simple job in his settlement. The representative gave Rinzin work in the carpet factory. Since then he has been without psychotic symptoms and functions well socially and professionally. He still performs religious rituals for his condition and says that this helps him a lot.

TPO-Tibet treats *psychiatric patients* through their acute phase. After a stabilisation of symptoms they are followed up medically and usually they receive counselling together with family members or close friends. A problem with this group of patients turned out to be that often psychiatric medication is given as long as the patient is in crisis, but discontinued as soon as the crisis seems to be over. Therefore counselling is complemented with health education so that patients and their attendants learn to understand the need for long-term medication. Also they are encouraged to learn to recognise the first symptoms of a crisis as well as the triggering factors in order to be able to seek immediate medical intervention, thus preventing an exacerbation of the condition. Rehabilitation within the family is followed by reintegration within the community.

The settlements have responded very obligingly to our suggestion to provide adapted jobs for patients and ex-patients. It has been realised that being able to contribute to the family or community increases a patient's self-confidence, which helps to improve his condition. Families have been guided to hand over small household responsibilities to their retarded children or mentally disturbed family members. Thus the community has the positive experience of seeing patients become active members.

Another category of patients visiting our clinic is people with psychosocial problems. They include: newly arrived single mothers, monks who have disrobed and married, old people who worry about their future and young Tibetans born in India who have to plan and define their future. These patients are usually successfully treated by providing with insight and problem resolving counselling (Box 3).

This story demonstrates a typical case of psychosocial problems. Traditionally Dolkar Tsering would have been helped and advised by family members but being in exile she had to rely on herself and find support through other channels.

In the Tibetan context problem resolving is a collective task carried out within the family. It can only function in a situation where the social network is intact. Yet in the refugee situation the social network has been disrupted and

---

Box 3. Dolkar Tsering

Dolkar Tsering, age 30, is a mother of three children and works in the carpet factory of her settlement. She heard about our clinic through friends. For the past two and a half years she has been suffering from severe headaches daily, mainly in the night, and has already spent a lot of her little money to consult different doctors and to pay for medicines. Physical reasons for her headaches have been ruled out. She came to India four years ago with her husband and daughter. Because her husband had been politically active they decided that it would be safer to live in India and start a business there. They soon had a second child and Tsering was pregnant with the third one when her husband went to Tibet for business. Tsering suspected he might have gone for political reasons. She has not had any news from him since he left three years ago. When we asked her what she thought had happened to her husband, she said that she was very confused. One day she worried that he might have been imprisoned and that he was suffering terrible hardship there. On that day she offered 10 Rs to the nunnery and asked for prayers for her husband. The next day she thought he had died and she felt very sad. Another day she thought he had a new wife and had abandoned her and the three children. This made her very angry. She never tried to find her husband. Through counselling she found out that she felt anxious to know the truth about his whereabouts. At the same time she understood that this confusion of thoughts and emotions was causing her headaches. She decided to face the truth and we guided and supported her through the inquiry. Meanwhile her headaches disappeared. It was eventually confirmed that her husband was living with another wife and children in Tibet. She became very angry and entered a process of mourning during which she frequented our clinic twice a month for four months. Subsequently she told her children the truth about their father and we helped her to cope with their reaction. She still has big economic problems but is able to seek and accept help from the Tibetan Government. Recently she even expressed the wish to get married again.

problem resolving is not any more done within the family or the immediate community. Due to this, especially newly arrived young Tibetans are often not able to analyse their problems and they are not prepared to make decisions concerning these problems. In such situations the clinic substitutes for the lack of trustful relationships and counselling has the aim to empower patients to make their own decisions. Also young Tibetans who are born in India and live with their parents often experience that they do not find help or advice at home. These young people who are mostly better educated than their parents have to cope with the responsibility towards their families, they have to compete professionally with the Indians and they have to be active in the freedom struggle as well as in the preservation of Tibet's culture. Some of them, who get overwhelmed by these kinds of expectations, end up doing nothing and in the worst case start using drugs. For this group of patients problem-resolving counselling has a quick and lasting effect.

Training

One of the aims of the Tibetan TPO project is the introduction of mental health care into the primary health care system. For the Tibetan exile community this implies training of the primary health care level which is the level of the health workers. They are the ones who visit patients and families in their homes and are able to detect and prevent mental health problems if they have adequate knowledge. The training of health workers focuses on mental health education and counselling skills. As we are dealing with people at the grass roots level, the scope and the approach of the training is kept simple. By giving priority to counselling methods we are not going back to complicated psychological issues or sophisticated western techniques of psychotherapy. Counselling is easily perceived as supplementing conventional ways of dealing with people and their problems.

Initially it was decided to train all the health workers employed by the Department of Health. A Train-the-Trainer approach was not possible in the beginning due to a restriction by the Minister of Health not to employ any new staff and to work with already employed ones. Although the Department of Health felt that it was important to provide all health workers with basic training in mental health issues it was decided not to expand the training before the need for an implementation of the project had actually been assessed. During the first mental health training workshops which we conducted from March 1997 to December 1998 in Dharamsala and in the South Indian settlements, 130 health professionals received training. The workshop sessions lasted for 9 days and were initially taught by us. We used training material provided by TPO-Tibet together with a training manual, which had been written by us during months of extensive preparatory work prior to starting the program. In the beginning while we were still conducting the training ourselves the Tibetan staff translated the manual simultaneously. At the same time they developed the Tibetan terminology. In the course of the training sessions the terminology and the content of the training manual were adapted to the language and educational level of the trainees. An English and Tibetan version of the training manual will eventually be produced.

It was the aim of this approach to pass the responsibility of training others on to the Tibetan staff in a gradual process. We succeeded in doing so with the result that the last 3 training sessions were fully conducted in Tibetan by the Tibetan staff alone. The trainees' response was very positive. They perceived the training as important and stimulating and in the evaluation they suggested longer training sessions and more workshops. They also helped us to understand that they found the workshops more efficient than simply theoretical information. We tried out different approaches of training and eventually decided to give a theoretical introduction to one topic before doing workshops in small groups. During the workshops the groups dealt with specific case examples, role-played and practised listening and questioning. Personal experiences of the health workers were discussed as well as special cases they had come across.

With the positive response of the health workers and the improvement of patients, activities involving mental health issues increased in the Tibetan community. At that point the Minister of Health gave permission to apply the "train-the-trainer" approach and we chose health workers who had shown particular interest and talent during the general training. Furthermore it was decided to focus on eight big settlements for the implementation of the training. In 1999 a six week "train-the-trainer" course was conducted in McLeod Ganj. After that the trainers returned to their settlements to train the health workers with the help of the manual. The trainers' responsibilities were redefined as follows: the trainer is in charge of supervising the health workers doing the home visits, of assessing social problems and mental symptoms of patients, of setting up treatment plans and of guiding the counselling. The trainer also guides meetings of all the health workers of the settlement as well as of the surrounding settlements. The trainer continues to be supervised by the TPO staff.

Initially we thought that training the health workers would not have a lasting impact but in retrospect we realised the soundness of this approach. We learned that the "train-the-trainer" approach can only be implemented if an awareness of mental health problems has been established in the field and on a government level. Both were achieved by providing services and by proving that the clinical interventions are effective, by creating awareness through training, and by setting up a mental health network.

We are pleased to realise that our training has furthered the mental health issue at least to the point that people with mental problems can be detected in the community and that trainers are able to diagnose symptoms of different categories. The need for and the benefit of counselling have been recognised but skills and techniques are yet to be further developed and established. In order to do so, continuity in supervision is necessary as well as accepting the fact that training is an ongoing process. To reach the intended level of knowledge and skills the supervision structure should be continued until September 2002. By that time health workers are expected to be familiar with mental health care and the mental health network will function, so that the incorporation of mental health care into the primary health care structure will be fully accomplished.

Meanwhile mental health training has become part of the general basic health worker training which is conducted once every two years by the Department of Health.

Interventions in the Settlements

The Tibetan settlements are scattered all over India and their size in terms of population ranges from about 80 Tibetans (Sataun) to about 12,000 (Mundgod).

Concerning mental health issues there are not many newly arrived refugees in the settlements and therefore no recent survivors of torture. The mental health problems prevalent in the settlements are mostly psychiatric diseases such as schizophrenia, recurrent psychosis, major depressive disorders, conversions, functional complaints, obsessive compulsory disorders, epilepsy, mental retardation, alcohol and drug abuse. Before the mental health care training was conducted in the settlements most patients with mental health problems were not even known in the primary health care centres as most of them were looked after by their families at home. These patients usually received traditional Tibetan medicine and their families performed prayers on the advice of a lama. After the Tibetan TPO mental health training had been conducted, health workers went into the settlements and looked for patients with psychiatric problems. They assessed the patients' symptoms and their socio-economic condition as well as how the families were coping with mentally affected members. Within 6 months of the mental health training the TPO-Tibet staff visited most settlements and all the patients were examined together with their respective health worker. The patients and their attendants were informed about the possibilities of treatment and a treatment plan was established for each patient.

Some families did not want to seek psychiatric treatment for their patients for a number of different reasons. Often elderly parents take care of the sick ones while other family members live elsewhere to work or study. These old people are mostly not able to travel outside of their settlement and a mental patient will therefore not be taken to a hospital. Old Tibetans do not speak Hindi and communication with Indian doctors is difficult. Many families are poor and cannot afford the travelling expenses or the cost of medication. Some families are so distressed by living with a sick and often even violent family member that they start having psychological problems themselves and therefore are no longer in a position to attend to their sick or take them to a psychiatrist. Tibetans often consult a lama before they seek help from allopathic doctors to find out whether the treatment will be helpful or not and sometimes the lama advises not to take allopathic medicine.

However, there were many families who did seek help from a psychiatrist once or twice but all of them stopped the treatment soon after the patients' symptoms disappeared. These patients often relapsed within a few months. Their families felt that the psychiatric treatment was not very useful since mentally sick people were not completely healed and consequently they did not return to the psychiatrist for follow-up meetings. The regional Indian psychiatric hospitals are generally facing difficulties with the big number of outpatients. One psychiatrist sees about 80 patients per day, which implies that there is no time for an elaborate presentation of a patient's symptoms. Yet to be able to prescribe the right kind of medication an assessment must be precise. For Tibetan patients however, a short presentation of symptoms is difficult because of their insufficient knowledge of Hindi as well as because of their traditional concepts of symptoms. In order to make the visit to the psychiatrist effective we emphasise the importance of a concise presentation of symptoms (disorders of thinking, feeling and behaviour) during our training. Furthermore government mental hospitals provide medication without prescription, although free of charge. Therefore patients or their attendants have to return to the hospital every month to collect medicine. This appeared to be a critical factor because medication was often stopped after one or two months due to the inconvenience of having to return to the mental hospital. To overcome this problem the TPO staff and the health co-ordinator visited the Medical Director of the nearest Indian government psychiatric hospital to discuss the problems of treating Tibetan patients. We requested prescriptions for the Tibetan patients so that the settlement hospital could keep certain medicines in stock. It was agreed upon that the settlement doctor would see the patients every month. Thus the follow up visits to the mental hospital could be reduced to every three to six months. In the meantime the settlement doctor would refer patients to the hospital if they do not respond to the treatment.

The policy of the Department of Health in the settlements focuses on prevention within the Tibetan primary health care system while curing is delegated to local Tibetan or Indian hospitals. Concerning mental health, prevention starts with the identification of symptoms at a very early stage and with a quick referral to a doctor or psychiatrist, if necessary. Prevention of chronicity is helped by continued long-term medication or depot. Prevention also includes keeping patients active in their family and community, informing patients and their families about the course and prognosis of the disease as well as the future expectation of the patient. This kind of intervention focuses in the first place on the prevention of disability of patients and on the secondary effects on family members.

With the younger generation having to leave the settlements for economic opportunities the traditional family structure does not function any more. As described before, chronic or retarded patients often live with their elderly parents.

Once the elder generation dies or has become too old to look after sick family members, these patients are left without care at a time when they would need even more care as the disease is progressing. Sooner or later the settlements will face the problem of having to look after patients needing 24 hours care. In order to tackle this problem the following plan has been set up together with the health co-ordinator and the Medical Officer of the settlement hospital. The Department of Health approved it.

The Implementation of the Primary Mental Health Network. All the patients referred to the Indian psychiatric hospital get a letter from the settlement hospital requesting the Indian psychiatrist to write down his diagnosis and to provide a prescription for medicines. In order to create a good relationship with the Indian government hospital we advise the TPO-Tibet trainer or health worker to accompany the patients on their visits to the psychiatrist. In this way the presentation of symptoms will be to the point and any unforeseen problems can be discussed on the spot. The patients will be followed up by the Medical Officer of the settlement hospital and provided with medicines from the pharmacy of the settlement hospital, which will keep a stock of psychiatric medicines. Usually the same medication is given for 3 months to 1 year so that regular psychiatric check-ups can be reduced. If a patient gets worse, he/she will be referred back to the Indian psychiatric hospital. A separate file will be kept for each patient and relevant notes made after each visit. If the health worker faces any problems or has questions concerning counselling, contact is made with the TPO-Tibet trainer for advice or referral of the patient back to the Medical Officer.

The counselling of psychiatric patients focuses on the identification of triggering factors and on understanding how to prevent a deterioration of mental symptoms. Counselling also encourages the patient to re-establish his/her functioning in everyday life as well as in social relations and responsibilities. Having the opportunity of doing little jobs and earn a small salary, can boost a patient's self-esteem and thus support mental stability.

Hierarchy of the Functions of the Network. *The health worker* assesses the symptoms of patients in the context of their socio-economic situation. The findings are discussed with the TPO-Tibet trainer and together they establish a treatment plan. The health worker does the patient's follow-up, which implies home visits and counselling of patients as well as their families. The health worker is also in charge of staying in contact with the TPO-Tibet trainer in order to define the aim of counselling, to present new cases to the TPO-Tibet trainer and to discuss their management.

The TPO-Tibet trainer who has had training in psychopathology and counselling from the TPO-Tibet staff during the six-week course in McLeod Ganj differentiates psychiatric diagnoses and is able to apply counselling. He/she monitors the health worker's interventions, trains the health worker in the presentation of new cases to the Medical Officer and the psychiatrist, and attends the visits to the psychiatric hospital. The TPO-Tibet trainer is also in charge of calling the health worker and the Medical Officer for a meeting once or twice a month to discuss all the cases and to arrange strategies for their further treatment. Any problems that the health worker may face will be discussed and the TPO-Tibet trainer will supervise him/her while visiting and counselling patients in the field. The TPO-Tibet trainer should know the patients personally, keep their individual files and check on their follow-up visits to the Medical Officer. Every three months he/she sends a report on each patient to the TPO-Tibet office in McLeod Ganj. In case of urgent problems the TPO-Tibet trainer can take instructions from the TPO-Tibet staff by telephone (if available). During the TPO-Tibet staff's field visit every six months the TPO-Tibet trainer receives additional training based on patient cases. The TPO-Tibet trainer discusses the social problems of patients and their families together with the health co-ordinator. Altogether the trainer is the contact person between the Medical Officer, the psychiatrist, the social network, the health worker and the patient.

The Medical Officer sees all the psychiatric patients once every two months and monitors the continuation of medication. He sees patients with deteriorating symptoms and makes the decision whether to treat them or refer them back to the Indian psychiatrist.

The health co-ordinator checks the health workers' attendance at the meetings, makes sure that the hospital pharmacy has sufficient psychiatric medication in stock, supervises the financial administration and is the adviser for social problems. The health co-ordinator keeps in touch with the Department of Health and provides feedback on the progress of the program. As a member of the settlement's health committee the health co-ordinator presents patients for social rehabilitation to the health committee.

The TPO-Tibet staff based in Mcleod Ganj supervises the TPO-Tibet trainer by telephone and responds in writing to the monthly reports. During the supervision field trip the TPO-Tibet staff discuss the management of the cases and if necessary see the patients together with the TPO-Tibet trainer. The TPO-Tibet staff take part in establishing the mental health network and help to find solutions for all kinds of practical and administrative problems.

This supervision structure will be continued until September 2002 when mental health care is expected to be familiarised to such an extent that it has become an integral part of the primary health care structure. From this point onwards refresher meetings of the TPO-Tibet trainers once in two years should be sufficient to update their knowledge. In case of urgent problems the TPO-Tibet counsellors in the McLeod Ganj mental health clinic will be available for consultation.

Development of Funds and Sustainability

With the gradual expansion of the project, financial needs also increased. From the beginning the Department of Health intended to run the project with a budget it would be able to sustain in the long run. Therefore TPO-Tibet did not employ any new staff and has been very concerned with managing within the granted budget.

The Mental Health Network has started to function but needs constant adaptation. During one of the supervision field trips for example the health coordinator pointed out that most of the expenses were going to the transportation of patients to the nearest psychiatric hospital and that a consultant Indian psychiatrist visiting the settlement once a month would be less expensive. These considerations were discussed with the medical director of the regional mental hospital but it was concluded that new out-patient clinics could not be set up due to a lack of staff. To resolve this issue following has been decided:

1. For an assessment the patient can attend an out-patient clinic, which is only a three-hour drive from the settlement (the regional hospital is a six-hour drive away and implies an over-night stay).
2. For admission and crisis intervention the patient has to go to the regional mental hospital.
3. For the follow-up one health worker can present all the patients to the psychiatrist.

With this arrangement the transportation costs can be reduced substantially. Adaptation concerning budget, rehabilitation interventions and referrals is still an ongoing process because the increasing number of patients requires a broad variety of solutions.

The full implementation of the project is not yet achieved as knowledge about psychopathology and counseling skills are still to be further familiarised. It appears that supervision of the TPO-Tibet trainers and network in the field by qualified staff is necessary for a period of at least two and a half more years. Consequently two more Tibetan supervisors should be trained so that the Tibetan staff can eventually run the project on their own.

TREATMENT AND TRANSCULTURAL ASPECTS OF THE PROJECT

Mental Health in Tibetan Medicine

Before dealing with transcultural matters it is useful to give a basic introduction into the concepts of mind, consciousness and mental health in Tibetan medicine. Medical theories and practices came to Tibet along with religious teachings between the eighth and thirteenth century. Tibetan medical theory, which is rooted in Buddhist philosophy, is based on a holistic approach to psycho-physiological processes. In Buddhist medical philosophy mind and body form an integrated unit. According to this philosophy ignorance is the root cause of all suffering because it leads to a misapprehension of reality. This gives rise to the three mental poisons desire/attachment, hatred/anger and confusion. These three poisons evolve into the three humours—wind (rLung), bile (mKhris-pa) and phlegm (Bad-kan)—on which the Tibetan medical theory is based. Desire brings wind, hatred brings bile and confusion brings phlegm. Once the humours are produced, their balanced circulation maintains the health of the organism, while their imbalance causes disease (Tsultrim, 1999).

The main diagnosis in Tibetan medicine is done by feeling the radial pulse to determine which humour flow has been blocked or is excessive. In general diseases can be classified into four categories:

1. karmic disorders that are caused by actions performed in this or previous lifetimes. Their cause is spiritual and their treatment has to be spiritual too. Only a spiritually advanced lama can detect these causes and prescribe the appropriate religious practices. These include the recitation of mantras, prostrations performed by the patient or rituals and meditations done by the lama for the patient. When regular Tibetan medicines are not effective, the disease is often attributed to a karmic cause.
2. immediate disorders which can be compared to what is defined as "self-terminating illness" in medical terminology. These disorders come and go quickly and do not require any medical treatment.
3. disorders involving evil spirits. They are generally treated with religious medicine and rituals in combination with herbal medicine and other kinds of treatment. Spirits are the main cause for severe psychiatric disorders.
4. life disorders that can be caused by humoral unbalance due to wrong diet, inappropriate behaviour, intoxicants, environmental factors and psychological factors. These diseases can be treated with traditional Tibetan medicine (Clifford, 1984).

In order to understand the Tibetan concept of mind or consciousness and its disorders, it is necessary to understand the significance of rlung, one of the three humours. Rlung is the Tibetan term for the movement of energy, which is a vital force pervading the human organism. This life force which moves in channels throughout the body, is believed to dissolve in death, to be blocked or disrupted in disease and to be controlled in the practice of meditation. According to the Tibetan medical theory, rlung, which is the leader of the three humours, serves as the physical base of consciousness and as a medium through which the mind is linked to the body. An imbalance of rlung, caused by an alteration of its flow, produces mental and emotional disturbances particularly when the life-bearing rlung, one of the five types of rlung, is disturbed. The life-bearing rlung, called srog rlung, on the gross level provides the base for the sensory consciousness, on a subtler level serves as a base for conceptual mental consciousness and on a very subtle level supports the subtle mind that passes from one life to the next. The disorders of rlung are numerous and depend on the severity of the alteration of the flow of the humour. A disturbance of the flow of rlung in its natural channel gives rise to the initial disorder. If there is an aggravation of the disturbance, rlung is beyond its normal range but still in its natural channels. When rlung reaches a critical point, it overflows its natural channel and disrupts the other two humours. In the same way the circulation of rlung can be affected and a rlung disease can become manifest if one of the other two humours is disturbed beyond range. There are two main categories of mental disorders: madness (smyonpa) and rlung disease (srog rlung).

For the explanation of madness Tibetan medicine relies on the Tantric theory of subtle energies and channels. There are seven types of madness. According to this theory it is the subtler form of life-bearing wind which is disturbed and gives rise to madness. The subtle life-bearing wind is placed in the heart and is the basis for the conceptual mental consciousness. When this subtle life-bearing wind is forcefully invaded by another energy (mostly a spirit but also an overflowing humour), then psychosis develops. This explanatory model of madness implies that certain predisposing causes and immediate precipitating external conditions have to act together to develop a severe mental disorder. The predisposing causes can be sadness, mental discomfort or excitement, a weak heart, poor diet, wrong behavioural patterns or intoxication. The precipitating conditions can be the interference of harmful spirits or a primary disturbance of humours. The Tantric texts describe in detail how and through which channels and doors this disruption evolves, and how blockage and reversion of the subtle life-bearing wind create a dysfunctioning of mental processes.

For general rlung disorders the medical texts list sixty-three different types of diseases and specific mental and physical symptoms are defined as suggestive of a disturbance of rlung. Most of the mood disorders are included in the categories of srog rlung. The general causes of srog rlung disorders include improper diet, dysfunctional behavioural patterns and mental strain of different kinds. When the external circumstances are very unstable and fluctuating, a disturbance is more likely to develop. A specific kind of srog rlung disorder is described as a complication of an improper meditation practice. According to Tibetan medicine there are four different methods for the treatment of rlung disorders: through diet (such as high-protein intake), through behavioural guidelines (such as keeping warm, avoiding a bright environment, cultivating friendly speech and nice company, rest and relaxation), through medication (with a variety of herbal medicines specific for each kind of disturbance) and through secondary therapeutics (such as massage, moxabustion or enemas).

Disorders which are considered to be psychiatric diseases or mental disturbance such as stress associated symptoms and functional complaints from a western point of view are always diagnosed and treated as a disruption of rlung by Tibetan doctors. By treating depressed and psychotic patients together with Tibetan doctors we have learned that Tibetan medicines and western psychopharmacological medication work synergistic. In the acute phase of a psychotic crisis for example Tibetan medicines have no effect but as soon as the symptoms have been reduced by neuroleptics and a combined treatment with Tibetan medicines has been started, the recovery seems to speed up by the Tibetan medicines. If a karmic cause of the psychosis has been diagnosed, which is frequently the case with patients who have a positive family history of schizophrenia or depression, a Tibetan doctor does not have any effective medicine and the patient is referred to a lama for spiritual practices and rituals.

Counselling and Explanatory Models

While counselling Tibetan patients we always ask their own ideas about the cause of their disease. Tibetan refugees living in Mcleod Ganj come from many different areas in Tibet. Although Buddhism is their overall belief system, there are many variations in terms of worshipping as well as a great diversity of deities and spirits that families attribute power to. In addition, individuals have their personal interpretations of traditional concepts. The knowledge of underlying concepts of disease is necessary to be able to translate traditional thinking into psychological terms during counselling. Consequently it is possible to remain within the personal explanatory model while applying psychological interventions.

Patients and practitioners hold explanatory models in all healthcare systems. They are basically the notions about sickness, offer explanations and give indications for treatment (Kleinman, 1980). Explanatory models of western and Tibetan doctors, lamas and healers show us how they understand and treat sickness. Patients' and their families' explanatory models tell us how they make sense of episodes of illness and how they choose and evaluate particular treatments. In this sense an explanatory model is more than the patient's own interpretation of the symptoms and causes of his/her illness but reflects the whole cultural paradigm.

In our clinical work we have come across a great variety of explanatory models which are often juxtaposed to the afore mentioned etiological categories and which can be divided into different groups. *Physical explanations* refer to diet, climate, certain diseases such as TB, unbalanced elements in the body such as an imbalance of lung, physical damage due to imprisonment, torture and conditions during the flight from Tibet. *Psychological explanations* include tension during studies, stress due to everyday chores or strict discipline in the monastery, frustration due to the feeling of inability to continue the freedom struggle from exile, missing prison mates, homesickness and suffering from the memories of traumatic experiences in Tibet. *Social and economic explanations* include lack of economical resources, the absence of relatives in India, lacking relationships with compatriots and lacking good communication between old and newcomer refugees. *Traditional beliefs* are for example the concept of mental pollution, karma and the influence of spirits.

In order to integrate traditional ways of problem resolving as much as possible we give priority to the patients' own idea about the cause and kind of their illness. While counselling we try to remain within their chosen believe system. To solve their problems Tibetans usually first consult lamas who are considered to be specialists for certain problems, such as the pacification of spirits or divination (Box 4).

Box 4. Lobsang Dolma

Lobsang Dolma was a nun who had arrived in India four years ago. In her school of Buddhist studies for nuns she was known to be silent, shy, very intelligent and always the first of her class. She was very happy for the opportunity to study and did not seem to be troubled with homesickness. She was presented to our clinic because of a drastic change in her behaviour. She had started to speak loudly and in an uninhibited way, she quarrelled with her friends and her behaviour was not appropriate for a nun any more. She became very agitated, had auditive hallucinations and experienced delusions of being a high reincarnation. When she was asked about what she thought the reason for her behavioural change could be, she explained that she felt it was due to a lha (god). We asked her which lha she thought was involved and she said it could be the lha of her home in Tibet who was affecting her. When we asked her how this lha could affect her after being away from home four years, she told us that she had received a gift from her family in Tibet three weeks ago through which this lha had been passed on to her. It was decided that she should quickly see a particular lama who performed a divination and confirmed the possession of lha. He advised her to return to Tibet immediately as well as assured her complete recovery. She got permission to leave and some money to return to Tibet. Within hours she recovered from her symptoms and left the same evening.

Patients holding explanatory models refering to a god who belongs to their native place in Tibet, are usually suffering from homesickness and/or inability to adapt to the new situation in exile. Returning to Tibet proves to be an effective remedy while religious rituals and prayers usually have a short-term effect on symptoms of this kind. In the above-mentioned case it was unusual that the nun was affected only after four years of successfully staying in India. From a psychological point of view a possible interpretation of her delayed reaction is a dissociative defense mechanism which became active in order to cope with the painful feelings of homesickness. The gift she received from her family in Tibet was such an undeniable sign of reality that the emotional distance created by the dissociative defense mechanism could not be sustained any more in a functional way. In cases where homesickness becomes a predominant emotional disturbance, psychiatric symptoms generally manifest themselves early, soon after the arrival of a person and reflect the inability to adapt to the new condition in exile.

Counselling and Buddhist Philosophy

Psychological concepts and the theory of mind in Buddhist philosophy bear many similarities. The introduction of counselling offers a problem solving strategy which is different from any kind of traditional Tibetan intervention.

According to the traditional way of solving problems in private life the younger people would receive advice from the elder ones concerning all important decisions. On the social and professional level the respected high-ranking members of the community would suggest to the common people ways to solve difficulties and conflicts. Since the family and other traditional support structures are much less available in the refugee situation, in particular recently arrived refugees cannot delegate problem solving to a superior. This change in the social organisation in exile has created a need for a different kind of problem solving strategy on a more individual level. From this perspective we have experienced that for many this need could be answered by counselling.

The hierarchical structure of Tibetan society is also reflected on the level of the health workers. They were usually trained to advice and teach patients. For many health workers the training of counselling was like an eye-opener. They realised the potential of listening to a patient in a different way and learned to understand the range of possibilities counselling could have on their daily work with patients. They often experienced that patients' symptoms were connected to stressful conditions in their lives but they were not aware of the fact that help in solving the problem would be sufficient to heal 'physical' symptoms. This was due to the fact that they did not yet have the knowledge and the skills to listen carefully and to ask information in a way that encourages patients to describe their thoughts and feelings regarding different life domains and to observe how symptoms influence their daily life. While implementing the project we observed that learning counselling skills requires a change in deeply rooted mental attitudes. This implies a slow gradual process of familiarisation with the new knowledge.

Coping Strategies and Mechanisms

The aim of counselling is to help a person find his/her own way of coping with the demands in life. For many Tibetans life changes drastically with becoming a refugee, being separated from family members and other supporting structures or being mentally isolated by traumatic memories. They are suddenly challenged to apply coping strategies in a different way. In our experience we

> **Box 5. Tashi Lhamo**
>
> Tashi Lhamo grew up in an extended family of nomads in a remote area of Kham. She came to India alone as a single mother with her one-year-old daughter four years ago with the idea to provide her child with an education in a Tibetan school in exile. When she tried to gain admission she was told that she had to wait for the child to turn six. For four years she took care of her child all by herself, facing many difficulties and at the same time developing a strong bond with her. Finally her daughter was admitted to a boarding school far away from her working place. Two weeks later she came to our clinic complaining of fatigue, headache and the feeling of "missing something". During counselling we were able to help her realise the link between the separation from her daughter and her feelings of loss.

observed that Tibetans prefer problem solving to emotional coping: in general they tend to face stressful situations by first solving problems in a practical way while avoiding expression of their feelings. This implies that they often do not allow themselves to recognize and elaborate their feelings related to the stressful situation, especially at the time of having to act. Consequently, after a critical decision is made, the person has to face the emotional consequences of this decision. At this stage symptoms may develop and the person can overcome them with the support of the family or a lama's rituals without necessarily having to go through a process of acknowledgement. In some cases symptoms can persist, especially when the traditional support structures are missing. For these patients the acknowledgement of the emotions through counselling proved to be effective to resolve the symptoms (Box 5).

Tibetans are rightly proud of their traditional collective coping and spiritual mechanisms that help many people. In general these coping mechanisms are mostly cognitive and spiritual. The following are the most common ones: reciting mantras, visualising H. H. the Dalai Lama, and focusing on karma, impermanence, and the suffering of others. Traditional mechanisms tend to work especially well for coping with loss, death, and other events within the usual range of life experiences. However, traditional, cognitive forms of coping do not always reach tortured refugees because severe emotional arousal and re-experiencing of traumatic events cloud the access to the cognitive and spiritual coping system. Without access to the collective coping mechanisms, the refugee is left isolated—especially since display of emotion is discouraged. During treatment we try to provide space for emotional expression and to bridge between the client's emotional experience and the available cultural forms of coping. The coping strategies we come across which are especially applied by victims of torture suffering of PTSD, can be divided into two groups:

There are coping strategies, which are used at the time of traumatic experiences. These include visualising H.H. the Dalai Lama, reciting mantras, meditating on karma, impermanence and the suffering of others, focussing on the usefulness of the suffering for Tibet's freedom, for the support of H.H. and the freedom of religion, concentrating on the will to survive in order to be able to spread the truth to the Tibetans in exile and to the international community, and feeling determined not to disclose the identity of other freedom fighters. Some patients reported that they cultivated a desire for revenge or a readiness to die as a way of coping. Some thought of their families, and others tried not to think at all and ignored emotional reactions. Ex-prisoners told us that feeling supported by other prisoners and co-operating with prison guards also provided a way of coping.

The second group of coping strategies deals with present problems. We noted the following strategies in our clinic: performing rituals to pacify spirits or purify karma, spiritual practice such as meditation or Dharma studies, seeking the guidance of elders or teachers, trying to be in contact with family members and friends, seeking the contact and company of people who have come from the same area in Tibet or who have also been politically involved and/or imprisoned, concentrating on the aim of keeping one's political commitment alive, reminding oneself that other people are suffering more, sharing one's problems with people one feels close to, discussing political issues and past experiences in a group, distracting oneself with physical activities, isolating oneself and trying not to think at all. We have observed that old comer refugees profit more from religious coping strategies than newly arrived refugees.

CONCLUSION

In this chapter we present the Tibetan TPO Project from the point of view of its development. Many other aspects of the project such as different anthropological perspectives, community interventions, technical sides of the implementation, evaluation strategies, human rights and political issues have not been addressed.

We want to point out that the interpersonal relationships in the Tibetan TPO project, which were established over many years, were the base for implementation.

The research results and the open dialogue were the stepping stones for the introduction of mental health care and counselling into the existing traditional system. At that stage neither the Tibetans nor we could foresee how this implementation of mental health care and counselling into the existing system was eventually going to work out.

The trust we established by adapting our interventions to the Tibetan planning policies together with our genuine respect for the traditional belief system turned out to be very conducive to the support and encouragement we received from the government, health professionals and patients. The implementation structure proposed by TPO-Tibet is based on a long experience with Mental Health Care in an established democratic welfare system. The Tibetan democracy, born in exile, is still young. The present government is working toward self-sufficiency and cannot yet afford to set up services, which it does not consider a priority. Therefore the government made a commitment to support our project and invest in it only after the need for Mental Health Care had been assessed through research, first within the group of newly arrived refugees and ex-prisoners and then through our clinical work with the whole refugee population. We for our part committed ourselves to try to find a way of implementation, which was in accordance with the needs, and resources of the Tibetan government. As a result the project developed only gradually and step by step. This had a definite advantage of allowing adaptations to be made at any stage. For the trainees too the learning process was a gradual one and gave them time to deal with a variety of problems and to apply and try out new methods. This opportunity which they had over a period of a few years will provide them with sufficient experience to carry on and to hand knowledge and skills on to the next generation of health professionals. The disadvantage of this approach proved to be primarily the restriction to employ new staff, as the Department of Health could not guarantee a long-term employment. For this reason the project needed altogether more time for its implementation than initially planned.

The aim was to make the project self-sustainable within four years, so that our presence and professional skills would not be required any more by September 2000. This plan initially included the training of four staff members as counsellor, social worker, trainer, supervisor and co-ordinator who would also be able to advise the policy making. To this day there are only two Tibetan staff members who have been fully trained and are available for the community. Tenzin Buthi, who has been with us since the beginning of the project, has acquired all the skills to apply counselling to different kinds of patients, to train with the manual and to function independently as supervisor. Kelsang Phuntsok who has administrative functions, co-ordinates the implementation in the settlements and is adviser to the Department of Health. Two more counsellors are expected to be competent for independent counselling, supervision and training by the end of 2000.

Another difficulty that we came across while developing the project was having to initiate activities on various levels. There was no mental health expertise structure apart from the traditional one. There was no mental health structure on government level, nor were there mental health professionals in the health care system. Even with the awareness in the community that mental health problems were a burden for many families there was no awareness that these problems could be addressed with psychosocial and mental health interventions. Activities had to be developed on all these levels to create a condition for the integration of mental health care into the primary health care. These are additional reasons for our commitment to exceed seven years. The implementation of the project has become increasingly complex. In order to ensure long-term sustainability the necessity for an extension of the project has been realised.

ACKNOWLEDGEMENTS. We want to express our gratitude to Prof. Dr. J. T. V. M. De Jong as it was his idea to implement transcultural counselling and mental health into the Tibetan context in India. He did not only help us to negotiate with the Tibetan Government in Exile but played a crucial role in funding the project and in providing support and help whenever we needed it. We also address our special appreciation to Dr. C. D. Kaplan, who taught us the necessary knowledge, skills and attitude to perform qualitative field research. His ideas and suggestions have been inspiring us throughout the process of the project and will remain with us beyond it. Many other people have contributed time and effort in various ways to implement this project. We are grateful to all of them for all their support on many levels. Sincere thanks are due to SIMAVI for granting generous funds and to COV (Meeting Centre of Peoples for Development, Peace and Justice) for employing and supporting us. We are obliged to the Tibetan government-in-exile for their genuine co-operation and commitment to our work. Our counsellor Tenzin Bhuti has not only been showing dedication and motivation for her work but has been of inestimable assistance throughout our time of working together. The health workers and the staff of the Tibetan Department of Health have been providing substantial support and we are indebted to them and to all involved in the fieldwork. Final thanks are due to Felizitas Fischer for her help in compiling material and for her admirable patience in correcting our language.

REFERENCES

Clifford, T. (1984). *Tibetan Buddhist medicine and psychiatry: The diamond healing.* York Beach, ME: Samuel Weiser.
Crescenzi, A., Ketzer, E., Van Ommeren, M., Phuntsok, K., Komproe, I., & De Jong, J. T. V. M. (2001). *Effect of political imprisonment on recent Tibetan refugees in India.* Manuscript submitted for publication.
Dalai Lama. (1982). *Collected statements, interviews, and articles of His Holiness the Dalai Lama.* Dharamsala, India: Information Office of His Holiness the Dalai Lama.
Kleinman, A. (1980). *Patients and healers in the context of culture: An exploration of the borderland between anthropology, medicine, and psychiatry.* Berkeley, CA: University of California Press.
Planning Council, Central Tibetan Administration (1994). *Tibetan Refugee Community Integrated Development Plan-II 1995–2000.* Dharamsala, India.
Tsultrim, L. (1999). *Tibetan medicine: Perspective on mental health.* Lecture given to TPO trainers meeting.

FURTHER READING

Avedon, J. F. (1985). *In exile from the land of snows.* Boston: Wisdom Publications.
Dönden, Y. (1986). *Health through balance: An introduction to Tibetan medicine.* Ithaca, NY: Snow Lion Publications.

Epstein, M., & Topgay, S. (1988). Mind and mental disorders in Tibetan medicine. In *Mind and mental health in Tibetan medicine*. New York: Potala Publications.

Kelly, P. K., Bastian, G., & Aiello, P. (Eds.) (1991). *The anguish of Tibet*. Berkeley, CA: Parallax Press.

Rapgay, L. (1988). Mind-made health: A Tibetan perspective. In *Mind and Mental Health in Tibetan Medicine*. New York: Potala Publications.

Tibetan Centre for Human Rights and Democracy (1999). *Torture in Tibet: Tales of terror*. Dharamsala, India.

Torture Quarterly Journal on Rehabilitation of Torture Victims and Prevention of Torture, 1a/99June 1999.

Van Walt van Praag, M. C. (1987). *The status of Tibet: History, rights and prospects in international law*. London: Wisdom Publications.

7

Community Mental Health as Practiced by the Gaza Community Mental Health Programme

SAMIR QOUTA and EYAD EL-SARRAJ

POLITICAL AND SOCIAL HISTORY OF GAZA

The Gaza Strip is a small piece of land stretching between Israel and Egypt on the Mediterranean coast (Figure 1). It is fifty kilometers long, and its width varies from five kilometers in the north to twelve in the south. Inhabited by more than a million people, it is one of most densely populated areas in the world; the average population density is 2,150 persons per square kilometer. Two thirds of the population are refugees, of which over 300,000 live in eight refugee camps. About 50% of the population is under sixteen, and 20% is five years or under.

When armistice lines were drawn up between Israeli and Arab forces in 1949, the strip became, along with the west bank of the River Jordan, one of the two parts of Palestine left in Arab hands. Originally administered by Egypt, Gaza was occupied by the Israeli army after the 1967 war and Israeli forces governed the strip for nearly three decades of occupation.

On December 9th, 1987, a mass movement of civil disobedience—the "Intifada"—broke out in Gaza and the West Bank. Initial protests over the deaths of four Gazans in a traffic accident involving an Israeli military vehicle escalated into mass demonstrations. Thousands of Gazans took to the streets to erect barricades and throw stones at the occupying troops. The Israeli response was to intensify its campaign: thousands were arrested, schools and universities

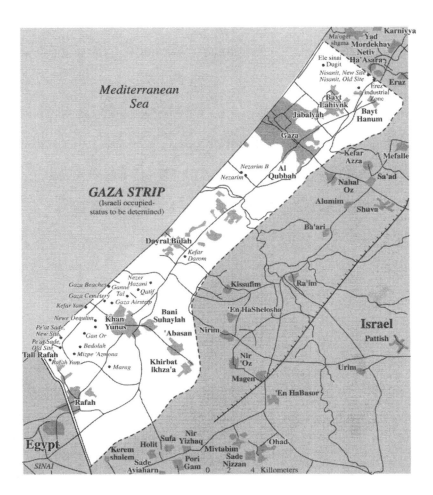

Figure 1. Gaza Strip.

were shut down, and economic restrictions were intensified. In the first thirty-three months of the Intifada, 1,100 Palestinians were shot and killed, of which 54% were children under the age of 14, 2,200 were physically injured and 55,000 detained (Nixon, 1990).

The signing of the Declaration of Principles by Israel and the PLO in September 1993 marked the first step toward a solution to the longstanding confrontation between Israel and the Palestinians. However, violent clashes between Palestinians demonstrating against Israeli settlers and military personnel continued to occur as a consequence of stalemate in the peace process and the continued Israeli drive for settlement in the occupied West Bank and Gaza.

The Declaration of Principles, the Gaza-Jericho agreement of May 1994, and the Interim Agreement as of September 1995 led to partial Israeli withdrawal and military redeployment in the inhabited area of the Gaza Strip and 3% of the West Bank. Civil affairs within Palestine, including health, education, infrastructure, and agriculture, were placed under the jurisdiction of a democratically elected Palestinian self-rule Legislative Council for an interim period of five years. The mandate of the Palestinian Authority covers 58% of the Gaza Strip and 3% of the West Bank. Until a permanent agreement on the status of Palestinian self-rule has been reached, Israel retains responsibility for external security, borders, foreign relations, and overall security of military zones, settlements, and Israeli citizens.

This partial transferal of authority has presented a great challenge to the Palestinian National Authority (PNA). The governmental, judiciary, and administrative structures, including the health care infrastructure, have suffered from years of developmental neglect under Israeli administration. The situation has not improved due to the loss of employment in Israel, the Gazan GNP has declined over the last five years. In periods of tension, Israel has shut off the border at Erez, forcing unemployment within the Strip up to 70% in cases of strict closures.

HUMAN RIGHTS SITUATION

Israeli Occupation

Israel is a member of the UN and also party to a number of the UN legal instruments, including the Convention against Torture. In 1998, the Israeli High Court prohibited maltreatment of detainees and use of torture to extract confessions. However, Israel had followed a systematic policy of torture and maltreatment of detainees in its prisons and detention centers prior to the court ruling. Since 1987 the use of "moderate physical pressure" against Palestinian prisoners has been "officially" accepted by the Israeli government in the cases of those who may have committed or have information about acts of violence. The exact forms of permissible pressure have been declared secret by the Landau Commission of Inquiry. Hooding, forced standing or squatting for long periods of time, prolonged exposure to extreme temperatures, tying or chaining the detainee in contorted and painful positions, shaking, blows and beatings, confinement in small and often filthy spaces, sleep and food deprivation and threats against the detainee's life or family are regularly reported by human rights organizations. In 1992, Amnesty International reported that interrogation procedures as a matter of course included systematic physical or psychological torture.

Since the Israeli occupation in 1967 more than 400,000 Palestinians have been detained or imprisoned. A Gaza Community Mental Health Programme study of 477 ex-prisoners, who had spent between six months and ten years in prison, showed torture to be commonplace. A large majority of the subjects had been tortured by beating (95.8%), as well as many other methods: exposure to extreme cold (92.9%) or extreme heat (76.7%), forced to stand for a long period (77.4%), threats against personal safety (90.6%), solitary confinement (86%), sleep deprivation (71.5%), deprivation of food (77.4%), pressure applied to the neck (68.1%), forced to witness the torture of others (70.2%), electric shock (5.9%), and an instrument inserted into the penis or rectum (1.1%). The study also showed that 41.9% of the subjects found it difficult to adapt to family life; 44.7% found it hard to socialize; and 21.1% had sexual and marital problems.

Since the 1970s Israeli torture of Palestinians has been carried out primarily by the Israeli Army and the General Security Service (GSS). Israel maintains that torture is not condoned, but acknowledges that abuses do sometimes occur and are investigated. The results of these investigations are not made public. In 1996, Israel conducted 60 investigations into 83 complaints received from Palestinians; in each case, the government concluded that the findings did not justify any steps being taken to punish the interrogators.

In addition to torture, organized violence related to clashes between Israeli armed forces and Palestinian demonstrators took place on a large scale during the Intifada from 1987 to 1994. During 1997, violent incidents between soldiers and demonstrators resulted in 10 Palestinian deaths, of whom at least five were below the age of fifteen.

Palestinian Authority

Since the establishment of self-rule the mandate of the Palestinian National Authority (PNA) covers internal security, law, and order in parts of Gaza and the West Bank. However, it has no full control over the land or resources. In the last three years, the PNA has launched several collective imprisonment campaigns directed mainly against opposition parties, particularly focussing upon Hamas and Islamic Jihad. The number of political prisoners was estimated to have reached approximately 1,600 (Palestinian center of Human Rights, 1997).

The PNA has officially committed itself to principles of democracy and rule of law, as well as the prevention of human rights violations. However, reports both from local and international NGOs and human rights organizations indicate that human rights violations and undemocratic practices are found within the Palestinian Police and governmental administration. There have been allegations of PNA torture and violence against Palestinians in most branches of the Palestinian Police.

Methods of torture and violence vary widely. Some methods, however, show striking similarities with Israeli methods recorded against Palestinian detainees. Common interrogation practices include hooding, forced standing or squatting for extended periods of time, prolonged exposure to extreme temperatures, and sleep and food deprivation.

PNA prison conditions are generally very poor. Prolonged detention and lack of due judicial process are common problems, while prison facilities and institutions often lack the basic necessities for humane physical prison conditions. Palestinian detainees have been recorded as held in detention without any form of communication for over a month. There has, however, been a noted improvement in the last two years.

Other factors in the prevalence of torture and abuse of detainees include the political pressure from Israel and the United States to fight terrorism (which leads to a large number of arrests), and the rapid expansion of the Palestinian Police which has had to rely on untrained officers in positions of authority. There are also suggestions that psychological factors contribute to human rights violations. The combative past of many Palestinian police, including experiences of Israeli suppression and periods of imprisonment before and during the Intifada make Palestinian officers identify with Israeli security officers and adopt practices experienced in Israeli prisons as a subconscious psychological self-defense mechanism.

MENTAL HEALTH SITUATION

Effects on Societal Groups

The past and present social and political environments have adversely affected all Gazans. But this situation has held different meanings for the different sections of society, depending on their traditional and cultural roles. It could be said that the entire Palestinian Society suffers to varying degrees from collective trauma. Some of these groups within the society and their responses to the trauma are discussed below.

Ex-political prisoners. During the time of the occupation, and particularly during the Intifada, many political prisoners sacrificed parts of their lives and underwent intense physical and psychological suffering in the name of a cause they believed in. Feelings of disappointment and frustration at the lack of political resolution are therefore common among the survivors of torture. Victims of torture and ill treatment have been shown to experience some of the classic symptoms of PTSD in proportion to the severity of their trauma (El-Sarraj et al., 1996). But other research conducted by GCMHP suggests that positive coping styles can emerge from the prison experience. Qouta and El-Sarraj (1997) discovered that many prisoners found the prison experience a catalyst to develop growth in personal insight, a sense of heroic fulfillment or to see it as a necessary and positive developmental stage in their life. Only older and severely tortured prisoners viewed the experience with suffering and disillusionment.

Children and Youth. Frequently cited problems include lack of respect and guidance in parent-child relationships, especially father-child, where the powerlessness of the father in the eyes of his child has changed his traditionally powerful image. Young people lack belief in the future, or do not see the worth in struggling or striving for anything. Thabet et al., (1998) estimate that each Palestinian child experienced 3.2 traumatic experiences during the period of the first Intifada, ranging from inhalation of tear gas to witnessing beatings and killings of close relatives. The perceived powerlessness of elders in the face of external pressures leaves children without role models, without hope and without any real vision of the future.

Research conducted by GCMHP explicated the negative psychological impact on children. Children who witnessed violence during the Intifada were unimpaired in certain cognitive abilities relating to organizing symbolic material and creativity, but did have impaired abilities to concentrate and remember. Those who participated in the violence were less effected than those who witnessed it passively (Qouta, Punamäki & El-Sarraj, 1995). Other research uncovered negative impacts on parenting styles of parents whose children had witnessed violence (Punamäki & El Sarraj, 1997). The Peace Treaty with Isreal lowered neuroticism and increased self esteem among children but residual neuroticism and self esteem problems remained among children who did not accept the treaty and participate in festivities following the signing (Qouta, Punamäki & El-Sarraj, 1995). Structural equations modeling conducted by Punamäki, Qouta, and El-Sarraj (1997) related to some of the earlier studies. Trauma in children effects neuroticism through two mediating paths, parenting and participation in political activity.

Women. As the image of the man as dominant and powerful in Palestinian society breaks down under the intensity of outside pressure, women find themselves occupying changing roles. As the men lose faith and confidence and suffer the symptoms resulting from their traumatic experiences, women often find themselves the victims of their frustration, manifested as physical abuse or withdrawal from responsibilities. In addition, husbands are often absent (working in Israel, imprisoned, dead) or are suffering from their experiences as political prisoners. As well as having to struggle with their own personal reactions to the overall situation, women must compensate for the changing role of the father in order to give the family a life as normal as possible.

Families of ex-Political Prisoners. The families of ex-political prisoners have suffered many different types of traumatic experiences. These included night raids, witnessing the brutal arrest of the father, brother, or son, long separation from a loved one, absence of a father figure, worry for the welfare of the imprisoned person. Since their release, many ex-political prisoners have suffered a variety of torture related psychiatric symptoms such as depression, anxiety, and psychosomatic illness (El-Sarraj et al., 1996). All of these factors naturally affect all individual family members, as well as the dynamics of the family unit as a whole. The ex-political prisoners' feelings of alienation can also lead to outbursts of anger directed at their loved ones. All of these factors threaten the harmony of the family, communication channels, and the structure and support traditionally found inside the family system.

The Need for Treatment and Support in Gaza

It is very difficult to conduct a precise measure of the need for treatment and support related to torture and organized violence committed against Palestinians. An estimation made by the Research Department at the GCMHP of the mental well being of adults in Gaza (16–60 years) suggests that 32.4% of a random sample of suffered from stress-related psychiatric disorders resulting from direct exposure to violence (including torture 15.4% and imprisonment 16.1%), and witnessing traumatic events (including clashes with the Israeli army 35.1%, killing of a friend 21% or a family member 20.1%). Twelve and a half percent suffered from anxiety, 8.3% from depression, 10.7% from psychosomatic disorders, and 3.2% from paranoia (Abu Hein, 1992). It was found that the traumatic experiences affect children's memory and concentration, and also children's relationships with their parents. Traumatized children started to perceive their parents as more disciplining and rejecting (Qouta, 2000)

Up to the end of 1999, GCMHP clinics have treated 11,742 patients from all parts of the Gaza Strip. 75% of the total are refugees who come from camps that are poorer and pose more social and economic hardships than towns and villages. Over the past two years, 2,208 (1,088 in 1998 and 1,120 in 1999) new cases were treated, excluding the number treated in the new clinic in Deir El-Balah (opened in August 2000). Of this total, 40% were children under 18. The ratio of male (56% in 1998, 52% in 1999) to female (44% in 1998, 48% in 1999) new cases is very close to the gender ratio in the Palestinian community, thus demonstrating the success of GCMHP efforts to reach Palestinian women. The total number of clients—new and follow up—treated in 1998 was 2,337. In 1999, the total number of patients rose to 2,386. Sixty-three percent of the cases in 1998 and 1999 were treated free of charge.

The vast majority of cases are self and family referrals, which comprise 81.6% of the client intake over the past two years. This percentage is slightly higher than the 1996/1997 figure, which stood at 80.3%. This reflects the decrease in the stigma attached to mental illness in Palestinian society. In addition, it is an indication of the increasing awareness of the importance of therapy as a result of the extensive public awareness and community outreach activities conducted by GCMHP professionals. Figure 2 summarizes the diagnostic categories presented for treatment in the most recent year that figures were available.

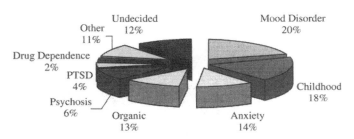

Figure 2. Diagnoses of clients who presented themselves for treatment in 2000.

The clinics continued to experience an increase in cases of mood disorder over the past two years. This increase stems from the rising depression associated with the deteriorating social and economic situation and frustration resulting from the political complications affecting the Palestinian people. On the other hand, there is a decrease in the number of cases with organic disorders treated in the clinics from 20% in 1996/1997 to 14% over the last two years. This is partially explained by the fact that many chronic cases are now being referred to other specialized service-providers.

The Union of Palestinian Medical Relief Committees (UPMRC) confirms this result: they suggest that 25% of the Palestinian population could benefit from psychological treatment as a result of past and present political turmoil. This figure includes Palestinians suffering from stresses from the Intifada and continued socioeconomic and political pressures.

Mental health is one of the least acknowledged areas of the Palestinian health system. The 1998 Mental Health Plan of the Ministry of Health acknowledges the need for rehabilitation but does not suggest methods of implementation. There are currently two psychiatric hospitals in the Autonomous Territories, one in the Gaza Strip and the other in the West Bank. They have limited staff, and offer bedside care without any community services. The 32 beds in the Gaza Psychiatric Unit represents 0.04 beds per 1,000 people, in a region that has some of the most acute psychological problems of the world.

THE GAZA COMMUNITY MENTAL HEALTH PROGRAMME (GCMHP)

Background

The GCMHP is a Palestinian non-profit making non-governmental organization. It was established in April 1990 by a psychiatrist, Dr. Eyad El-Sarraj, to provide comprehensive mental health services to the Gaza Strip. The need for such services became apparent during the Intifada, and is increased by the subsequent frustration and disappointment. Focusing on direct clinical work with both adults and children, in particular ex-political detainees and their families, the GCMHP aims to diagnose and treat the effects of violence and other human rights violations. Specific projects highlight the condition of women, and work for their empowerment in society. GCMHP also provides multi-disciplinary training to meet the need for qualified professionals in the field of mental health. In addition, it has launched public awareness campaigns to combat the ignorance and stigma associated with mental illness and the effects of torture. Our outreach includes a broad range of therapy and counseling services in four clinics: in Gaza City, Jabalia, Deir El-Balah, and Khan Younis.

The Program was established in the midst of the Palestinian "Intifada" against the Israeli occupation. The last ten years have witnessed the end of the Intifada, the Oslo Accords and subsequent agreements, and the establishment of the Palestinian National Authority (PNA). Such broad-sweeping changes, with all their psychosocial implications, highlight the need for substantial and sustained planning and development. This decade has seen GCMHP grow from three staff members at the time of its establishment to 100 full-time staff and 52 part-time employees at the end of 2000.

As the pioneer community mental health service-provider in Palestine, GCMHP has a rich record of achievement. Up to date, Approximately 13,000 patients have benefited from our therapeutic services. The Program has four clinics serving the Gaza Strip, the last of which was opened in August 1999 in Deir El-Balah to serve the central part of the Strip. GCMHP professionals have held hundreds of public awareness workshops, lectures, meetings, and seminars to educate professionals and the general public in mental health and related concerns. The Program has organized scores of specialized training courses for mental health professionals. In the field of research, GCMHP has been the first organization to conduct extensive scientific research on the psychosocial problems prevalent in Palestinian society. The research results are published in international journals and serve as the reference for mental health information on Palestine. Furthermore, the Programme publishes the only local bi-monthly specialized Arabic mental health magazine, "Amwaj."

GCMHP's Mission

GCMHP's purpose is to serve the Gaza community in particular and the Palestinians at large, especially the vulnerable groups, by improving the situation regarding mental health and human rights.

The promotion of democratic change within the society based on respect for human rights and people's dignity can best be achieved through developing a strong, professional, and transparent institutional model that is responsive and sensitive to community needs and local culture.

The many facets of GCMHP's work reflect the firm belief in the link between sound mental health and the respect for human rights, democracy, and freedom. Recognition of this link is vital in building a healthy civil society. Thus, the Programme is active in torture prevention and human rights advocacy locally and internationally. Consequently, networking and lobbying are an important component in the Program's work. This is clear in the ties established with local, regional, and international governmental and non-governmental organizations. For example, GCMHP is a founding member of the Palestinian Non-governmental Organizations Network (PNGO) and the Network of Centers for Rehabilitation of Victims of Violence and Torture in the Middle East and North Africa (AMAN). Through this network, the Programme actively participates in establishing centers for rehabilitating torture survivors in other Arab countries. In addition, the Programme is a member of the International Rehabilitation Council for Torture Victims (IRCT) and associated with TPO.

As the context of the Palestinian community is greatly politicized, it is difficult to separate politics from mental health of the people. This is why the philosophy of GCMHP take into consideration the issue of human rights violations and the historical context as important components affecting people's psyche.

Long-term Objectives

The mental health situation in Gaza has worsened due to three local factors. First, a population that is particularly vulnerable to mental health difficulties having undergone, and continuing to undergo, a high level of trauma and stress. Secondly, a culture that has traditionally stigmatized mental illness and its sufferers. Thirdly, traditional spirit healers who complicate the delivery of mental help services to the community. If a professional wants to examine help-seeking behavior in the Palestinian community, he or she would find two models. The first one is the traditional one in which the people go to traditional healers in order to solve their problems. These healers use some quotations of Quran or other methods like herbs. The second model is the medical model where the people go to primary health care centers complaining of physical symptoms. They continue to visit physicians without achieving positive results.

In order to improve this situation and contribute to the development of the Palestinian society as a whole, the Programme's immediate objectives encompass the following priorities:

- Enabling Gazans to cope with their traumatic experiences through (a) public awareness, (b) social support, and (c) individual treatment.
- Strengthening professional expertise in the areas of mental health and human rights through the training of professionals from the health, social services and education sectors.

- Working towards preventing further abuses from occurring and towards building an atmosphere of respect and openness.

Strategy

Immediate Objective 1: Enabling Gazans to better cope with their traumatic experiences through public awareness, social support, and individual treatment.

As indicated above, the coping strategy of the project consists of three mutually reinforcing levels of intervention that meet the different needs of the Gazan population exposed to trauma.

Public Awareness

At the community level, public awareness activities are initiated to provide the Palestinian people with the language and concepts with which individual victims, and the community at large, can address and understand their traumatic experiences in ways that do not stigmatize those suffering from traumatic experiences. Understanding the symptoms of trauma and practical ways of dealing with them is an important aspect of coping, and a way to ensure that relatively minor symptoms of trauma do not develop into more severe suffering. Public awareness activities are also initiated to make those in need of further assistance (social support and individual treatment) aware of the GCMHP and other services. The following initiatives are designed to reach a large public audience, across all sectors of Gazan society:

Amwaj. One thousand copies of the magazine 'Amwaj' (Waves) are published and distributed throughout the Gaza Strip on a bi-monthly basis. This magazine is free of charge and is distributed to the general public mainly through Ministries, schools, women's groups, NGO's and a variety of other public institutions. The magazine is specifically designed for the local population (as opposed to the professional or international communities), in an attempt to make mental health issues understandable and approachable. In addition to working towards the destigmatization of mental health problems, the magazine provides information about the mental health and social resources available in Gaza.

Video Centre. GCMHP established its video center to produce documentaries about pressing psychosocial issues as well as training films. Films are used in public awareness activities as they reach a wide audience more efficiently. Therefore, high quality, professionally produced films are an important facet of any public awareness campaign. The Video Center produces an average of three films per year by the GCMHP Video Centre, to be shown in public venues both locally and abroad. Since it started work in June 1996, the Video Centre has produced 15 documentary films dealing with issues of mental health and human rights, which have been aired in workshops, conferences, film festivals and training courses both in Palestine and internationally. Video Centre films have also been aired on Palestinian and European television.[1]

The Video Centre is currently engaged in three projects:

- Carrying out and recording a series of interviews with people uprooted in 1948, from towns and villages throughout Palestine. The subjects of the interviews range from 70 to 80 years old, and talk about their experiences before, during, and since their uprooting. Seventeen interviews have been conducted so far. This project seeks to preserve what is seen as an important Palestinian national resource-the narrative history of the Palestinian Diaspora-before it is lost forever.
- Documenting the lectures that comprise the Diploma in Community Mental Health (see below). The objective is to create a video resource library which would contain all necessary stages of the Diploma, to consolidate the lectures and seminars.
- Training women to shoot and edit on film. In August 1998, the Video Centre trained twelve women from the Women's Empowerment project during a three month course. Other training courses will follow. This documentary becomes a visible object lesson for suppressed Palestinian women that there are other possibilities besides passively accepting a traditional role.

Other initiatives. One public meeting is held per month, attended by approximately 50 people, on issues of mental health and human rights. These meetings are held in different venues in the Gaza Strip and are publicized through letters, posters and the local press. The meetings are also generally sponsored and publicized by local community groups.

At least four interviews for local television are conducted each year.

At least one article per month is written by GCMHP staff for local newspapers on issues of mental health and human rights.

Social Support

At the family level social support, such as family counseling and strengthening of the economic and social structures available to clients, are important means of reinforcing the coping abilities of those affected by experiences of torture or organized violence. Such support may, for example, take the form of

---

[1] In July 1997, the video team received an award for the film 'Near to Death' at the Cairo Third International Film Festival for Television and Radio in July 1997.

information and counseling of relatives on how to support and cope with their traumatized family member(s). The support may also take the form of referrals to vocational training that may help the client to find a job, or—in cases of severe economic and social problems—referral of clients to economic relief programs or social support carried out by other NGOs.

Individual Treatment

The majority of the work of the GCMHP is done with individuals, treating torture survivors, traumatized children, women victims of violence, and drug addicts in the clinics. Since 1990, about 13,000 people have visited the clinics for advice and treatment; we see between 80 and 100 new cases each month. Methods of treatment include psychoanalytic therapy, behavioral therapy, play therapy, cognitive therapy, occupational therapy and visual therapy.

GCMHP's multi-disciplinary teams utilize numerous forms of therapy. Counseling remains the most common form. Supportive therapy is second and is provided mainly for cases with chronic disorders. In addition, the staff provides cognitive therapy for patients with depressive conditions and cognitive-behavioral therapy for those with PTSD. Behavioral therapy is used mainly for clients with obsessive-compulsive disorders, phobias, and tic disorders. Children receive different forms of therapy, mainly behavioral, drawing, and play therapy.

Occupational therapy (OT) is another form of therapy provided to patients with chronic conditions. OT aims to enable patients to function as independently as possible in their daily activities and work environment. During therapy sessions, patients develop their skills in recreational and vocational activities. The OT unit conducted a total of 1,162 sessions in 1998 and 1999. The majority of clients were cured, improved, or had their conditions controlled.

The physiotherapy unit works to meet the physical as well as psychological needs of survivors of torture and organized violence. Locally, it is less stigmatizing for clients to seek physical therapy alongside psychotherapy rather than pure mental health services. Thus, the unit contributes to decreasing the stigma attached to mental illness while providing an important aspect of therapy. In 1998 and 1999, the unit treated 244 cases in 2,044 physiotherapy sessions. The unit staff also conducted 1,753 home visits.

Other services available to clients include a pharmacy and an EEG unit. Whenever necessary, medication is prescribed to patients, and is sold to them at cost price. Clients who are unable to bear the costs are given the medication at a discount or free of charge. In 1998 and 1999, clinic pharmacies provided medication to 7,866 clients. Of this total, 55% received it free of charge. The EEG unit is also available to the public and assists in the diagnosis of organic disorders. Like the pharmacy, this service is provided at cost price, or free for those not capable of paying fees. Nine hundred and eighty-six clients benefited from the EEG service in 1998 and 721 in 1999, with twenty percent of the total number free of charge.

There are also specific initiatives:

The Women's Empowerment Project (WEP). It seeks to improve, through education and training, the lives of women who have been victims of violence and unrest. The project started in 1994 and runs six-month rehabilitation courses for female victims of violence. These courses include social, psychological, health, and legal counseling, therapy, and vocational training in a variety of skills including literacy, ceramics, and embroidery. There are also more advanced courses in computing skills.

The project is based in Gaza City with centres in Rafah, Deir El-Balah, and Beach Camp (Shati). 30 women attend each of the four centres for the rehabilitation courses. There are also shorter vocational courses for women who are not necessarily victims of violence.

The Beach Camp centre holds one public meeting each month to discuss the role of women in Islamic tradition and society. Every two months, there is a meeting about the child/parent relationship, specifically looking at the different treatment of girls and boys within the family. These meetings take place with the cooperation of community and religious leaders.

Immediate Objective 2: Strengthening professional expertise in the areas of mental health and human rights through the training of professionals from the health, social services and education sectors.

GCMHP research carried out before we began the Programme indicated that 73% of those who visit primary health care centers in the Gaza Strip also suffer from psychiatric symptoms. This percentage demonstrates the need for a large professionally trained mental health workforce. Our training programs aim to create that workforce. The in-service training gave us the expertise to design the short courses and then the Diploma. Our staff also frequently attends international conferences, in order to build academic links with other organizations and to raise the international profile of the GCMHP. The ultimate intention of the GCMHP Training Department is to create an Arab Institute of Mental Health Sciences based in Gaza, with the cooperation of international universities.

In-service Training

GCMHP staff have also attended a range of courses within the Programme to enhance their expertise in the field of mental health care; the psychologists and psychiatric staff regularly contribute to seminars, workshops, study days, journal clubs, and case conferences, courses in (group) psychotherapy, as well as courses in child care, nursing, and computing.

Short Courses

The Programme also runs a series of shorter courses to train Palestinian health care providers in various mental health skills. In 1993, twelve nurses from the Palestinian Health System completed a three-month comprehensive course in community mental health nursing. In 1994, the department conducted a one year course in community mental health. Twelve social workers, psychologists, nurses, and doctors from different governmental and non-governmental organizations completed the course. Due to the success, we repeated the course in 1995 for another fifteen professionals. Upon completion of the course the Palestinian Ministry of Education employed all of the students as mental health professionals in health institutions and as school counselors.

In 1996, the department organized a six-month training course for women community leaders in coordination with the Women's Empowerment Project. Twelve women took the course, and are currently running their own women's community center in southern Gaza. To improve communication skills and to enable kindergarten teachers to instruct children and their parents, the training department organized two six-month training courses for child care providers in 1997. Forty participants from different kindergartens throughout the Gaza Strip attended these courses.

Post-Graduate Diploma in Community Mental Health and Human Rights

This Diploma is the first of its kind in the Middle East. A two-year, culturally sensitive, community-based course designed to encourage professionals to explore the theoretical concepts and practical applications of community mental health and human rights. The first year of the course provides participants with training in state of the art theories, principles and strategies of treatment and prevention. Under the guidance of international and local trainers, students complete ten core modules:

- Child/Adolescent Mental Health
- Social Psychology
- Clinical Psychiatry
- Communication and Counselling
- Culture and Mental Health
- Trauma, Stress and Coping

- Clinical Psychology
- Research Methodology
- Community Mental Health
- Mental Health Education

During the first year, students are also gradually exposed to clinical experience, interacting with clients to offer support and emotional containment without the demands of a structured therapeutic encounter. These experiences are aimed at facilitating the integration of theoretical and clinical work and the development of professional identity.

During the second year, participants receive a series of supervised clinical placements to explore the application of their knowledge. Students carry an outpatient caseload of 4–6 patients and provide therapy according to the needs of the patient. Over the year, the students also complete six two-month rotations. Four are core rotations conducted by all of the students in the areas of child/adolescent, adult, community, and family mentalhealth and well-being. The remaining two are elective rotations, in which students choose to focus on women, geriatrics, children, or other areas that interest them. The program culminates with the completion of a final project, in which the students integrate their theoretical and clinical training by writing about a clinical experience or community issue in which they were involved.

Following the GCMHP philosophy of community-based mental health care, the Post-Graduate Diploma emphasizes the shift from segregated and self-contained treatment systems within institutions to community-based therapy and social involvement in health related issues. The course seeks to move psychiatric therapy away from a traditional Freudian focus on the individual and his unconscious motivational conflicts towards an emphasis upon the role of environment and social interpersonal care. It also emphasizes the change in the role of mental health professionals from being providers of treatment to facilitators of treatment, helping individuals to solve their problems using the resources of family and community institutions such as schools, mosques.[2]

International Conferences

One of the traditions of the Programme, begun in 1993, is to hold international conferences in Gaza, both to raise international awareness of the problems faced by Palestinians, and to benefit from the academic dialogue with

---

[2]Seven international universities, including Edinburgh University (UK), Oslo University (Norway), Tel Aviv University (Israel), Tunis University (Tunisia), Flinders University (Australia), and Utrecht University (the Netherlands) contribute to the curriculum and teaching of the Diploma. Since it began training in February 1997, 37 people have completed the Diploma course.

foreign professionals in the field of mental health. The conferences allow professional cooperation resulting in education, research, and funding opportunities.[3]

Research

Research activities improve knowledge of the mental health and human rights issues facing the Gazan community; the publication of research documents is a valuable tool in raising the profile both of GCMHP's work, and of the current situation in Gaza. The work of the Research Department is therefore central to the work of the Programme. There are four areas of focus for GCMHP research:

Children. The impact of violence and traumatic experiences on children's psychological adjustment, child-parent relationships, and academic performance.

Human rights. The experience of torture, and psychological and social problems among ex-political prisoners.

Women and families. Families were the main target of Israeli military reprisals. The family also plays an important role in the protection of children, and is a vital factor in the social environment of victims of violence.

Epidemiology of psychosocial problems. Palestinian society in Gaza is engaged in rebuilding a peace-time environment and creating ministerial activities for social affairs, education, and primary and psychiatric health care. Gazan society therefore needs basic information on the epidemiology of health problems, illness behavior, social problems such as drug abuse, domestic violence, and mental illness and on cost-effectiveness of its interventions.

---

[3]In 1993, the GCMHP organized a conference on "Mental Health and the Challenge of Peace". This was the first international conference to be staged in Gaza; by chance, the date of its opening, September 13, coincided with the signing of the Declaration of Principles. Since 1993, the GCMHP has hosted another four conferences: in 1995 on "Palestinians in Transition: Rehabilitation and Community Development", in 1997 on "Health and Human Rights," in 1998 the Programme hosted the 6th IRAP conference on forced migration, and in 1999 on "Women in Palestine." In 1999, over 800 health professionals, scholars and activists from 24 countries came to Gaza to discuss the relationship between health, human rights, democracy and other ideals which form part of the individual self and community spirit. The fifth international conference is planned for 4–6 November 2001, with the title "Democracy and Arab Culture." The conference themes will include: Democracy: definition, roots, and history, Democracy and Mental Health, Religion and Democracy, Media and Democracy, Socialization and Democracy, Democracy and the Family, Role of Civil Society and Intellectuals, Democracy and Human Rights, Women, Equality, and Participation, The West and Democracy in the Arab world, Democracy and Rule of Law, War, Trauma, and Democracy, Economic Development and Democracy, Democracy in Politics, Education and Democracy Building, Democracy between theory and practice, and Democracy and the Struggle for Liberation.

Other Initiatives

The continuing activities of the GCMHP to prevent further human rights abuses, and to promote an atmosphere of respect and openness include:

- Since 1997, the GCMHP have been cooperating with the Palestinian Police in the training of their officers, to improve their communications skills and awareness of mental health disorders.
- Increasing activities and cooperation with local and international human rights organizations who are already working in the prison system.
- Increased cooperation and exchange with other initiatives involving the security forces and the prisons.
- Regular prison visits (possibilities: treating prisoners with mental health problems, interviews with prisoners, interviews with prison staff, evaluation of prison conditions, etc.)
- Material assistance for prisons (i.e., help in setting up a library for prisoners, providing limited amount of basic equipment such as table, chairs, overhead projector for Gaza prison training hall).

Staff of the GCMHP

Over the past ten years the staff of GCMHP has grown enormously. In 1990 we started with 11 fulltime staff and one temporary staff member. By 1995 these figures had grown to 47 full-time and 39 temporary staff. In 2000, GCMHP has 100 full-time staff members, and 153 temporary workers.

CONCLUSION

The GCMHP is one of the leading mental health organizations in Palestine. We believe in community mental health principles. Sound mental health is the product of the subjective feeling of harmony between man and the environment: man can therefore never have real mental health in an oppressive environment.

We believe that mental health workers have an important role to play, along with all sectors of the community, in the struggle for democracy and peace.

REFERENCES

Abu Hein, F. (1992). *Mental health of Palesstinian Children*. Gaza, Palestine: Gaza Community Mental Health Programme. Presented in the Third European Conference on Traumatic Stress, Bergen, Norway, June 1993.

El-Sarraj, E., Punamaki, R, Salmi, S., & Summerfield, D. (1996). Experiences of torture and ill treatment and posttraumatic stress disorder symptoms among Palestinian political prisoners. *Journal of Traumatic Stress, 9*(3), 595–606.

Nixon, A. (1990). The state of Palestinian children under the uprising in the occupied territories. *Swedish Save the Children report* (pp. 21–39).

Palestinian Human Rights Information Center (PHRIC). (1991). *Report 9*. Jerusalem: Author.

Punamaki, R. L., Qouta, S., & El-Sarraj, E. (1997). Relationships between traumatic events, children's gender, political activity, and perception of parenting styles. *International Journal of Developmental Behavior, 21*(1), 91–109.

Punamaki, R. L., Qouta, S., & El-Sarraj, E.(1997). Resiliency factors predicting psychological adjustment after political violence among Palestinian children. *International Journal of Behavioral Development, 24*(0), 1–12.

Qouta, S., Punamaki, R. L., & El-Sarraj, E. (1996). The relations between traumatic experiences, activity, and cognitive and emotional responses among Palestinian children. *International Journal of Psychology, 30*, 289–304.

Qouta, S., Punamaki, R. L., & El-Sarraj, E. (1997). Prison experiences and coping style among Palestinian men. *Journal of Peace Psychology, 3*(1), 19–36.

Qouta, S. (2000). *Trauma, violence and mental health: The Palestinian experience*. Unpublished doctoral disseration, Vrije Universiteit, Amsterdam.

Thabet, A., & Vostanis, P. (1999). Post traumatic stress reaction in children of war. *Journal of Child Psychology and Psychiatry, 40*(3), 385–291.

8

Walks in Kaliti, Life in a Destitute Shelter for the Displaced

LEWIS APTEKAR and ROB GIEL

INTRODUCTION

Since the end of the Second World War the frequency of wars has increased, and there have been more and more civilians casualties. Nearly 90% of the war related deaths during the last decade occurred to non-combatants and of them more than half were children (UNICEF, 1986). In last dozen years more than two million children have been killed in wars, and nearly 5 million more had been disabled. Add to this another 12 million children who were made homeless and another million orphaned or living without their parents (UNICEF, 1996). Furthermore the horrors of these wars where rape and decapitation of children and women were documented as a purposeful war policy have increased. Far from being senseless or irrational, war had become more rational, at whatever human costs it is designed to win. These costs include targeting health workers to prevent heath care, destroying schools to prevent education, and ruining places of religion to prevent a spiritual life.

In the small corner of the world where we worked the statistics were grim. More than a million and half Ethiopians died from 1974 when the late Emperor was deposed until 1990 when peace seemed to be at hand, most of them civilians (Endale, 1996). There were also 400,000 Ethiopian war returnees from the Sudan and nearly a half a million Somali war refugees living in Ethiopia. Add another half a million Sudanese refugees and 110,000 Ethiopian returnees from the wars in the west with Sudan. Then figure an additional 350,000 Somalian refugees and 450,000 Ethiopian returnees from the wars in Somalia and the Ogaden in eastern Ethiopia (UNICEF, 1996).

Of this massive group, some 57,381 people comprising 14,000 households were displaced Ethiopians living near or in Addis Ababa (UNDP, 1993). Over the course of next two years we would get to know these people at a level of intimacy which placed the statistics in the perspective of particular people facing their own very difficult circumstances. This meant that some of the problems that service providers who work with large numbers of people could deal with in abstraction or only logistically while we were forced to work fact to face with people who we knew. This created many moral dilemmas for us. For example, should we give material assistance? If so to whom, should we give help to our friends or to the people chosen unjustly by the powerful in the camp? Another dilemma our work posed was political. (TPO has a politically neutral stance, but realizes that politics are always part of the work that is being done). How could we not lobby for Kasu or Zewde, only two of many people we became close to, and who were essential to our work, and finally who were denied services because they were unfairly taken off the census list? If we did lobby would this not involve us beyond our expertise in mental health and beyond what we had promised the government we would do? But if we didn't, would this not be a betrayal of relationship to them?

Another problem that knowing people up close posed was to what extent should we use local people to help us? We knew that international organizations routinely promoted local ownership of programs, in large part to keep the project going after the expatriates and their money left. Our experience however suggested that it was far more effective to use people who were not tied or committed to the local society. We also found that money from international sources was far more important in keeping a project going than where a person was born. Even in a more psychological context, where positive memories and relationships might endure, we found that it was more likely to come from expatriates than local people (the reasoning of these points follow).

The problems of the people in Kaliti stemmed from living in Eritrea at the time the Eritreans were successfully concluding the war that led to their independence from Ethiopia. Many of them had lived in Ethiopia, now Eritrea for decades. They had made a decent living as civil servants in the ports of Aseb and Massawa, or in the provincial capital of Asmera. At the end of the war, their wives, usually Eritrean women, were given a few hours to choose either Eritrean or Ethiopian citizenship. If they chose Eritrean citizenship they could stay close to their families of origin, but they would not be able to stay with their husbands and children because they were considered enemies. If they accepted Ethiopian citizenship they could continue their lives with their husbands and children, but they would have to leave their families and homelands. The one's we came to know in the project described in this chapter left their past to start a new life with their husbands and children.

To get to Addis many were forced to trek through the hostile Danakil Depression, arguably the most inhospitable place on earth, where temperatures reached 50 degrees centigrade, (122 Fahrenheit) and where there was absolutely no water (Hancock, Pankhurst, & Willetts, 1997). Because they were forced to leave with only what they could carry in their hands, they made this march with insufficient water. Almost everyone witnessed relatives and friends who perished from thirst. Nor was this the end of their tribulations. When they arrived in Ethiopia they found that the Derg government (meaning military council) that had supported them, when they were in what became Eritrea, was no longer in power. The new government, the Ethiopian People's Revolutionary Democratic Front [EPRDF]) had overthrown the Derg. The EPRDF were not happy to have these former Derg supporters back in town.

At the time we began to work with them they had already spent six and a half years in camps for the displaced where their shelter had been primitive, and where health care had been inadequate. They were allowed to work in the public domain, earning 3 kg of wheat per day per family. Most families had as many as eight people. This meant that they not only lived near starvation, but because the ration did not always come on time, they lived with the fear of starvation.

It is important to note that they were not alone in these circumstances. Not only were there some 53 camps in and around Addis, but these are just a small number of the ones that now exist in nearly all cities of the developing world and in increasing numbers in the developed world. Because these shelters are so difficult to serve, by which I mean to show improvement to donors in quantitative figures that they are becoming more and more under served, including such primary needs as water, shelter and schooling. In fact as we discuss in the conclusion, our work in Kaliti is an example of what might be accomplished and not-accomplished in places of near absolute deprivation.

AIMS OF THE PROJECT

The Transcultural Psychosocial Organization (TPO) of Amsterdam had been in contact with the Department of Psychiatry of Addis Ababa University for several years, during which time they worked together to solicit funds for a research and training grant that would help this group with their psychosocial problems. The TPO, a World Health Organization (WHO) Collaborative Center has organized a cross-cultural study to assess the prevalence and types of mental disorders among war traumatized populations. They wanted to find out if there were any cultural differences that led to increased or reduced incidences of mental disorders and to find ways to support and build upon existing and successful coping strategies.

From the experience of the research that TPO had already accomplished they believed that the existing Western taxonomy of psychosocial responses to war trauma was unclear and inadequate (de Jong, 1996). They suggest that although the symptoms for Post Traumatic Stress Disorder (PTSD) and Acute Stress Disorder (ASD) are part of the Diagnostic and Statistical Manual (DSM-IV) another psychosocial disorder labeled Disorder of Extreme Stress Not Otherwise Classified (DESNOS) is more appropriate in situations of continuous traumatic stress. People diagnosed with DESNOS have difficulty modulating their anger. They tended to feel victimized or to victimize others. They had difficulty modulating their impulses, and found it hard to trust others. Amnesia, dissociation and somatizations were common symptoms.

The TPO research plan called for an epidemiological survey with the long-term aim to adapt its interventions to the evaluated need of the population. One part of the protocol, the Composite International Diagnostic Interview (CIDI) 2.1, was designed by the WHO to assess different types of psychopathology along the lines of the DSM-IV and ICD10, and it yielded specific diagnostic information. The CIDI had been tested in several cultures and was shown to be diagnostically reliable (de Jong, 1996).

The CIDI was composed of a set of questions followed by what was referred to as probe questions. For example, did you tell the doctor about your symptoms? If the person said yes, the following question would be, did the symptoms interfere with your life or activities? Before the reader rushes to judgement both the WHO and the European institute were aware of the immense difficulties of translating this information, (doctor, professional, medicine, etc) into culturally appropriate words and concepts.

Other standardized tests in the protocol included the ninety item Symptom Check List (SCR-90). This was a general standardized measure of psychopathology, particularly as an indicator of general neuroticism, as well as a measure of change in psychopathology. It had been used in various cultures indicating its cross-cultural applicability.

The Life Events and Social History Interview and the Hopkins Symptom Checklist (HSCL) gave demographic information, and the degree and type of trauma(s) experienced, and the subject's type of stress responses to them. The Social Support/Social Network Instrument gave information on the subject's social support and how much they took advantage of it. The Coping Style Scale, which indicated differences between trait, (commonly used coping mechanisms of an individual), and state, or specific coping strategies for particular circumstances. All of these were paper and pencil tests.

TPO recognized that it was necessary to go beyond paper and pencil data, and to collect other forms of data collection. The qualitative data was to be collected to yield specific information not likely to be found in the more impersonal testing. Focus groups were used to discover how people felt about their own mental health, including the ways in which they talked about it, that was their cultural concepts, the choice of words, etc. Key informants were to be chosen, because of having a special view of the community, to talk of their experiences (teachers, parents, children, and the elderly). Snow ball sampling, finding a subject with a particular characteristic and asking the subject to identify others with the same characteristic, so that insiders would add their point of view about particular topics, also helped in getting information from particular points of view. And data was to be collected from the use of participant observation and from narratives from various people. These kinds of data would help TPO discover how people had been able to cope, and therefore provide an avenue with which to work.

In addition to research, the TPO project included training a Core Group of people in mental health so that they would be able to train non-professionals to give mental health services in communities where trauma was prevalent.

What follows in this paper is a discussion of the information gleaned from the qualitative data and the problems and promises of training a Core Group. Most of the information that we report on here comes from the work we did in a single shelter, Kaliti.

THE SURVEY

To begin to assess the psychosocial problems in Kaliti we had planned to start by numbering each household, but before we could do that we had to define what we meant by a household. We listed the characteristics of a household as the physical place where people slept. It had to have demarcated boundaries. In some cases one wall of a household was the tent wall, while the other three were made from cardboard, but whatever their construction they still served as walls, they were used by the occupants to define the boundaries of their home.

Using these criteria we found that almost no households had their own separate four walls, by far the majority of them shared more then one wall with their neighbors. In more than a few cases all four walls were shared so that to get into the household it was necessary to walk through another household. Since, we defined households by these physical dimensions and included all the people who slept in the space, we found that many households had more than one family in them. Who slept where, and who could be considered, as a member of a household if they slept in and out of the camp was often difficult to determine.

We had also to deal with the fact that some people who said they lived in the camp were not always there. Some were visiting family and routinely left and returned, others lived outside of the camp for a time, then came back. There were also many kids who were fostered in Addis by relatives or friends of relatives, and these children returned on the weekends or on holidays. Some came back to stay in the camp. These were in fact coping strategies that the people of Kaliti used, and because on the guiding principles of TPO is to build upon existing coping strategies we were particularly interested in pursuing our understanding of this.

There were also many people who were in the hospital. Some of them came back, others came back after time, and some did not come back. People left to take the holy waters and did not return for a month. Even faster than the people left and came to the camp, were the far too common deaths. On the other side of life and death were the many newborn children.

It was also problematic that the physical structure of the households changed over time. As time progressed and people's financial statuses changed for the better or for the worse their household changed. In some cases new households were built, although more often people made improvements on their existing households by changing a wall of newspaper to a wall of cardboard, or moving an old wall to make a larger space. In cases where financial situations worsened, people had to downslide their spaces.

One thing we did was to take the census twice. After we numbered the households and made their first count of the people who were living in each one we made plans to come back and recount. The variability between counts gave us an additional reliability check. When we did the second count there were instances when we found someone who was there on the first census, but not there on the second. The opposite also occurred.

In spite of our efforts we were never able to eliminate problems. These were mostly related to the displaced being caught between trying to be honest with us because we knew each other, and having to inflate their numbers in fear of being left out of getting what was their due. All we can say is that we made several attempts to reduce this bias as much as possible while realizing that it was in part a way of their coping with their poverty.

In our second census we found a population of 2,076 people in Kaliti. There were 218 households. The average household size was 9.55. This was not the same as the average of people in a family, which was 3.86. Since we defined a household as a give space demarcated off from another space and the people in the household were the ones who slept in it, then it became obvious that people of different families were sleeping in a single household.

We then measured the perimeter boundaries of the camp, as well as the dimensions of the tents and the households within them. With this data we obtained information on population density. The approximate size of Kaliti camp including the living and non-living areas was about 4,125 square meters, or slightly less than an acre (4,840 square yards). The density of living space (including private living areas, public buildings like the schoolhouse, latrines, and stores, and public walkways) was about one person per 1.98 square meters. This meant that if a step was taken in any direction a person would either bump into someone else or be forced to take a side step.

We could only guess at what their current incomes were, because like getting the names of who lived in the camp getting the amount of money they had or earned was fraught with similar issues, including the fact that they used this as way of coping with their situation. I knew that daily laborers were jumping at the chance to work for 4 birr per day, which amounted to about 80 birr per month (at the time there were 7 birr per US dollar). Because of the esteem in which these jobs were held we thought that this was a high-income figure for the camp.

THE MATERIAL CONDITIONS OF THE SHELTER

There were four types of living accommodations in Kaliti. The camp had originally been built by the UN to house Sudanese refugees. These structures were made of mud and had tin roofs and were divided into small apartments. They were the first to be taken when the displaced arrived. Next were three large tents donated by the European Economic Community (EEC). These were supplied soon after they arrived in 1991. They were 25 meters by 12.2 meters, or 305 square meters. One of these tents, much like the other two, had been subdivided, in this case into 26 households. Each household had 11.7 square meters of living space. This meant that each person in the tent, which had a population of 247 people, had 1.23 square meters of living space). There was no electricity, no water, and no toilet facilities in these tents.

Most of the 26 households contained more than one family. Tshenish a chronically ill woman for example, shared her household tent space which was 3.5 meters by 2.8 meters (13.8 square meters or slightly more than 40 square feet, the size of a five by eight foot American prison cell) with a family of four. She lived on a bed made of dried mud mixed with straw. It was covered with the same blanket she received when she arrived. The other family had a slightly larger bed, also made from mud and straw. Newspapers and cardboard boxes composed the walls, as they did in most households in the camp. And, similar to almost every household in the camp, there were decorations on top of the newspapers. In this case there was a copy of a religious painting in bright pastels, and several figures of attractive young white women cut out from newspapers and magazines.

There was a plastic five-gallon container for water, and a black long necked ceramic coffeepot with six small, white ceramic coffee cups. All of her personal belongings were stuffed into one corner in two cardboard boxes, each large enough for a single person to use as a stool. Her single set of extra clothes hung from the Eucalyptus pole tent rafters. The households had no roofs, save the single roof for the whole tent, so that conversations and cooking odors were communal.

From June to September it rains every day in Addis Ababa, often excessively making the public health problems severe. The mud combined with the sewage and flowed into the public spaces. Drinking water should have been boiled, but this took fuel, which cost money. Carrying water was not easy so it was difficult to wash adequately. Using the latrine because it was a walk from the tents was problematic for the weak, and most children did not go there, particularly at night. Instead they relieved themselves in buckets, or on the ground in front of the tent. It was not much better in the dry season, because the heat inside the tents became intolerable, and the flies intrusive. Whatever the season, every night, the noise from painful tubercular coughing rumbled throughout the camp.

Injera, the local bread, was made from *tef*, (*ragrostisis teff*, a very small kernelled grass indigenous to Ethiopia and related to an ancient wheat species) an ancient wheat species that was milled, boiled and fermented, then poured into large pancakes and cooked on coal fires. In the morning the people ate *injera* with *wat* (*wat* is the stew or sauce, made of onions, garlic, pepper, and meat if possible). There was no lunch, except at times left over *injera* without *wat*. At night it was *injera* again, maybe with lentils. Many meals were no more than sweetened popcorn.

At first families were given grain rations of 500 grams per day per person by the government, which in turn received the grain free from international donors. The grain did not always come on time, perhaps a few months late. After this stopped a new program, the Food for Work Program allowed one member of each family to engage in a public works project, usually repairing roads, cleaning sewage lines, or the like. The family was paid in grain. When food was earned this way it created incentives for families to disperse so each person could get more to eat.

Many Ethiopians felt that the wheat each displaced family received from the Food for Work (FFW) program was too much. As we said the people in the camps around Addis had been displaced for six or more years. As time passed the amount of relief aid was diminished. At first there were food handouts of 15 kg of grain per person per month. Later it was reduced to 12.5 kg per person per month. The FFW program then replaced the food handout. At the start of the FFW program, every capable person could participate by working on public projects, like fixing roads. This was modified so that only one person was allowed to work from a single family. At the beginning FFW was paying 4 kg per day to a maximum of 100 kg a month. Even at this higher amount it wasn't much. The value of 100 kg per wheat was between 120 and 140 birr. This was about $20 per month in food per family.

In fact the grain was not a gift from the government. The grain came from donors who gave it as international aid. The Ethiopian government from Haile Selassie's time to the present periodically told donors that they had to pay an import tax on their donations before this aid could enter the country, but more of that later. For the time being as painful as it was to accept the argument that the displaced were getting too much assistance the people offering it might have had a point, particularly if the displaced were compared to the overwhelming number of Ethiopians who made up the impoverished masses. The Ethiopian infant mortality rate of more than 11.4% meant that more than one child in ten died before the age of two. Only 85% of children survived to see their fifth birthday and half of them were underweight which was defined as more than two standard deviations below the median for weight given age. Two thirds of the children who lived to be five years of age were stunted meaning that they were more than 2 standard deviations below the median for height given age. Two thirds of the population was below the absolute poverty line, defined as not having enough family income to buy food even at the lowest level of nutrition. Life expectancy was 49 years of age (UNICEF, 1997). In comparison, life expectancy in India was 62 years of age, while stunting and infant mortality in India were half of what it is in Ethiopia.

SURVIVING IN THE SHELTER

As soon as we started going to Kaliti we came to the realization that each time we went we were brought to see a person who was either gravely ill, or we were invited to attend a ceremony for a person who had just passed. This was becoming so common that the greater part of my days was being taken over by going from one to the other of the acutely ill or by attending funerals. Furthermore it was not simple to help them.

Astra, a small dark skinned woman in her mid 30's was so acutely ill that she could not raise her head to acknowledge us when we came into her space. She had a fever and was dehydrated. Her friend Checkla said that she had not eaten for several days. By her side was her eight-year-old boy, Frazier, who we were told was her only living relative. He had remained with her night and day.

Astra, as we were to learn from the other acutely ill in Kaliti, coped with their illnesses by waiting until they got better or died. After we sat down to try to get Astra's attention Checkla helped her change sides to face us. When she did the plastic grain sack that was her blanket came off her body, revealing her thread thin legs and a pair of red bikini underpants. Checkla held her gently while we tried to take her history. Her immediate concern was that she didn't have enough food to take her medicine with so that each time she tried to medicate herself she vomited up the medicine. With a grunting physical effort that was more eyes than words, she pleaded for money for injections, because injections could be taken without food.

We were told that in spite of having the referral paper to see a specialist she had not gone to the doctor, because she did not have the money for transportation.

We were to hear this over and over again. She had already spent all of her resources on medicine, which in fact was bought with the money that was supposed to be used for food. This was the reason why she was not eating.

There were three ways for her to get money, each revealed the stark reality of how they had to choose between coping strategies. One was for her to borrow from a family or a friend. She had no family except her boy Frazier who had been contributing a few pennies by shining shoes. Her neighbors had already loaned her some money. They had no more to give without jeopardizing their own lives. The second was for her to borrow against her future grain rations, which she had already done once. She knew if she did this again she would have no hope of being able to retire her debt and in her demise the debt might pass onto to her son. Third, she could get money from us. We knew that short of success on one of these options she would die.

Being white and foreign meant that she, and the others in the camp, thought we had a lot of money, which in comparison to Astra and the others we did. Although the parameters of our wealth were probably substantially exaggerated in their eyes, it is sufficient to say that we had enough to give her and many others adequate care. On the other hand what we did have, even if we were to give it all to them, would never cure all of their problems. We did have to accept that in Kaliti (as in Ethiopia) we were wealthy, not even solidly middle class as we were in our countries. The question was how to act given our newfound status. We did not have an easy answer; indeed much of what transpired over the next couple of years was in great part trying to figure out a moral and comfortable way to answer this question.

What was our responsibility as wealthy people? Should we give money to Astra? If we did what would be our rationale for giving in this case and not another? If we started giving to Astra or to anyone when would we stop? Should Astra die, which seemed imminent would we have wasted the limited available funds? When she did die should we pay for her funeral, given its much higher importance in this culture than in ours?

How would the act of helping materially alter our role as mental health experts? Any material assistance given would also have to take into account that our program had already tried to come to terms with the camp on this issue. We had agreed that in return for our work we would give some of them training in mental health, the services of a nurse, a teacher for a school, and psychiatric care at the hospital. If we gave Astra money, what would this mean to our previous agreements and how would the people in the program look upon my efforts?

With Astra in front of us we also thought about how the displaced people in the camp might help her. At what point would Astra's friends and neighbors stop giving her money, would it be at the point when they thought she would die with or without it? Once they made a commitment to her would they follow through until she was buried and her death properly mourned? What about Frazier her boy, would there be any effort from the community to help him? Did they talk about these options openly, or was there some other way they dealt with these decisions? Obviously, how they came to make or avoid making these decisions would shed a light on the mental health of the community.

We would continue to go on these daily rounds and see the sick and dying. Our giving or not giving material aid was not just an economic or theoretical problem; it was a therapeutic issue. Coming to an acceptable agreement with them about what it was that the program had promised, and how we would deal with the inevitable situations that were outside of this domain, like the problem with Astra, would be an on going trial. This was a struggle of no less significant outcome than who would live and who might not.

It was impossible to come to a judgment between their constant need to get what they could from us, and in our continual desire to draw the line and prevent them from becoming dependent upon us, outside of the Ethiopian context. There was something in this akin to the Ethiopian beggar asking for alms. In each case it was stark reality of their coping choices. Still it was difficult for us to understand (and for Westerns generally) that the beggars were working in God's service by asking people to help. On the streets the more persistent the begging, the more the beggar asked for, and the worse the presentation of the beggar's self (elephantiasis and leprosy being common), meant that the beggar was actually creating a favorable situation for the benefactor. Because the more in need the beggar was in the greater the opportunity the benefactor had to demonstrate his religious generosity. What was happening in the camp was not dissimilar to what was occurring on the streets. In the cultural context it was our duty to share out wealth.

Astra finally was admitted to Mother Teresa's home for AIDS victims and her friend, Checkla, who took her there was staying with her because Astra needed constant care. A problem emerged over what to do with Checkla's two children. Several people were gathered around to talk about this problem. Before long the conversation became heated. A flamboyant stout middle-aged woman, Amharich, screamed at us to get out of the camp. We were not helping them, she said, only causing more problems. Why should she give up her *teff* (her grain ration) for these two children when we, the *ferenji* (the foreigner) could give them money? An argument immediately broke out. Yeshe disagreed with Amharich and told her about the teacher at our school, our offer to give them psychiatric care, and our effort to get a nurse. A few other people came forth to support us, but it was clear that the woman was not alone.

On the face of it the reasoning was clear, we had a duty given our wealth. But there were other factors to consider. The crowd felt we were closer to Yeshe than anyone else in the camp, and thus believed that she must have been getting something material from us. (Another aspect of Ethiopian culture is that patrons take care of their help [Pankhurst, 1990]). They were not able to feed any more children, and they thought that it was Yeshe's or our responsibility to take over this added burden.

We also had to consider that the motivation of Checkla for taking care of Astra in the hospital was financial. She might have calculated that she would be able to get extra money by earning a profit on what we would give her, and therefore have something left over for her family. It was also possible that part of the anger from the camp was coming from their frustration. Each time they saw us coming they became agitated, it was almost a physiological reaction. As if seeing us was the stimulus that provoked their recurrent worry of the uncertainty of whether or not they would get help.

REVIEW OF MENTAL HEALTH PROBLEMS, PTSD AND THE HORRORS OF THE CAMP

Over the course of our work we had many visiting European experts on post-traumatic stress disorder (PTSD) come to the camp. They had been in Cambodia and Rwanda, and other places. Usually they commented on the lack of PTSD in Kaliti. The central symptoms of PTSD, which they felt were not apparent, included unwanted mental interruptions of images and thoughts. At night the afflicted person had bad dreams, during the day he or she were not able to control troubling thoughts. In short, people with PTSD were plagued by what they were trying to forget. We came to believe that the visitors did not see PTSD because the people in Kaliti were preoccupied with getting something to eat and obtaining medicine, often for death threatening illnesses, and so the visitors were not able to separate their mental health problems from the "real world" problems.

Yet, in spite of the obvious needs of the displaced in Kaliti, the trauma they had lived through paled (at least by our standards) in comparison to what the Europeans told us about the highly traumatized people. Pol Pot's regime murdered more than a third of the population, often with the family's participation. Among the inhabitants of Kaliti only a few had seen their loved ones murdered, and no one that we knew of had been made to maim or kill their relatives in order to survive. Nor, had they been through the kind of genocide that was associated with Rwanda.

What characterized the people of Kaliti was their march across the Danakil, and their poverty. (A paper yet to published by TPO on the results of the epidemiological survey will show that the march more than the poverty predicted what PTSD that was found.) Their poverty meant they were able to eat only one meal a day. This meal was no more than a threadbare *wat* and *injera*. They were also familiar with non-existent or nearly non-existent medical care that forced them into a demeaning posture to even obtain the minimum service.

Having been promised compensation for what they had to leave behind, or perhaps more succinctly holding on to the possibly of what they thought they had been promised, they also lived with the fear of giving up what claims they had. Thus they were unwilling to leave Kaliti because they knew it would certainly mean forfeiting any of their claims and therefore of the possibility of being able to return to the style of life they had had. Some of these people remained in a deadly state of a psychological waiting. They were unable to look back and resolve their grief or make a decision to move forward. This was what separated the resilient from those who were likely to succumb. It also helped us realize that there was probably a selection factor of the people who were now seeing at Kaliti. In the physical reality of Kaliti there was some question about how long a person with a severe psychosis could last. This helps explain why over the time that we were working there were less than expected cases of psychosis. We found no one who was mentally retarded. This might well have been because psychotic people did not live through this type of ordeal. (We should be clear, acute psychosis was more common, but much of it probably came from HIV infection, untreated epilepsy, and TB).

We never were able to get an accurate assessment of how many people left the camp. I would not be surprised if over the years, the better functioning people left. What we were seeing was not a random sample of all the people who marched through the Danikil. We were seeing a narrower distribution, as if the ends of the normal curve were truncated. In this middle, the people stayed afloat, barely, but for the most part clearly. They usually found resiliency from attachments to other people, most commonly this was family, but it was also between young men and women, and also from administering and receiving care for the illnesses that were always present. Also, in many ways they were like Job, in spite of being tested above and beyond what life should bring, they maintained and found solace in their faith. Resilience also came to some extent by preexisting biological factors.

Another explanation for the visitor's observations was that PTSD might have had different symptoms among the people in Kaliti. We wondered if the horrendous of the common was what the experts visiting Kaliti missed and therefore this was why they did not see the people of Kaliti as bona fide psychologically traumatized? In Cambodia nearly 40% of the population was killed, and in Rwanda 14% of the population had been slaughtered in three months. In Mozambique 48% of the health care facilities and 45% of the schools were destroyed. Did the trauma in Kaliti, much more a feature of the 45 million refugees and displaced in the world, fade by comparison so that the visiting experts from the worst stations of Hell could not find the manifestations of trauma in the more common spaces of Hell?

Over the two years we worked with them we could not help but imagine the mental health of the people who shuffled through a day and then another day leaning against the weight of promises and possibilities made and broken. It was not possible to accept them as psychologically functional as we saw them being forced to bend again and again to the vagaries of the on going weather of despair and hope. In fact, throughout the study we went from believing they were suffering from PTSD, to believing they were not, and later coming up with a broader, and we believe more accurate assessment of PTSD, one that would encompass their psychosocial problems, which finally we could not dismiss as benign. These subtler, yet still debilitating, psycho-social manifestations of trauma, their manner of coping with their problems, included many physical symptoms, difficulties of facing new challenges, and problems associated with engaging unnecessarily and often self destructively in petty disputes. All of these symptoms overrode the process of coming to terms with the larger issues of grief and recovery that the people would have to face. They were therefore serious symptoms of mental disorders.

It was almost as if the people found that the symptoms were too frightful to bear. Instead of being able to cope directly with them, their problems were released in constant bickering between different factions seeking help and in being too demanding to those who were trying to help. There was also a terrible void in the civic body. No public health efforts were made even though the community had plenty of time to care for one another. Poor sanitation and nutrition led to preventable illnesses that reduced the people's capacity to function, which in turn led to further community health problems, and so on, all of which added to the stress of life in the camp and to mental disorders. In fact the cycle had placed them at such a low level of morale that many people, particularly those who were outside of the traditional kinship system and those with particularly strong stressors to deal with, were not able to meet their basic mental health needs.

What we found was that there were cultural differences in the symptoms of psychopathology. For example elective mutism, hysterical blindness and other dissociative disorders like shaking and falling down were far more common in Kaliti than in the West. These unsuccessful coping strategies, which we rarely faced, seemed in our encounters with them to stake out the bleak degree of what they were dealing with. In fact it was difficult to know if people were possessed by spirits, or physically or mentally ill, and to go one dimension deeper past our Western cultural beliefs, it was difficult to know if there were any differences between the three. What we did find important was that all the above disorders were related to anxiety, which is also considered the source of post traumatic stress reactions. It might well have been that this was the way they showed their post-traumatic stress, rather in the more typical symptoms defined in the DSM-IV.

We also found that not everyone in the camp suffered or coped in the same way. There were the physically ill who were emotionally strong like Tsehenish, who before her illness was able to roll over her less than righteous job as a bar-girl into the ownership of her own bar. This strength helped her cope with her fatal illness and in coming to terms with the death of her husband and the loss of her daughter. Also in this category was Solomon, who died a slow death from HIV infection, which reduced him from thinking of a career in theatre to thinking about suicide.

Another category was the physically ill who were also emotionally compromised either by intense environmental factors like Yodit whose losses mounted almost beyond what was imaginable, or by existing mental disorders. In this category there were psychiatric patients, including those with AIDS and AIDS related dementia (it was impossible to distinguish without laboratory testing AIDS related dementia and some other mental disorders). There were far too many like Traz, who were not ill themselves but who had to treat and deal with the loss of their loved ones who were ill. Grief was as rampant as the lack of health.

There were also the resilient like Mama Zewde who had buried three children since being displaced, but who danced in public ceremonies. And, Ato Abdu, the one legged man who fostered an orphaned girl. And Mulu, whose stepfather spent his days with her two-year-old hemiplegic daughter on his lap. And, there was Lumlum who found pleasure from fostering the orphaned boy, Frazier. And there was Shama who never stopped working to find health care for Mengistu, her eight-year-old epileptic boy.

There were the overqualified who hadn't given up like Mengistu Asefa, the former captain who had led a Division in war, but could do no better than sell chat in a local kiosk. And Afwak without work raised his family to succeed (his oldest daughter was at the top of her high school class). And there were many under qualified like Abana, a woman with eight children who could not feed any of them. She could only survive by getting assistance. Not much could be done to help her or others like her, save building a strong community, one capable of taking care of its lowest functioning members.

TRYING TO INTERVENE, CONCEPTS AND MISCONCEPTIONS

Each couple of months, the Christian Relief and Development Association (CRDA), a self styled mega-NGO of all the groups working with refugees and the displaced in Addis held a meeting. The CRDA wanted to coordinate programs, thus avoiding duplication and serving as a focal organization for donors and the government. They had produced a document on the displaced that they were going to discuss today. They were hoping to take a vote and come to a final position statement. We were asked to make comments.

As soon as we convened, and there were representatives from all the NGOs, we started talking about how difficult it was for the NGOs to continue working in the camps. Donors were offering relief but not rehabilitation funds. (Relief funds come immediately after a disaster and are for food, shelter and immediate medical care. Rehabilitation funds, which come at least six months after a disaster, are for more long-range assistance, including job training. These funds are more difficult to get and become even more difficult as time progresses).

It was the opinion of many in the meeting that the government did not want the NGOs to continue. They thought that what the government wanted was to worsen the situation in the camps and therefore make it easier to close them down and get people out. This made more sense than the other position, which was that the government wanted to destroy the camps by using bulldozers. We thought it was more likely for the government to use an approach of benign neglect than out right hostility. They would just stop giving aid and let the displaced live where they were going to live, which was what happened in most parts of the developing world where squatting had been the way that the poor got a start with a home. It could happen here so we were more optimistic. In fact this might be used as a good negotiating stance with the government—you stop giving us food, we keep the shelter. The government could shed its responsibility and the displaced would keep their place and their community. By negotiating this rather than just letting it happen it would at least make things clear and allow people in the camps to get on.

The CRDA report began with the background information about the displaced, which stated that there were 52,927 displaced people in Addis. This was twice the figure of the second registration, which came without warning. Some people in the room thought the real number was closer to 24,000 and maybe even less than that. They argued that the inflation of the numbers was "a coping strategy" that the displaced use to get more aid. We didn't think it was a meritorious coping strategy. It was too much like fraud, because given a limited amount of funding for the displaced the ones who increased their numbers received more, thus cheating the honest people, or causing everyone to lie. It was a matter of citizenship, of the importance of working toward the communal well being over self-interest. While others continued to see it as a legitimate way of dealing with a corrupt government policy we thought that what happened in the government registrations was that people without families were being pitched against families, while the government was winning the war of not caring for its own.

The report focused on giving priority assistance to the women and children. In fact it was our opinion that it was men who needed the most help. The women were working in Food for Work (a public work project funded by donor countries), and had continued with their traditional roles in child rearing and being in charge of the household. They were too busy, but better off than the men who sat and played cards, chewed *chat* and were out of work, but desperate for it.

Although it was easy to view the men who were only drinking tea, gambling in card playing, and not taking care of their families or communities, as part of their cultural gender roles, we saw these men as emasculated from their gender specific roles and clinically depressed.

As young men they moved from their rural homes into the cities, competed successfully to gain access to the miniscule salaried economy, some in the military and many in what might be referred to as the military industrial economy. In this new life they worked in teams on tasks that were far greater even in imagination than they had ever dreamed of. They learned to be mechanics for tanks, transport vehicles, and some worked on airplanes and naval ships. In the civilian sector they refined oil, learning and becoming in command of the technology that it required. They earned enough to buy homes, electrify them, have refrigerators. They had children and the children were fed and clothed, and attended school. The family had medical care. They were a part of the Ethiopian middle class.

It was in the tearooms where they sat like patients in a hospital day care recovery room, rather than as men (most of them were young and hardly any of them were too old too work) relaxing and celebrating their accomplishments. They had lost the power to support their families, their wives were doing what minimal and menial work in the Food for Work program that was available. They were no longer warriors or providers, nor part of team of men working together to reach a challenging goal. They were war victims, not physically wounded, but certainly injured and deserving of attention. Giving priority to children and women would make men even more withdrawn and less involved. This would place yet more stress on their families, even the families that were able to make it intact through this would only find themselves more in stress and disharmony.

We thought it prejudicial (and wrong) to say as many in the meeting did, that the men walked off with money that was given to them, while the women actually would used it appropriately. What was being said was that Ethiopian men, (and also by implication men of the third world) were not responsible. If there was any truth that men were not responsible would this not be even more reason why they needed help before women did?

In fact it was prejudicial to favor any group over another, but this was what came out of central planning. It worked to reduce individual initiative. It was better to take things case by case. We told them about Abdu, the one legged man who had adopted his deceased friend's daughter. Here was a man without a family, the lowest on the scale, yet he might be the most worthy and the best investment for funding. Why shouldn't he be given priority? Why not meet everyone on his or her own merit?

We ended up thinking that it was not wise to cultivate inter-NGO support. The NGOs wasted too much time and money by the need to make communal decisions or in spending money on offices, equipment, vehicles, etc. On more than one occasion we had seen $35,000 dollar vehicles, being driven by salaried drivers, running errands to accomplish a $1.00 task, like getting photocopies. Consensus building tended to work toward continuing the past, rather than trying the new. At the ground level the job of helping the displaced didn't need political consensus.

There were plenty of other problems to deal with (Aptekar, in press, a). Based on our Western training we wanted to start by using the family as the basic level of social interaction, but we could not stay with this for long, because most people in the camp no longer had traditional families, and their traditional families were changing quickly. In fact the balance between the traditional the modern was always a difficult act to understand.

There were, for example, long standing Amharic descriptors for mental illness, including people who wandered naked on the streets and whose language was unintelligible, who were aggressive and talked to themselves (*ibd, kewes*). *Wofefe* referred to rural people whose mood fluctuated suddenly. *Bisichit* described people who were greatly irritable, intensely gloomy or severely anxious. *Abshiu* referred to people who were aggressive because of being intoxicated. The reader can see Araya and Aboud (1993) and Kortmann (1987) for additional terms. The main point here was that in the West mental illness was assumed to come from childhood experiences, ongoing mental stressors, and physiological dispositions, while in Ethiopia mental illness was believed to be caused by evil spirits, the main ones being the *buda*, and the *zar* (Vecchiato, 1993a,b).

In Ethiopia it was estimated that 2.6 million adults and about 3 million children suffered from psychiatric disorders (Araya and Aboud, 1993). Very few of these people would be served in secular offices. Almost all the mental health services were provided in the church or in an area, which were designated for its spiritual value.

Our philosophy was secular humanism and our counseling practice was democratic, while in Ethiopia the practitioner was religious and authoritarian. When an Ethiopian went to Church or to a traditional healer for psychological problems they supplicated themselves to God or to other forms of the supernatural. For us it was more common to form a professional alliance and to expect healing to come from secular theories based on natural scientific principles.

Our therapeutic expectations involved occasional emotional arousal. But it was mostly well thought out recollections of past and current events, while among Ethiopians counseling clients were expected to be taken over by what we might refer to as a "hysterical" or dissociative trance or what they referred to as spiritual procession by for example a *Zar*. While we were expecting the clients to listen and contemplate they were expecting to pray and to follow directives.

On one occasion we were presented with a 40 year-old woman who like a few others in the camp was living with non-relatives. She never had had any children, and no money of her own. As she said, she had no relatives, no blanket, no clothes, and no friends. The couple with whom she was staying had just had a new baby. We were taken to see her because the noise in the house and the crying of the newborn were driving her as she said, crazy. She cried uncontrollably. While she was crying the new child's aunt came out and held and hugged the woman. One of the Ethiopians with us told her in no uncertain terms that in spite of the noise she should stay in this house where she was loved and where she would be missed if she left. She agreed, stopped crying, became more animated, and we left. Counseling in Ethiopia was often done when a person of higher status lectured and gave direct order to a person of lower status.

We began our intervention by starting school for the children, and beginning supervised sports activities. We also organized some adolescents in the camp who were interested in the performing arts. We found that beginning with children helped the community come together because they were able to put aside their differences to help their children. We also believed that as the children learned more and became more active, their self-esteem would rise. And as the children's self esteem rose the community would feel better, and this would result in having more energy to tackle the long list of other problems they faced.

Our first training began with four young men and four young women who were identified by the Kaliti community as having high character. We paid them a small stipend and enlisted them as students. They accompanied us on our daily rounds, and listened to us as we talked about what we were doing. In spite of the possibility of being ethnocentric (and modern) we demonstrated to the community with these eight people that we were willing to collaborate with them.

Trust between us loomed as a serious problem in this particular cultural context for the reasons we have suggested, but also because of their particular history. They were displaced persons and they had been traumatized. They had become too efficient at understanding how they should respond, they said only what they thought needed to be heard. For us to penetrate this barrier we had to drop the draping of conventional professionalism and open up to a much more personal approach. Our work with the eight camp students helped us in this, and in coming to terms with the differences of our cultures.

What we found was at the heart of the resilience in this community was the value they received from their spiritual beliefs. They were actively religious. Even after they came to grips with the loss of their loves ones and the demise of their material lives, with faith and philosophy they were able to endure. We should acknowledge that these very two factors were commonly the focal points of criticism of life in the West. On the other hand their civic politic, a strength in the West was particularly weak in Kaliti.

We could not move forward without a way of knowing if their mental health was improving. In the case of the children we could look to see if our work was improving attendance or performance in school. But there were less tangible but important parameters. These included the balance between religious and civic life. For example, we wanted to improve their camp committees so their duties would be more fairly carried out. We wanted to help them form new coalitions as situations demanded so that adolescents or widows or orphans for example could work together for a common goal better met by collective than by individual efforts. We wanted them to become stronger when relating to the political process that so scared them. We hoped that they would work on their own sanitation problems instead of waiting for someone to help them, or that they help each other with resources like pooling money to buy food communally.

We wanted to help the community get to the point where they were ready and able to make a decision about staying or leaving the camp. If they chose to stay we wanted them to acknowledge that they would continue living with the onslaught of programs offered by the government to get them out. They would also have to live with the decreasing amount of assistance by the NGOs, including the increasingly lack of adequate health care, food and shelter. Their food was coming later and less regularly. The governmental offerings to get them out of the camp were coming more frequently and were coupled with stronger threats about closing the camps and taking away all services.

If they chose to stay we wanted them to realize they were facing only the hope of getting a better compensation from the government, and we wanted them to dig into camp life and make it better, instead of spending all their energy asking for help. What was important was that they acknowledge the reality of their circumstances, and make a clear decision—either take one of the options offered to them, with the realization that it was not as good as they wanted or perhaps even deserved, or stay. If they chose to stay we hoped they would do something more than wait, we hoped they would become involved in improving their lives.

WORKING WITH THE CORE GROUP

To reach this end we began a 15-week training of a Core Group of 18 mid career Ethiopians who were working for NGOs, the international associations like the UN agencies, the Ethiopian government, and from Churches. These institutions were the ones that were involved with refugees and the displaced, although they did not have mental health programs. What we discovered was that while these professionals began their careers working in the field they had long ago moved into the office. If they had been to any of the camps it was on a quick, "official tour", which meant they rarely had more than a perfunctory view. Most of them really had no idea about what life in Kaliti was like.

After the first week when the students came back with their first written histories, they said that their clients did not have mental health problems, only physical health problems, and problems of poverty. One man from the Ethiopian

Orthodox Church for example began counseling a chronically ill woman. She asked him for medicine. A week later he brought it to her, and then he was ready to change clients, because he saw no reason to continue seeing her. Yet, he understood that counseling could be of help to her if for nothing else than preparing her for her demise and death.

Another of our students, Makde, interviewed Yodit, a young woman who lost her child and her husband last year, as well as being chronically ill. After her initial interview she did not think that Yodit had a mental health problem. We wondered if the reactions of these two students, and of several others, was not a form of mutual denial. For example, Yodit denied the intense loss of her husband and child by thinking that her return to her mother would resolve these losses, while Makde contributed to Yodit's denial by avoiding thinking how these problems might cause her mental duress. The same for giving medicine to the chronically ill. Our student thought she would be better and have no problems, an idea as unrealistic as it was foolishly hopeful.

Eventually, we were able to overcome this problem by asking them to think of Yodit. She was barely 21 years old, had been married, left, remarried and had a child who had since died. She also was a chronic TB patient and probably was HIV positive. She obviously had a lot of grief and worry and also probably very little idea of herself as an adult woman. There were many ways that counseling might be of help to her. This suggestion was not difficult for them to understand.

We also noticed that when the mid-career students began counseling they did not have a clear idea of what the outcome of counseling might be. For example, Nesibu, a serious young man who was one of the growing number of Ethiopians brought up in the Orthodox church who converted to Protestantism, was counseling Getachew, a 28-year-old Amharic man whose wife left him with their boy who was then a toddler. Since then he had been bringing up this boy, who was now nearly six years old. Getachew complained of sleep disturbance since his wife left him. He also had a chronic health problem that eventually led to his demise. Nesibu brought him some medicine and gave him clothes for his son. Nesibu explained his work as "spiritual counseling" in order to change Getachew's "life style". He didn't think he was successful because after two weeks his client continued to have vices, meaning he smoked cigarettes and chewed *chat*. It was as if the goals of counseling could be accomplished miraculously, as if there was no psychological aspect to it. Did this work? I think it had temporary benefits. It was in line with their customs so it was easy to digest and getting the material comforts also was uplifting, but I never saw that it changed character.

The student's traditions gave them information about what behaviors were considered mentally ill. These included acting strangely or having severe anxiety or depression. They were aware that some things in the camp were morally wrong. They knew that some people took advantage of the weak, either by lending money at exorbitant interest or by charging for services like administering medicine that should have been given to the abject for free. They did not consider these issues of people's psychosocial well being. We tried to point out that to a great extent the level of a person's psychosocial well being was what separated those who succumbed to those who survived. When we made our rounds of the sick, it was clear that there were differences in their will to live. It accounted for determining the energy they had to compete for the daily struggle of getting food and getting health care when it was needed. The amount of fear about what would happen next was also important to predicting who might survive and who might succumb. Rest at night and some peace from anxiety in the day, kept people physically healthier. Constant distress wears the body down. With serious illness so close this too was dangerous.

Over the course of our work we were beginning to see some changes. What broke the door open to understanding was a remark by one of the mid-career students. He said that although his client was getting sicker and sicker, and there was nothing more that he could do for her physically, he thought talking to her had helped her feel better.

Several people over the next several class sessions mentioned a few practical feats we had accomplished. We were able to get health letters from the Kebele for people who were not properly registered. We were able to get the TB patients reregistered for extra rations after they were taken off the list with the second registration. We were able to increase the numbers of people from the camp who could go to the clinic each day from 10 to 15. We had a meeting in which the displaced and the government talked directly to one another, and even though it was not a pleasant meeting, both sides agreed to meet again. We also agreed that we were more educated about the problems of the displaced, and that we had raised the awareness of others in the NGOs, in the government and among the international organizations. Among ourselves we were thinking about the fact that in many ways these successes were political in nature.

This coupling, the connection between impacting the government and improved mental health posed a professional dilemma, in the West mental health practitioners did not become involved in this way. On the other hand, while it was true that these were tangible results we pointed out that in the field of mental health it was very difficult to know if or what progress was being made. We said that rather than see someone make a significant change in his or her life, it was more likely to see someone see old problems more deeply and complexly, and to question old themes more subtly. Then Almaz a student in the class said that she had been working with a woman who had no food and was about to die. She didn't know what to do. Finally she thought of going to see Sister Mary's feeding program. She went and was given food to give to the dying woman. After the woman ate, she said her wish was that her only son would know his father before she died. She gave Almaz some details and she began to trace his whereabouts. Although the woman died before she could find him, Almaz said that the search itself had given the woman hope and she died knowing that it was still possible for her son to meet his father.

It was apparent that they had been counseling clients who had died while they were working with them. Most of these deaths had been from preventable diseases, meaning that the students had watched the people suffer from sicknesses that could have been avoided by public health efforts, often with just a little bit of money, sometimes no more than the transportation needed to get them to the hospital.

It was obvious that we were asking a great deal from these students. We were telling them to work without being able to give much if any material support to their clients who were in dire need of it. We were telling them to get and give solace solely from the psychological help they could give. We were also saying that they needed to do this in the face of death, in fact in the face of preventable death.

It was highly unlikely that any of us would find a definitive pleasure or *raison d'être* from out work in Kaliti. Like most of our clients the progress of the mid-career students would be subtle and complex. Just as the mid career students were beginning to see some changes and the more involved they became, the greater the emotional difficulty of working in the camp became so that in the end the biggest problem was to prevent them from dropping out due to frustration.

DISCUSSION AND CONCLUSION

One European woman who had been hired by an NGO to ascertain how their organization might help the "poorest of the poor" came to class to talk about her work. She said the two major assumptions of her organization (and indeed this was true of the NGO's in general) were first not to give direct assistance to these people because this would produce aid dependence, and would in the end be spent foolishly without making long lasting changes. The second assumption was that local people should be used as much as feasible and that as soon as possible local people should replace all expatriates. In a lively discussion we disagreed with both of these points.

She encouraged the generally accepted idea among most donors that as soon as possible the donors should turn their organizations over to local people. This was in our position usually a mistake. The turnover policy transferred money from the middle class in the developed countries to the aspiring middle class of the developing countries. I wanted her to know this was not in itself immoral or unwise, but it was a far cry from helping the poorest of the poor in the best possible way.

The usual career path for local personnel was to start out at the lowest level of helper, for example as assistants to people collecting data on health or vocational programs. As soon as they entered the NGOs, even working in entry level capacities they received, relative to their compatriots employed in local organizations, far better pay. If they continued with the NGOs, putting in time, and receiving some training by ex-patriots they moved up to mid-level employees, such as the data collectors for our epidemiological survey. As they moved up their income would be in a higher income bracket that further separated them from their countrymen in the local market, even when the latter also moved up in rank. Then, with another level of expatriate training, possibly including a trip to a workshop or conference in a developed country, they would get to point where they would be working under the expatriate administrator of the program. At this point they would be on the edge of entering the local middle class. Finally, with additional time and exposure (and comfort) with the employees from the donor country they would be ready to take over the program.

We were impressed that the Ethiopian people who had been in Kaliti and who were on this employee track were very moved by how badly the displaced were living, but they all nevertheless had a reason not to contribute. Their reasons for not helping the displaced in Kaliti invariably included the fact that working with the displaced would disrupt their careers because the displaced were not favored by the government. They had built up or were building up some middle class security and they became very careful not to lose their perch. This was apparent across cultures, but seemed to shine more clearly when the stakes, like they were in Ethiopia, were higher and the potential fall from grace more profound. There were very few middle class options in Ethiopia and those at its precipice knew how important it was to look after one's own welfare. It was imperative not to make a mistake. The result was that people in this position did the same of what had been done before, usually with more gusto.

Once in the position of being responsible for a project and a budget the local person had two camps to please. One was the foreign donors and the other was local people who the person would live with far after the donors packed up their bags and left for home. Thus once in power, there was a strong tendency to look in both directions. From the local viewpoint it was necessary to take care of one's own, giving favors to friends, to others who might be helpful in the future, and to those who had been helpful in the past. This was the local cultural way of sharing wealth. It was the obligation of those who had some income. This meant making sure that the right local people were able to share the largess. In the case of our project, the university was receiving considerable overhead from the project, and would inherit the cars, computers, and other capitol equipment. They expected that the local director would see to it that these extras were not jeopardized. At the same time the local director had to make sure that his own accomplices were taken care of, lest he be considered a turncoat. If he were they might have reason to accuse him of irregularities, like how the funds got into the country.

As more aid came into the country, and because in this case aid had been coming into the country for many years, there was a privileged group of people who owed their special advantages to the foreigners who had placed them in their positions. The burden that was placed on them, of trying to keep what they had, and to take care of those who they needed or might need and those who had former claims from friendship or family invariably contributed to problems. At the same time they had to do the work the donors demanded, which often relied on a completely different set of cultural expectations. Given all of this would it not be better to have a foreigner pass out the scarce but highly needed resources that assistance program brought to the poorest of the poor?

At the same time this was not to blame the local people. It was not easy to get any job, let alone have a decent level of income. Ethiopians have had to live under several governments. In each case making a mistake could be quite costly, either in economic prospects or in civil liberty. Add to this the importance Ethiopians gave to family and friendships. It was important to consider before donors hired local people to run their programs.

In fact there were many comparisons that could be made with how the people in the camp were coping. Their strategies laid on a continuum; on the one end they were self-defeating. These people were retreating from their problems like the young men in the tearoom who were playing cards instead of taking care of themselves. Or the constant bickering between different groups in the camp, like the people from Asab and Asmara, which took away the energy to gather together and work in common. Somewhere in the middle of this continuum were the people who put their names on lists unfairly to inflate their chances of getting aid, thereby serving themselves but possibly depriving others in equal or more need.

At the highest end of the continuum people's coping strategies provided them with a resilient shield that we wanted to learn about. For example, Zewde after losing three of her children on the march expanded her remaining family by including Mulu's family, and the orphaned Soloman. She became known by the moniker "Mama". The way Soloman coped with his illness was also an example. He started out being suicidal but later became the first person in the camp to come forth with the fact that he had AIDS. Or when Mengistu, the unemployed middle aged electrician came to terms with his losses by finding comfort in helping his daughter reach her academic potential.

The comparison that I wanted to make to the woman was that the continuum did not only exist in the camp, it was also part of the culture, and was part of our argument against automatically hiring local people. Both the local hires and the people in the camp shuffled up to expatriates. Like poor Ethiopians for centuries they asked and expected their patrons to help.

The demands that the local hire would have to face were also not qualitatively different than the strategies for coping that Astra employed in the face of her death. In her case she had three chances to live. She could continue to borrow from friends even though she was overdrawn with them, or continue to borrow from a loan shark and sell her son's future because he would inherit her debt. Or like the local hire she could hope to get money from an expatriate or an expatriate funded group.

Another common method of coping common to both groups was they tended to inflate their own needs. When Checkla figured she might be able to charge us a little extra for the transport for Astra, she was figuring out how she might be able to earn something for her family. It was not dissimilar to the common exchange between Ethiopian and *ferenji*. This had served to reduce the income disparity between them, and was one reason why the woman I was talking with, like the NGO's she represented, wanted to give the money to local people. So did Checkla.

Persistently asking for help and over estimating your need for it bothered people from the West. We in the West are more likely to favor independence over asking for help, and explicit accuracy to vague boundaries. But their coping strategies had often proved to be of value. Asking for help gave a person of relative wealth a way to find grace with God. Being less than straightforward about needs reduced the need to say no. In a culture on the fringe of physical well being this was an effective coping strategy.

There was a better way to help the poorest of the poor by trying to ingratiate oneself with the local populace by hiring puppet leadership or establishing a situation that was deemed at the moment to be politically correct. Instead, hire an expatriate to lead the project, but only if during the interview they said that instead of buying vehicles from the donor country and developing an office to meet donor country standards, they had other ideas like avoiding overhead and caring for the needy. But these were only some things to look for, there was another important one, accepting the coping styles of what people were accustomed to was another.

While we thought it was impossible to work with the truly poor people without addressing their immediate needs immediately. We wanted to find a way to help them directly with their basic and immediate needs but to link this assistance with their own coping strategies, and that in the end would help them.

The woman argued against giving material benefits. She thought that this could not be sustained, which was another holy word among the NGOs. But what did sustainability really mean? How long would the effects of an intervention have to endure to be considered sustainable? If a program existed for a period of time that was equal to the time of the funding would it be considered sustained? Would it be sustained if it existed as long as the government itself? Another way to look at sustainability was to see it as part of a person's life cycle. If a displaced person got a needed boost like medicine given to a sick boy or girl, at the very moment when it would be most helpful, and therefore never be forgotten, would that be considered sustainable?

To help them be sustainable it was necessary to join them if they coped successfully. There was one way in particular that the camp coped with their circumstances that moved the whole community forward. It was an example of the kind of change that once adopted might well be sustained. This was the community's openness in allowing a nontraditional life style particularly with young females who were allowed to become adults fully and with legitimacy without having to subsume the traditional subservient role of women (Aptekar, in press, b).

This allowed the young people to open up to each other. In spite of their antecedent trauma and current conditions many of the adolescents were able to see their lives in less than dire terms. They did this by taking an historical perspective of youth and women and realizing that they had the opportunity to take advantage of the expanded role of mixed gender relations. The conspicuous absence of delinquency, child abuse and neglect in Kaliti was one positive outcome of this. Perhaps, the largest evidence of their resilience was that they took care of, and enjoyed each other. Young people were in love, and their love shed an embracing light over the poverty of the community. They danced and sang both constant reminders to everyone that happiness was still possible (Aptekar, Paardekooper, & Kuebli, 2000).

There were other signs of resilience in this camp. One by one they may not have been impressive, but in total it was possible to envision supporting their coping strategies so that counseling could become viable. Although all the households were poor, they were cleaned every day. Beds were made. Each item they had, from the red plastic buckets which were used to wash feet and clothes, to the spoons needed to stir the *injera* were either being used, or elaborately cleaned before being hung in their proper place. In spite of the difficulty of carrying water people continued to bathe, even if it was just their feet and their faces it was evidence of persistence in surviving. People found ways to earn money in spite of the lack of employment opportunities. One man bought discarded cotton, and made mattresses from it. Some older women bought raw wool from sheep, spun and wove it. Young women made beer, or sold *injera*, onions, garlic, or peppers. Life went on.

With every meal, no matter how meager it was followed by the coffee ceremony. A few strands of freshly cut grass were lain under white cups, the grass and the color of the cups were subtle signs of life. Then incense was roasted with coffee beans and the smells served as a sensual reminder that pleasure was still possible. Three cups were always served offering a lengthy reprieve from the outside world and which mandated conversation and intimacy. Each time they shared the coffee ceremony, which in some cases was several times a day, they had a palpable sign that life was better than it had been. They derived the same comfort from other ceremonies. They celebrate birth through birthdays and paid homage to death and burial, and the mourning that followed. These were common events, almost everyday many people would have a chance to participate in their history, and a place to practice their culture.

The fact was that almost all programs ceased as soon as the funding stopped. What kept aid sustainable were new funds or the memories that the recipients reflected upon, many of which came from the long moments they had together over coffee, or in celebrating or mourning the passage through life. It was the memory of conversations that led to new understandings, and relationships between people that kept thinking about the future possible. These events led to actions that changed the direction of a person's life. These were the important (and most sustainable) aspects of any program. Yet, these difficult to measure phenomena were rarely considered part of a program, which was more often measured by the more easily defined nuts and bolts, like number of meals served, numbers of people in job training programs, etc.

From local ground zero we could see that programs came and left but what made them important were not their longevity but their impact during their existence. This often depended on the character of the person in charge and that person's freedom to make decisions on the spot. What kept programs sustainable were usually the skills of a single person and his or her commitment of living among the improverished. The mix of two cultures this provided, the spice of difference sparked unusual encounters between belief systems and ways of coping.

We were proposing a structure that placed a person of integrity in the middle of wretchedness, allow him or her to make decisions, and after time through the decisions made and the moral directives given become accepted by the community. The community would learn from observations how to confront difficult situations. Through this person's example a special space would be created, where people could find retreat, and meaning and hope in the midst of misery. This was why we were encouraging our mid career students to work with the young people in Kaliti. To give recognition and credence to the ways the people were coping and rejoice with them, so that the fun they had, the care they took of what they had, and the way they gave to one another. This showed the example for the community to follow and created a space that gave them all some reprieve from their difficulties.

On the other hand all the job-training programs which were getting much more funding, mostly to employ local middlemen and women were known for their high overhead, their short life spans, and their questionable results in getting people employed. Hardly anyone actually received a salaried position as a result of job training, indeed about the only reliable job skill that was needed in getting a well paid job was speaking English, and we never saw a training for this.

She asked what would happen if in fact the donors were willing to have an expatriate in charge, how would that person know what the indigenous people wanted? We said she had spent the last three months going from person to place observing and talking in order to see what was needed. This seemed like an adequate plan. If we added the next step, which would be to begin a program, and then to observe it, modify it and act again, would this not be sufficient?

We educated expatriates shouldn't underestimate ourselves, and our training and our abilities. We should also keep in mind that in many cases our history and experience of living and working successfully (at least relatively) in multi-cultural democratic communities was far beyond the experience of local people. In this case, we should not be blind to the fact that Ethiopia had been involved in a war that lasted for three decades and still appeared far from over. The way they treated one another had led to the very services that had brought us here in the first place. This of course did not mean to throw these points up in the face of our hosts, and certainly not to put down individuals, but we all were at least to some extent prisoners of our history and culture. In this case the history of feudalism and totalitarianism left its mark.

Initiative, a nearly sacrosanct characteristic in the West was not an attribute that was favored here, it was considered inappropriate even rude. While our Western upbringing had stressed making sacrifices at the expense of family and friends so that we could perform as well as possible in the work place, our Ethiopian counterparts were raised first and foremost to make sacrifices at work. Ethiopians would be expected to spend time taking care of extended family responsibilities including time off from work to attend marriages, funerals, religious activities, to speak nothing of the priority of talking with friends over coffee. While we in the West would be expected to find time to take care of these duties outside and after work, Ethiopians would be expected to do this before attending to work. In short we could not discount the fact that people from the West (as a rule and not always) were much more likely to work on getting the job done, than our local counterpoints.

One Ethiopian man who was working for an NGO got the job in part because he was displaced and orphaned. His father was killed in the war and his mother died in one of the camps. He was now in charge of his five younger siblings and was earning 300 birr per month (about 24 dollars, which was half the average yearly income of Ethiopians). He was obviously happy to be doing so well, and it was clear that he knew what he had. He was one of a group of people who were not normally considered dependent on receiving assistance, one of the local nationals working for an expatriate NGO. He was earnest and worthy and we were happy to see him get ahead, but we also thought that much of what we were saying in class was being shown to us in Kaliti.

Furthermore, we began to look more carefully at the term, "Aid dependency", which was frequently used to describe the displaced. It was a pejorative term that described them as being without initiative and unable to get along with the help they were receiving, which was only making them more dependent.

In fact Aid Dependency applied to the psyche of the donors more than it did the people in the camp that received the aid. It helped explain to us why we were having so much trouble keeping our mid career students in the field. Like the donors who were frustrated with not getting enough bang for the buck, our students felt "burned out" by trying to help and not being able to see results.

As the project came to a close we were aware of some particular problems that had to be left unsolved. There was the problem of coping beyond taking care of oneself and one's family. This contributed to the problems of governance, where people would have to learn to work for the common good instead of personal enrichment. There was the massive amount of illness, which was a test of will for the community, providing the awful drama of slow and tortured death, even though it gave them a chance to cope by showing their love and care. The latter being a force of empowerment which if coupled with their religion helped them deal with what we in the West could not imagine save for our most awful literary images of Hell.

Finally, our work was on one level, but there was work to be done on a higher level, one would have to consider counseling for reconciliation, not only for the victims but also training their children and adolescents. Only the next generation would accept ethnic differences, which in the end was the only hope to prevent the cycle of recurring war.

REFERENCES

Aptekar, L. (in press, a). Some cultural problems for Westerner's counseling in Ethiopia. In Bemak, F (ed).

Aptekar, L. (in press, b). The changing developmental dynamics of "children in particularly difficult circumstances": Examples of street and war traumatized children. In Gielen, U. & J. Roopnarine, *Childhood and adolescence in cross-cultural perspective*: Greenwood Press.

Aptekar, L., Paardekooper, B., & Kuebli, J. (2000). Adolescence and youth among displaced Ethiopians: A case study in Kaliti camp. *International Journal of Group Tensions, 29*(1–2): 101–135.

Araya, M., & Aboud, F. (1993). Mental illness. In H. Kloos, & Z. A. Zein (Eds.), *The ecology of health and disease in Ethiopia* (pp. 493–506). Boulder, CO: Westview Press.

De Jong, J. T. V. M. (1996). *TPO program for the identification, management and prevention of psychosocial and mental health problems of refugees and victims of organized violence within primary health care of adults and children* (7th version). Amsterdam: Transcultural Psychosocial Organization. Internal document.

Endale, Y. (1996). Ethiopia's mental health trampled by armed conflict. In T. Allen (Ed.), *Search of cool ground: War, flight and homecoming in northeast Africa* (pp. 274–277). Trenton, NJ: Africa World Press.

Hancock, G., Pankhurst, R., & Willetts, D. (1997). *Under Ethiopian sky* (3rd ed.). Nairobi, Kenya: Camerapix Publishers.

Kortmann, F. (1987). Popular, traditional, and professional mental health care in Ethiopia. *Transcultural Psychiatric Research Review, 24*, 255–274.

Pankhurst, R. (1990). *A social history of Ethiopia*. Addis Ababa, Ethiopia: Institute of Ethiopian Studies.

UNICEF. (1986). *Children in situations of armed conflict* (E/ICEF.CRP.2). New York.

UNICEF. (1996). *The state of the world's children: 1996*. Oxford, England: Oxford University Press.

UNICEF. (1997). *The state of the world's children: 1997*. Oxford, England: Oxford University Press.

United Nations Development Programme. (1993). *Human development report*. New York: Oxford University Press.

Vecchiato, N. (1993a). Illness, therapy, and change in Ethiopian possession cults. *Journal of International African Institute, 63*(2), 176–195.

Vecchiato, N. (1993b). Traditional medicine. In H. Kloos, & Z. A. Zein (Eds.), *The ecology of health and disease in Ethiopia* (pp. 157–178). Boulder, CO: Westview Press.

9

Terrorism, Traumatic Events and Mental Health in Algeria

M. A. AÏT SIDHOUM, F. ARAR, C. BOUATTA, N. KHALED and M. ELMASRI

INTRODUCTORY NOTES

Algeria is situated in northern Africa on the Mediterranean Sea. Its area extends over more than two million square kilometers consisting of coastal plains, high mountains and the Sahara. According to the National Office of Statistics its population was an estimated 29.3 million persons in 1998, of which around half are younger than 20 years (ONS, 1999).

In 1962, after a long struggle for liberation, Algeria gained its independence from France, which colonized the country for 130 years. Ever since, it has been governed by the National Liberation Front (FLN), with a succession of elected presidents, most of whom were colonels during the liberation war. The government followed a one-party socialist system until 1988, when the riots in Algiers and the constitutional referendum of 1989 opened the way to a multiparty system. Since then, many political parties with different orientations have appeared and disappeared. Three main poles characterize Algerian politics: The first is the conservative pole represented by the old party FLN and the recently formed RND. The conservatives still hold power and seek Arabization of culture and education, and Islamization of the country. The second pole is the Islamic pole, represented by a range of parties that seek the restoration of an Islamic state in Algeria: the FIS (Islamic Front for Salvation), Hammas and Nahdha. Finally, the democratic pole, represented mainly by FFS and RCD, calls for a democratic civil society.

Like the diversity of its terrain and politics, Algerian culture shows a wide diversity and coexistence of different, if not conflictual, beliefs and life styles.

Ethnic origins are varied and complex. Most inhabitants are Berbers, a generic term that includes all the original tribes inhabiting northern Africa, followed by Arabs which came to the area with the extension of Islam, and small numbers of European nationals, most of whom have left the country recently because of terrorism.

This diversity in itself has been the background of the current conflict. Islam seems to be the single, most important link between the different subcultures, and used to support all claims of Islamists, nationalists and socialists alike. Over the years however, there were several fluctuations in power and control by the different cultures, ethnicities and ideologies.

A century and a half of French colonial rule has created an ambivalent, strongly polarized relationship with the West and western culture, and made western French culture an essential component of the identity and social structure. Paradoxically, Algerian nationalism has been fostered by the confrontation with French colonial rule, and has been based on Islamic concepts and relations with a wider Arab-Islamic world.

This chapter aims to fulfil several purposes. First, to explain the current situation in Algeria after a decade of tragedy and to describe the origins and patterns of the violence. Second, to describe the unique outlines of a mental health model initiated by the Algerian Society of Research in Psychology (SARP) with the objective of alleviating the burden of this tragedy on the population. In the absence of systematic credible research, we had to limit ourselves to the data provided by the daily work of our team, complemented by the preliminary results of an epidemiological survey carried out in partnership with TPO (Transcultural Psychosocial Organization). Reflections on the implications of the available data will enable us to define priorities and specificities of the program, and orient us to the perspectives on the long run.

FUNDAMENTALISM AND VIOLENCE IN ALGERIA

Despite the tragic nature of violence in Algeria, Algerians have endured it in relative silence. Moreover, halting the elections in December 1991, which is seen by many as the starting point of violence in Algeria, was only the trigger that served to escalate and generalize a movement already building up for many years prior to that (Samai-Ouramdane, G., 1990). We can consider October 1988 a turning point in recent Algerian history. In fact, the events in this month forced the government to recognize the demand for political pluralism and to modify the constitution to make this pluralism possible.

On October 5, 1988, several riots started in Algiers. They rapidly expanded to other parts of the capital and to other cities in the country, such as Oran and Annaba, largely surpassing the capacities of the security forces to stop the protests. There were two indicators of the importance of this popular revolt: the state of emergency that was declared six days before the first riots and the building up of security forces to disperse the crowds and to stop the destruction and looting of public institutions. According to official estimates, this intervention resulted in 159 deaths and 3,500 arrests. The impact of the events of October 1988 on the political and social level was high. First, the revolt opened the political field to a multiparty system marking the end of the FLN supremacy. This change has been ratified later by the Constitution, which was adopted by referendum in February 1989. Second, it allowed a critical review of the socialist option so far considered a taboo. This second change has also been explicitly introduced in the 1989 Constitution. It is necessary to underline that this new constitution clearly prohibits creating a political party on the basis of religion, ethnicity or language.

Some Indicators for the Period Preceding October 1988

There have been many indicators even prior to February 1988 that point to the fact that fundamentalism did not emerge spontaneously. We will cite some events for the purpose of illustration, in order to facilitate comprehension of issues such as the appearance of fundamentalist violence and the democratic openness that the Islamists have used to their own advantage.

Berber Spring in February 1980. The prohibition of a lecture of Mouloud Mammeri, a writer and advocate of Berber culture, was the direct reason for a demonstration in Tizi-Ouzou. This demonstration rapidly transformed into a big riot, first in Tizi-Ouzou and later in the entire Kabyle region, and more modestly in Algiers. In order to stop the popular riots, which surpassed the capacity of the habitual security forces (police and national gendarmerie), the government at that time had to call for the army for help.

The assassination of a student on 2 November 1982. This assassination by Islamists took place at the law school during their opposition to a theatre play by Kateb Yacine. The scheduling of this play by the student committee of the university campus made some circles of fanatic students, who were firmly installed and strongly organized at the campus, feel offended. The assassination took place in the context of the struggle between Islamist and progressive students. Islamist students called for the support of militants from outside the campus, who arrived armed with knives, chains and sticks. On November 12, 1982, the fanatic students, as a reaction to the students' demonstration against violence, riposted by organizing a big demonstration to demand the release of their arrested militants. On that day, the demonstration at the University of Algiers and its surroundings gathered around five thousand Islamists who came to listen to their leaders Abassi Madani and the *Cheikhs* Sahnoun and Soltani. These three leaders were arrested the same evening and were put under surveillance.

Soltani and Sahnoun were released a month later, while Abassi Madani, suspected to be the principal inspirer of this meeting, stayed in prison until the end of 1984 (Rouadjia, 1991).

The Formation of the First Islamic Armed Group

Islamic fundamentalists begun their activities well before October 1988. At the beginning, these activities focused on controlling the mosques and building new ones where they could ensure the loyalty of *imams* of their choice. With the arrival of the Islamists in Iran, they started reproaching their chiefs for "focusing a lot more on preaches in the mosques than on action" (Rouadjia, 1991). Mustapha Bouyali was the first to start acting by creating his own group. The Bouyali group called Armed Islamic Algerian Movement (MAIA) was created in 1982. MAIA committed itself to using force against security forces. In 1983, the Bouyali group attacked a production unit at Ain Naadja (near Algiers) and stole the workers' salaries. Over the next years, the group attacked several other targets until Bouyali himself was killed during a fire exchange with the gendarmerie in 1987. On 20 June 1987, 202 members thought to belong to Bouyali's group were brought to trial. Three weeks later, four of them were sentenced to death, four to life sentences and seven to 20 years of criminal imprisonment.

Indicators for the Period After October 1988

The period after October 1988 was marked by a rapid evolution in the Algerian political situation, in which the interruption of the election process in December 1991 constituted an important element. Table 1 illustrates this rapid evolution during this period.

Evolution of Terrorist Activities

As was emphasized in the report of the United Nations Panel in June 1998, published in the daily newspaper *El Watan* on 17 September 1998, the terrorist movement went through four stages differentiated by the nature of objectives targeted by the terrorist attacks.

In the first stage, the FIS and its armed groups, benefiting from a large popular support, targeted only the security forces and public service employees, i.e. all persons representing the authority of the State. Partially, it was the absence of a strong legitimate state that made a part of the population lean towards supporting fundamentalism. The FIS, drawing from its divine legitimacy, had the advantage of attracting a large number of unsatisfied people. FIS gave them the hope of breaking with a painful past, which was replaced with the illusion of a perspective of a just future.

Table 1. Evolution of Events in Algeria from 1988 to 1992

Date	Event
October 1988 to January 1992	This period has been marked by the almost systematic recourse of the Islamic fundamentalists to the use of intimidation and threat in order to force the population to conform to the principles of Islam according to their own interpretation. This massive use of force went to the point of forming militia groups that where charged with repressing some habits and conducts in public life, which they judged contrary to their conception of Islam.
June 12, 1990	First pluralist local elections, which the Islamic Front of Salvation (FIS) won with 55% of votes. It is said that Islamist militias had forced people to vote for FIS by using intimidation and pressure.
June 1990	A general amnesty for political prisoners proclaimed by president Chadli. This amnesty concerned especially the Islamist fundam entalists who were fighting with Bouyali.
May 1991	The beginning of an open strike announced by FIS to protest against the election law made up by the National Assembly to benefit the candidates of the former single party, and to demand the resignation of president Chadli. After a bloody exchange between the militants of FIS and the forces of security, more than 700 fundamentalists were arrested, including the president and vice-president of FIS.
November 1991	Attack on the military camp of Guemmar in the south by Islamist fundamentalist groups. Victims were found mutilated.
December 1991	Organization of the first general elections in the context of the multiparty system. The FIS won, after the first round, 47% of seats in parliament. It should be noted that there were many reports of electoral irregularities.
January 1992	The dissolution of parliament, followed by resignation of president Chadli and the composition of a five-member High State Council (Haut Conseil d'Etat, HCE), nominated to ensure the functioning of a multi-person presidency. Mohamed Boudiaf, and the Ali Kaffi, were nominated as presidents of the State Council successively.
February 1992	A flame of violence led by the militants of FIS against all symbols of the state was launched and the HCE reacted by enforcing the state of emergency to stop the FIS leaders. FIS was dissolved by a decision of the Supreme Court in March of the same year.
June 1992	Assassination of president Boudiaf.

In the second stage, the FIS considered it necessary to attack every person who attempted to encourage the population to take a critical stand toward the archaic maneuvers used to manipulate the crowds emotionally. To illustrate the archaism of the procedures used, one example is enough. On 5 June 1990, on the occasion of the last meeting of the election campaign, the FIS used a holograph to write the expression *Allah Akbar* ("God is the greatest") on the clouds in Arabic script. Many people came to listen to the election campaign's closing speech by the president of the party. The appearance of the holograph on the clouds was presented as a miracle through which Allah gave his blessing to the actions of the FIS. The great majority of those who were present reached a state of trance by repeating the divine expression after the president of the FIS.

Intellectuals were especially targeted by the terrorists. Persons with very varied itineraries, sometimes youngsters not beyond the age of 15, have been enrolled to participate in the assassination of a big number of intellectuals, scientists, media professionals or simply citizens who had a certain credibility among the population and who refused to be speakers for religious fundamentalism. Among these target people some decided to leave Algeria, others preferred to hide, while others took the risk and participated in their own way to resist fundamentalism. The expansion of organized violence has gradually led to spreading doubt concerning the authenticity of the fundamentalist project, and to the first breaks in the popular support to the fundamentalist discourse.

We can interpret the tendency of the third stage (destruction of the country's infrastructure) as a panic reaction inside the fundamentalist core group, to confront the worries over early signs of split inside the movement. They then had to act, and by all means, to subjugate the state, even if they had to destroy all the country and its economic and social structures: bridges, vehicles, factories, schools, local administration settings, health-care units, etc.

The impact of this massive destruction on the citizens whose lives became impossible seriously harmed the fundamentalist movement. The popular support to the terrorists started to decline. This made the toughest of them angry, and therefore, they decided to launch the first "punishing operations" against some areas. They were aimed to serve as examples to warn against any failing in the support that the population was supposed to provide. To justify these operations and to involve the population, they promulgated a *fetwa* that considered any person showing resistance to their project as a renegade, committing a serious fault with regard to religion. However, contrary to the terrorists' expectations, the results of these operations led to the fourth phase of massive killings.

As a matter of fact, the inhabitants of some isolated areas were really frightened when the first population massacres occurred. Those who had the means began leaving their homes, others asked public authorities to give them arms so they could defend themselves. In another context, conflicts took place between different armed groups and between their political representatives. The reduction of the popular support was sometimes interpreted as a result of helping a rival group. Consequently, the punishing operations increased and took new forms. With the rapid decline of support to the fundamentalist groups, the scope of this reactive punishment extended. The number of collective massacres counted by the National Observatory of Human Rights (ONDH) was 299 until 1997 (cited in Benyoub, 1999).

These massacres claimed the lives of hundreds of people at a time. The brutality of killing and mutilations, the secretly told incidents of rape, the horror of children having witnessed the killing of their own parents are beyond description. In all massacres, maimed people and some children were left alive to tell the stories and deliver the message that this will be the punishment of those who betray.

THE IMPACT OF THE TRAGEDY: ASSESSMENT OF MENTAL HEALTH NEEDS

Due to the scarcity of systematic research, we will largely draw upon the clinical experience of our team at SARP to understand the situation of violence that Algeria has been going through for the last years. We will also draw upon the first results of the epidemiological research in mental health led by a team of SARP, which was focused on the impact of the current situation on the population's mental health. To formulate a coherent set of mental health needs in Algeria, the implications of several indicators should be assessed. These are: the implications of losses in human lives for the living; the implications of the destruction of life space, especially for the children; the future of children who find themselves, overnight, without any landmarks in their lives and without resorts, and the implications of the lack of assistance to all these victims for a very long time, i.e. for future generations.

The General Scheme: Neither War, Nor Peace

It is difficult to grasp from the outside the situation that Algeria is going through. This situation is neither a situation of war nor one of peace. It borrows characteristics from both. As a consequence, it has acquired unique characteristics.

During times of peace, the efforts of human societies are essentially invested in ensuring the well-being of the population. Situations of war, however, are essentially characterized by efforts of societies to face danger. Every social effort in society is oriented to this purpose. This orientation does constitute a certain regulation of activities of individuals and of social groups. The aspiration after well-being and the achievement of goals—studying, getting involved in one's family, developing leisure activities etc.—become synonymous to betrayal. This violation of the sacred human life and the glorification of its sacrifice in the name of an ideal is a powerful mechanism to make mourning easier.

The current Algerian situation is at the same time close to and different from these two archetypes. It borrows from the situation of war the risk of death and the violation of the sacred human life. However, it does not adapt, or it does so very badly, the discourse that attempts to justify this violation, and for this reason, it cannot release the regulating mechanisms that are characteristic of a war situation. Because of this absence, the dead leave lasting injuries within the living. Moreover, we have been able to observe particular reactions in many persons who suspected that their lost loved ones have somehow themselves been accomplices in their own death. They blame them, either for having had activities that have increased the risk of dying, or for having neglected to take some necessary protections to stay alive. This particular reaction consists of an anger of the living towards the dead, and this would run contrary to the survivor's feeling of guilt as frequently described in the literature.

The Algerian situation maintains the aspiration for possible happiness and supports the legitimate endeavor of pursuing goals that give sense to such an aspiration. However, the regulating mechanisms that ensure a certain stability, and the efficiency in such a search are greatly weakened. There are no specific social arrangements foreseen for the management of this situation, and there is no real possible psychological preparation to undertake it. If the case of persons directly involved in the management of the security situation can be understood in a certain way, because they are in a state of war, it is not the same case for the great majority of the population. For them, death is here, and it can strike at any time without knowing really why. At the same time, they are supposed to take care of life demands, those pertaining to peacetime.

To complete this dramatic picture, we add the effects of a deteriorating socio-economic situation. The mean income of Algerians was reduced to a fifth of what it was, and this was especially due to the fall in oil prices. It is in this situation that the Algerians live, that they are summoned to work, to make children and raise them. It is in these conditions that Algerian mothers have continued having children and taking care of them. This situation is demoralizing and traumatic in several ways. First, there is the sudden, meaningless loss of loved ones who were found tortured and mutilated; very few Algerians have not lost a relative or a friend since October 1988 until now. Also, there is the sorrow of watching loved ones disappear under mysterious conditions. Finally, there are the drastic limitations of every kind that one imposes on oneself, especially in aspects of social life like going out or visiting friends, which can also be traumatizing.

The Loss of Human Life

The number of victims officially declared by public authorities has increased since 1998. This is due to the fact that in earlier years, the government kept its silence about the number of killings. The new president of the Republic, who was elected in April 1999, mentioned the number of 100,000 victims. This is comparable to the estimations that are often used by political parties and the press.

In addition to the total number of people killed, there are many hundreds who have disappeared. Some of them were kidnapped, others left without a note and may have joined the armed groups, but the majority just disappeared without a trace. It is feared that most of these disappeared people have actually been killed, although little concrete evidence exists for this.

The Effect on Social Structure and Social and Family Values

Since the FIS won the municipal elections of 12 June 1990, the political situation in Algeria has been in chaos. Starting on this date, the FIS had access to the management of the country. After 1992 and following the spread of terrorism, armed groups of AIS (Islamic Army of Salvation) and of GIA (Armed Islamic Group) imposed their law on the region. Even before the collective massacres of Rais and Bentalha, the whole Algerian population has been under continuous and regular pressure and constraints from terrorist groups. In the absence of any collective and organized means to defend themselves, the social structure of Algeria rapidly eroded and many social and family values disappeared. This evolution took place in the absence of any system of regulation, as even the State abandoned the afflicted area. The collective massacres finished off the fragments of social organization that were still resisting this long process of deterioration. The results have been distressing.

In observing the situation in its complexity, we cannot help saying that the tragedy in Algeria is a tragedy that will have long-term effects on individuals and the society. An individual trauma which has not been worked through gets encysted like a foreign object in the psyche and forces the psyche to a progressive deviation from its own trajectory. Likewise, in case reconstruction work of ties and institutions has not been done, collective tragedies destroy gradually social regulatory mechanisms and dramatically affect attempts to reorganize society. It is important to note the effects of the co-existence of both victims and terrorists in the same community, and sometimes even in the same family. In many cases survivors of violent acts know the people who killed their relatives or friends. The tensions caused by this situation have destroyed the family and community ties that normally stimulate social exchanges and mutual support. It suffices to observe how, within an area like Sidi Moussa, a semi-rural region in the surroundings of Great Algiers, suspicion and social labeling (victim families/killer families) have replaced trust and social cohesion. In many instances, such splits have even taken place within the single family unit and created situations of extreme tension within a household (Box 1).

Box 1. Case Example Zina

Zina, an Algerian woman in her forties has two children who are younger than 10 years (a boy and a girl). She was raised in a rural family near Sidi Moussa, in which a young woman is expected to become a good housewife. Her husband was killed in 1997, after the terrorists demanded that he cooperates with them and come to the mountains. She was seen in the Sidi Moussa center by the social worker.

The husband, although religious and sympathetic at first to the cause of the Islamists in achieving social justice, refused to join them and showed his disapproval over the killings and violence. To the terrorists, his refusal was considered a betrayal to their cause and he was sentenced to death. A neighbor, a young man who Zina knew, was with the group that came to take her husband, who never came back. After a short period of intense shock and disbelief, she realized that she was left with two little children who needed nurture and care. According to her, grief and anger over the loss of her husband had to be put aside and the need to keep the family alive, the role she was prepared for, became her first priority...

She worked or received some assistance from neighbors and relatives, but the money was not enough to support two children to go to school. After the death of her husband, and with no older son to take his role in the family, as would normally happen in the rural setting, she found herself alone and with a responsibility that she was little prepared for. The rest of the families in the village, and those relatives who remained there, were too poor to take her and her children as an added burden to their own.

Later, when the law of *Concord civil* in effect since July 1999 and the truce between the government and the AIS gave full pardon to all AIS members who put down their arms and surrender to the authorities, the young neighbor came back to his home and children and was even receiving support from the government in the context of the *Concord civil*. *"He was well off and he had children of his own"*, so she expected that he would help her by testifying of the death of her husband. She went directly to this neighbor to beg him to come and testify to the authorities, nothing more! She was neither seeking revenge nor justice, she only wanted to get the necessary papers. Although her case was very obvious, and fitting all the criteria for a victim of violence, the necessary papers that confirm that her husband was killed by the terrorists were missing. She tried to get all the necessary papers, but it was impossible to obtain a death certificate for her husband, whose body has never been found. In such a case the official procedure requires that two witnesses testify that the husband was killed by terrorists.

According to the social worker, the woman seemed to be confused. She described the killing of her husband and the miserable state of her family in great details and with little emotions. To her, one night sound sleep was only needed in order to wake up the next morning strong enough to pursuit her search for help. She thought that the pains and aches in her body were the result of the long walks she had to take from one office to the other. Despite her apparent depression and poor sleep, she did not come to the center in Sidi Moussa to ask for psychological assistance, but because she had heard that this center provides *support* to victims of terrorism, a group she considered herself to belong after she learned the official terms. For her, support meant material, legal, administrative and social support and meeting people who have the time to listen to her story.

The social worker's advice emphasized the need of this woman to awareness of her legal rights, procedures and available services. Case management for such victims of violence is done through a multidisciplinary team. For this particular woman, it was necessary for the psychologist, social worker and legal advisor to intervene. The social worker coordinated the intervention.

The Variety of Traumatic Situations Experienced by Individuals and Families

If we would like to assess the impact of the violence on the mental health situation of the Algerian population, it is not enough to study the reaction of people who experienced or witnessed the death of family members, friends or strangers. Restricting this assessment solely to the number of deaths (according to the government 100,000 until 1999), will totally distort the evaluation since it focuses on a very small part of traumatic situations. The number of deaths and causalities constitutes only one parameter in the assessment of the impact of violence. The observations made from our clinical experience and the first results of the epidemiological survey allow us to order facts related to mental health into nine different situations. The people who have experienced these situations are:

1. Survivors of villages and areas where there were collective massacres
2. Families who have lost several members
3. Persons who have lost one or several loved ones and are going through a complex mourning process
4. Persons destabilized by the disorganization of their environment
5. Children and family members of people involved in terrorist activities
6. Raped women, especially those who got pregnant as a result of rape
7. Physical casualties after bomb attacks or collective massacres
8. Individuals, families and communities that lived under threat of assassination or serious terrorist attacks
9. Individuals who have been directly or indirectly involved in terrorist activities

A lot of human and material resources must be mobilized in order to proceed to the objective evaluation that is necessary to set a rational strategy suitable to meet the mental health needs of all these individuals. Professionals attempting this task must be well prepared. Part of this preparation is to gain familiarity with the local reality of traumatic situations, their effect on different social groups, and the adaptation of these groups to changes in their security situation. Also, these professionals should be competent in adapting and using different mental health evaluation instruments.

Survivors of Villages and Areas where there were Collective Massacres. As a result of the massacres, there are many Algerians who have lost everything, from members of their families to their most basic possessions. Nobody can give a reliable estimation of the number of persons who have experienced this situation. We can however say that there are hundreds of villages and areas that have experienced violent raids. As cited before, the number of collective massacres counted by the National Observatory of Human Rights was 299 until 1997. Many survivors of these massacres have lost all supportive structures and networks, and are deprived of the essential requirements for a basic social life. It is important to remember that although the collective massacres have stopped, mass killings of whole families or groups of people still continue to occur in some areas of Algeria.

Families who have lost Several Members. The importance of loss of human life for families is to be taken as a distinctive criterion. The sudden death of several loved ones totally unbalances a family. The impact of the loss is different however, depending on whether families have shelters and a minimum of living resources or not. In the case of destructed family structures, classical psychological help would not be enough. It should be combined with family-oriented multidisciplinary support.

The number of these families is great; probably there are several thousands. Only the Ministry of Interior owns reliable data, but for evident political reasons, these are not published. Not only is it important to know how many families experienced losses, it is also necessary to know what happened to them after the death of their family members. Although an important number of these families continue to live in the place where the tragedy took place, others have been scattered at random to shelters provided by the State. This does make strategies to provide support to them difficult to carry out.

Persons who have lost One or Several loved ones and are going through a Complex Mourning Process. Even in case the family structure keeps a relative coherence, at least with regard to its structure, people who have lost one or several loved ones might undergo a complicated mourning process. One should keep in mind that each death is at the origin of a grief situation that is difficult to cope with, given that the conditions of the unexpected death do not fit in schemes that individuals know and for which they are somehow prepared. The experiences of clinical practice show us, that persons who really need psychological help rarely seek consultation. Only an epidemiological screening can give an indication of the need for psychological support.

Persons Destabilized by the Disorganization of their Environment. In this group, we can include all vulnerable persons enfeebled by psychological, social or medical problems. These people normally would be greatly dependent on the functionality of a supportive environmental structure. Once this structure is disorganized, they will be the first to notice the effects. An example of this group would be the handicapped, the mentally ill, the children and the elderly.

Children and Family Members of People Involved in Terrorist Activities. Victims of this category risk being unrecognized or, if recognized, denied assistance. The situation of children and families of persons involved in terrorist activities is dramatic and complicated because these people find themselves not only deprived of solidarity and compassion, but are also subject to rejection. Especially the situation of children should be emphasized here. Many children suffer from the rejection by society. Some of them have lost both parents.

As they do not fit in the definition of victim of terrorism they have no access to the financial support the State provides for other victims.

Raped Women, Especially those who got Pregnant as a result of Rape. The tragedy of women raped by terrorists is very serious. The majority of rape victims are young girls and women with rural backgrounds, with little education or training. According to a press review of an independent daily newspaper, there were 2,084 recorded cases of women raped by terrorists from 1993 to 1998. Besides, the destiny of 319 women kidnapped by terrorist groups remains unknown (newspaper *Al Khabar*, 4 August 1998). To this, we should add a number (impossible to determine) of raped women who have not reported what happened to them to the authorities to avoid social prejudices. In order to solve the problem of those who got pregnant, the Ministry of Health has changed the law to include therapeutic abortion.

Physical Casualties after Bomb Attacks or Collective Massacres. Many people have attained different degrees of physical handicaps as a result of bomb attacks or collective massacres. Experience with such persons shows that their needs extend beyond the financial compensation given by the State. Only an assistance that ensures their psychosocial reintegration into society could alleviate their grief and enable them to function normally.

Individuals, Families and Communities that Lived Under Threat of Assassination or Serious Terrorist Attacks. People who have not (yet) been directly affected by a real assassination or an attack will be tempted to minimize the seriousness of their situation. They risk being unrecognized or, if recognized, denied assistance. Observation shows that living under threats of this kind is in itself a source of traumatic stress especially for those who are already vulnerable or deprived.

Individuals Who Have Been Directly or Indirectly Involved in a Terrorist Activity. According to some sources, especially the *Annuaire Politique de l' Algérie* (Political Yearbook of Algeria), there have been more than 34,000 prisoners arrested in the context of anti-terrorist campaigns. Among them, over 15,000 were accused of complicity and support of terrorist networks, according to the 1997 annual report of the Observatory of Human Rights. They may be repentants who have surrendered to the authorities after being involved in terrorist activities (several thousands), or members of armed groups of the AIS who have accepted the truce conditions between AIS and the government since 1997. They all share the characteristic of having participated directly or indirectly in the organization of subversive actions, classified by Algerian Law as terrorist activities. The necessity to differentiate this category is linked to the particularity

> **Box 2. Case Example: Woman who Lost her Son**
>
> Ms X. is a fifty-year-old housewife and mother of three, she came to the center complaining of poor sleep, which is interrupted by nightmares, sadness and weeping, loss of interest and pleasure in life. Her tragedy started when her son of 15 years old disappeared five years ago. The son was approached by the Islamists whom he met often in the mosque during prayers and religious lessons. The Islamists often asked him to join them, but his mother strongly opposed their request, and tried very hard to protect her son and prevent him from meeting these people. Although she always told her son stories about her father, a *Moujahid* (freedom fighter) in the war of liberation, she could not imagine him joining such fanatic youngsters who were terrorizing the people. One day, her son did not return home from school, she and his father looked everywhere but in vain: their son disappeared. She did not know if he was alive or not, she did not even know if he willingly joined the Islamists. She was left to her preoccupations and feelings of guilt. Maybe it was her overprotection that made the son leave home, or maybe he was kidnapped, or maybe he was killed... endless questions tormented her day and night.
>
> Her nightmares reflect her confusion, in some dreams he returns home, in other dreams he is taken away by the police or by the terrorists, yet in others he calls for help and she is absolutely paralyzed. She frequently thinks that if he would be dead, she could complete her grief and go on with her life, but this thought itself provokes deep feelings of guilt. Of course she wishes that he would be alive, but if so he might be in trouble needing help, worse yet, he might have joined the terrorists in the mountains.
>
> The sense of unfinished grief is not restricted to her, although she struggles to keep her thoughts and nightmares to herself. It permeates the whole family, her husband, who often tries to support her, retired early and the other two sons are jobless and not even looking for work, they tell her that life is useless.
>
> The whole family has been struck by the impact of the disappearance. A gradual decline in the family functioning was evident, the family members are no longer supportive enough to each other. Actually, new worries have been added to the old ones. She worries about her husband who is getting sicker and weaker, and about her two other sons who have lost hope in life. She even worries that the whole family structure is going to crumble.

of psychological and psychosocial interventions that are necessary to ensure their right to health: psychological interventions inside prisons, psychosocial reintegration programs for the repentants and for those who have benefited from the presidential amnesty or from the Civil Concord Law (*Concord civil*) in effect since June 1999. This task is inevitable, because these persons are seldom over the age of 30 and some of them are just emerging from adolescence (Box 2).

PSYCHIC TRAUMA: REFLECTIONS FROM THE EXPERIENCE OF SARP

General and Clinical Observations Regarding Trauma

General Observations. Our clinical observation of the Algerian situation since 1990 has led us to note the particular character of and highly individualized reactions to traumatic stress (Aït Sidhoum, 1997). This observation has also led us to take notice of the misleading character of classifications to describe these same reactions that clinicians have recourse to. Each time we attempted to use a dynamic approach which integrates these reactions into the psychic or 'psycho-somatic economy' (Marty, 1990), these classifications have regularly proved insufficient in describing the clinical realities. We realized how misleading the notion of reaction to trauma can be when it is used in an individual, circumscribed and time-limited way.

Observation of individual reactions to long-term trauma exposure leads us to realize the styles of coping and elaboration that victims have developed in the long run, which attempt to mobilize all their potential resources. The fact of living in Algeria since 1990 until now, can be called a situation of "high traumatic potential". Living with insecurity and the risk of death in themselves or because of the restrictions that they impose on daily life, can generate extreme stress that exceeds the coping capabilities of some persons. We use the term "high traumatic potential" to designate situations described regularly in the literature as traumatic events, emphasizing the relative character of the impact of external events on the individual.

Trauma is always the result of the conjunction of two types of facts. On the one side, there are events that strike the individual and the situation he finds himself in from the outside, temporarily or long-term. On the other side, there are internal means by which the individual has to face these events and to cope with these situations. Trauma appears when these means of coping are not sufficient to maintain the homeostatic balance of the subject in these situations and in face of these events; or when these means are not sufficient to restore this homeostatic balance in a short period of time without professional help.

Clinical Observations. SARP's experience with prevention and psychological consultation leads us to confirm several clinical observations. Traumatized persons seldom seek professional help by themselves. The nature and the characteristics of the posttraumatic pathology limit the victims' access to situations in which they can benefit from professional help or screening. Inhibition, avoidance, denial, suspiciousness of the other, helplessness and hopelessness, all these states of mind partially explain this attitude. There is a sizable number of traumatized persons who show an extraordinary capacity of denial or avoidance in order not to face grief resulting from traumas and confusing ideas that follow them. As a bio-psychological affection, trauma may develop quietly. Its existence may not be apparent until detected accidentally during an investigation requested for another reason, or when the aggravation reaches a stage where little can be done at the therapeutic level.

Observations From the Research Results

In this section we attempt to objectively assess the impact of the tragedy by drawing upon the results of an epidemiological survey conducted by SARP (Khaled, 2000). The survey sampled two representative areas in the Wilaya (department) of Algiers, Sidi Moussa and Dely Ibrahim. The total sample of 652 was equally divided, with 50% from the area of Sidi Moussa and the other 50% from Dely Ibrahim (Figure 1).

Exposure to Traumatic Situations. The main themes in exposure to traumatic stress were death, threat and loss (Table 2).

Nearly all respondents reported deaths of family members or friends during the crisis. In Sidi Moussa, 61% of the respondents reported killing of a family member or a friend during the crisis, and 26% of them actually witnessed the killing. Although the situation was less dramatic in Dely Ibrahim yet the corresponding figures are 33% and 12%. Considering the total number of deaths, 23% of the reported deaths in Dely Ibrahim and 32% of those reported in Sidi Moussa were attributed to the violence. We can easily say that grief over the loss of human lives is prevalent all over. This survey, sampling households, points to the fact that over one in two households in Sidi Moussa, and one out of three in Dely Ibrahim suffer the tragic loss of at least one family member or a close friend.

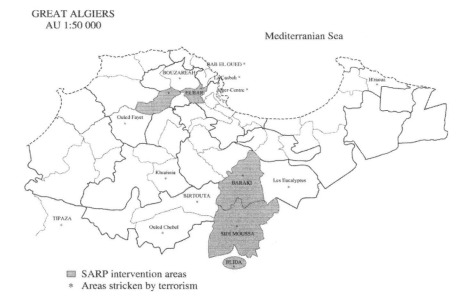

Figure 1. Map of the Wilaya of Algiers showing areas of SARP interventions.

Table 2. Exposure to Trauma (Epidemiological Survey, SARP, 1999)

	Sidi Moussa (n=326) Percent exposed			Dely Ibrahim (n=326) Percent exposed		
	Male	Female	Total	Male	Female	Total
Loss and deprivation						
Lack of food or water	30	40	34	14	11	13
Ill health	20	29	24	5	8	6
Lack of shelter	23	18	21	8	14	11
Lost house or land	16	9	13	2	3	2
Lack job or employment	32	11	23	17	19	18
Lost means of livelihood	11	6	9	5	2	3
Lost personal belongings	16	15	16	4	5	5
Imprisonment and torture						
Imprisonment	15	1	9	8	1	4
Torture	11	2	7	9	1	5
Witnessed torture	11	4	8	11	6	9
Solitary confinement	6	2	4	7		3
Death						
Death of family member or friend	53	44	50	53	48	50
Murder of family member or friend	31	18	26	19	5	12
Witnessed murder of strangers	47	24	38	31	9	21
Threatening situation						
Caught in combat situation	56	60	58	30	23	27
Witnessed curfew searching	78	83	80	52	32	42
Was close to death	65	63	64	46	27	37
Serious injury	20	11	16	22	12	17
Separation from family						
Separated from family	18	7	13	10	6	8
Witnessed other events	45	40	43	28	17	22

Exposure to threatening situations, like witnessing massacres and terrorist attacks, witnessing murder of people or the sight of decapitated and mutilated bodies, was reported by nearly every one in Sidi Moussa and more than a third of the respondents in Dely Ibrahim.

Regarding the loss of material resources, in Sidi Moussa 13% of the respondents reported loss of their house, 9% loss of source of livelihood (shops, stocks, jobs) and 5.8% loss of personal belongings. It is interesting to note that Dely Ibrahim, which was considered a relatively safe town spared of massacres, also witnessed high degrees of losses and life-threatening events.

Psychological Distress. The survey used the SCL-90-R (Derogatis, 1977), a psychological assessment instrument that measures the degree of current psychological distress measured on a Global Severity Index, and nine subscales. The results show that the degree of distress was high, with 38% of residents in Sidi Moussa and 27% in Dely Ibrahim scoring high on the Global Severity Index (GSI above 1). Distress was especially high in women and those of younger age. Most at risk were people who were exposed to traumatic separations from their family or to threatening situations and people who were deprived of basic resources.

The characteristic response of women in this sample were feelings of sadness, loneliness and hopelessness, and crying easily, accompanied by self-blaming and feelings of guilt. Males on the other hand complained very frequently of sleeping problems, poor concentration, nervousness and irritability and inability to trust others. Multiple somatic symptoms were frequent in both males and females.

The prevalence of DSM-IV psychiatric disorders: The survey used an adapted Arabic translation of the CIDI 2.1, Composite International Diagnostic Interview (WHO, 1993) to measure the lifetime prevalence of psychiatric disorders using the DSM-IV criteria (APA, 1994) (Table 3). The results are alarming.

There is an evident increase in the lifetime prevalence of all disorders, especially those like PTSD and major depressive disorder. Panic disorder and phobias are very prevalent: high rates of morbid fears of all sorts were found: specific phobic disorder, social phobia and agoraphobia. This was especially evident in young females exposed to threatening situations.

Table 3. Prevalence in Percentage of DSM-IV Psychiatric Disorders (Epidemiological Survey, Algeria 1999)

DSM-IV diagnosis	Sidi Moussa			Dely Ibrahim		
	Male %	Female %	Total %	Male %	Female %	Total %
Posttraumatic Stress Disorder	41	58	48	22	33	27
Major Depression	23	36	28	13	23	18
Specific Phobic Disorder	22	44	31	17	37	27
Social Phobia	4	7	5	2	2	2
Agoraphobia	4	20	11	4	9	6
Panic disorder	5	6	5	1	3	2
Generalized Anxiety Disorder	1	1	1	1	1	1
Obsessive Compulsive Disorder	1	3	2	1	5	3
Any somatoform disorder	5	22	12	3	6	5

The high prevalence of PTSD reflects the wide exposure to many types of traumatic situations. In general, females had higher lifetime prevalence of most disorders than males. Widows, divorced and separated women had even higher rates of prevalence.

If we consider the size of the population in both areas, we can imagine the enormous size of the problem faced by mental health workers. In Sidi Moussa alone, with a population of 300,000 people there would be more than 40,000 women who have ever suffered from PTSD, and 21,000 suffering from a lifetime major depressive disorder. Further calculations, taking co-morbidity in consideration, would point to the fact that at any point in time around 20,000 women in Sidi Moussa would have a current diagnosis of PTSD, and half of them would have an associated major depressive disorder. These two disorders, usually chronic or recurrent, have been shown to be associated with a high degree of distress and disability, making the sufferers more vulnerable to further loss and suffering (Wells et al., 1989). This association between depression and grief has first been noticed by Freud (1895). The rates described here exceed most rates reported in population studies on depression (Robins and Regier, 1991), but are comparable to rates reported for some third-world countries that went through civil wars or conflicts (Weissman, Bland and Canino, 1996).

Questions in Relation to the Clinical Practice

In face of the tragedy that Algeria is going through, the following questions need to be answered by Algerian psychologists:

1. What are the *urgent interventions*—psychological, psychosocial, educational—that professionals should organize or encourage in order to provide help for victims?
2. By what kinds of interventions is it possible to *complement and reinforce* the impact of emergency interventions?
3. Since the great majority of victims does not benefit from emergency interventions, and since there are tens of thousands of victims, by what types of interventions is it possible to *organize and develop* services on the medium and long-term in order to help the victims?
4. What *preventive interventions* should be organized or encouraged in order to provide prevention or screening? As we already know, the effects of tragedies such as that experienced in Algeria can be seen over several generations.
5. The worsening of the security situation in 1997 and the progressive increase of the number of mentally affected persons under the impact of various traumas, have led us to introduce necessary interventions to face the particularity of the situation. In what way can we *evaluate and monitor* the efficacy of these changes?

Clinical-Theoretical Reflection

In the face of these questions, our previous reflection on the diversity and the variety of traumatic situations has led us to attempt to grasp their effects on the persons who find themselves, directly or indirectly, in what we call the "range of action". The notion of range of action of situations with high traumatic potential, for instance displacement, has directed us to explore the similarities between traumatic situations and epidemic outbreaks. We will only point out here two parameters that, according to us, can make this comparison plausible.

1. Having been in contact with an epidemic source does not necessarily imply contamination. However, this contact indisputably increases the risk. In the same way, being in the range of action of a traumatic situation does not necessarily imply traumatization. The latter depends on the degree of exposure and the capacity of the individual to cope with it. This capacity in turn varies from one individual to another.
2. The notion of epidemic outbreak implies the idea of a germ transmitted by direct contact. But the disease contamination can result only when there is a favorable arena. Indeed, the idea of a transgenerational transmission of unresolved grief in particular, and of trauma in general is being addressed in the literature. In other words, clinical research has left no doubt that unresolved grief reactions in a mother can be transmitted to the child through the mother-child relationship, and later reactivated in adulthood after exposure to trauma.

Technical and Ethical Problems Linked to the Support of Repentant Terrorists

Providing psychological assistance to victims of terrorism implies recognition of their status as victims, as well as recognition of the malicious nature of the context that affected them. Although it is a rare occurrence, perpetrators can also seek psychological assistance, especially in the context of returning to their "normal" life. In such situations, difficulties arise when the psychologist discovers—in the course of therapy—that his patient has participated in terrorist activities. Such difficulties are both technical and personal. The literature on psychotherapy rarely mentions the techniques of dealing with such situations. This adds to the personal difficulties of a psychologist who would have to deal with feelings of fear and rejection to a patient who could have been his own killer.

Clinical experience with such cases leads us to underline that the right of clients to psychological help cannot be dissociated from the psychologist's right to have limits and to recognize his inability to work with people who put him in a state of emotional tension which surpasses his own capacities of restraint. It is then that the necessity of a keen preliminary investigation should be seen, because it is better to recognize one's limits in advance than to find oneself in a situation which will end up in a stalemate or failure. Our reflection leads us to assert that, first of all, it is important to recognize the psychologist's limitations in coping with such situations. It is also human to recognize the right of the psychologist to refuse to be involved in a treatment situation that exceeds his capacity and tolerance. However, the psychologist must not under-estimate his capacity to overcome the emotional tensions caused by such an encounter. Second, there is an urgent need to study the psychic processes at work within the psychologist in these situations, and to review the contributions of others that have studied this problem (Box 3).

Box 3. Case Example: Ex-terrorist with Impotence

Mr. M. is 35 years old. He asked for a consultation for impotence. The first thing he said was that he needed only a prescription because his occupations cannot permit him to come back for other consultations. He knew that the treatment of impotence would take a lot of time. Apparently embarrassed by the direct question asked by the psychologist: "Tell me about yourself", Mr. M. got up to make sure that the video recorder on the shelf was not on. His move was surprising, and we had the feeling that he was stuck between two tendencies. On the one hand wanting to talk about himself, to tell about his distress, to talk about his life so that we can help him, and on the other hand the impossibility to do so for a reason we did not know. He went back to his seat but a feeling of a frightening strangeness crossed the psychologist's mind. After a long silence, Mr. M. said that he had heard a lot about the psychologist, and that he was the only one who could help him. After that, he burst into tears like a child, and the psychologist, surprised, sighed and told himself there was no reason to be afraid.

Mr. M. dried his tears, got himself over and said "I do not know why I came to see you". After a silence, the psychologist said: "You have been told that I could help you but something prevents you from talking". He stared at the psychologist for a long time before replying: "You have understood. There are things which should not be said, you will not bear seeing me here again. I know that you do not like people like me, even if what I did is in the past... It is Ms. X. who pushed me to come... The fact that she is *moutahadjiba* (wearing the veil), and that her brother was in the *maquis* has not prevented you from helping him". During this time, the psychologist was astonished, stuck, he could hardly hear... Mr. M. went on talking but the psychologist did not understand anything. He only understood that the patient had married the sister of Ms. X., that he had a job and this reassured him.

We have learned from the remaining of the interview that Mr. M. has benefited from the law of clemency after having given himself up to the security forces, under pressure of his family. He did not want to say anything about the nature of the activity he was involved in before surrendering himself to the authorities.

The psychologist decided to end the consultation, which had lasted for 50 minutes, and suggested another appointment for the next week, because he felt that his ability of listening was declining gradually. Mr. M. only said that he was not sure to come back. At the time of the second appointment, Mr. M. did not show up and the team wondered if it would be wise to send the social worker for a home visit.

STRATEGY TO PROVIDE PSYCHOLOGICAL AND PSYCHOSOCIAL HELP FOR VICTIMS OF TERRORISM

Before presenting the experience of SARP and its strategy, we will give some indications of the Algerian prospects in the psychological and psychosocial fields. This paragraph describes the existing potential for psychological support to the Algerian population: an overview of the number of psychologists and their skills and a description of the organizations and networks currently providing services.

Human Resources

Algeria has an important human potential of mental health professionals. The State allocates 30% of the national budget for education. However, the educational policies of successive governments, among other causes, have limited the efficacy of the educational system. During the first three decades following independence in 1962 the main objective of these policies was the democratization of education. According to the data given by the Ministry of National Education, the educational system in Algeria counts today 15,000 primary schools, 4,500 high schools and 330,000 teachers. The enrolment rate is about 94% for children in primary schools. However, according to the latest statistics the illiteracy rate remains high at 31.9% at the national level (ONS, 1999).

Until now, with regard to technological fields, exact sciences and medical sciences, there is a misleading anachronism between university education and high school education. At the high schools, where students are prepared for the university, teaching is principally in Arabic. At the university level however, Arabization has practically not been implemented and all teaching is done in French. Subsequently, a great number of students who have chosen one of these three fields of study have great difficulties in following and apprehending the teaching content. However, despite the obvious limitations in the quality of education, we can say that this effort toward democratization of education at all levels has allowed the country to get out of an inherited situation of the colonial period—with an illiteracy rate of more than 80% - and to change the social setting of the country by providing professionals.

In the framework of this chapter, it is useful to give some numbers of workers in the health care system here. According to data provided by the Ministry of Health, Algeria had 24,103 health workers in 1997, among which 8,196 were medical doctors, 3,866 pharmacists, 7,837 dental surgeons, and 85,296 paramedics working in the public sector. Besides, there were about 12,000 medical doctors, pharmacists and dentists who work in the private sector. There were also 275 psychiatrists at work, in all sectors, besides those who left the country (about a hundred) because of insecurity and escalation of terrorism. (Ministère de la Santé et de la Population, 1998).

The case of psychologists deserves special attention. It is not easy to give the exact number of practicing psychologists in Algeria, in all majors—clinical, school, educational, occupational psychologists and speech therapists (a specialty of psychology in Algeria)—because they work in varied sectors and because many among them are currently out of work. However, some indicators permit the estimation of the importance of this profession in Algeria. The number of certified teachers with a graduate diploma working in the three psychology institutes—in Algiers, Oran and Constantine—is more than 250. The number of psychology students in all majors and levels at the Psychology and Education Institute at Algiers University was over 2,000 for the academic year 1997–1998. Moreover, the Ministries of Health and Social Affairs employ around 850 clinical psychologists. According to the data given by the Ministry of Health, there were 176 general hospitals in 1997, 13 university hospitals, 4 psychiatric hospitals, 455 polyclinics and 556 medico-psychological centers. Nevertheless, despite this human potential and the importance of this institutional network, no serious program has been provided to help victims of terrorism.

The availability of qualified psychologists is an important potential that should be considered when planning mental health services. However, it is also a potential that needs supervision, reinforcement of basic education and especially a program for continuous training and upgrading. Currently, the education of psychologists is essentially theoretical and is characterized by an almost absence of continuous training and perfection.

Proximity Cells ("Cellules de Proximité")

Special attention should be given to proximity cells, groups of professionals (in the medical and social fields) that try to provide services to the people. The nature, organization, composition and geographical setting of these cells allows them to play an important role in helping victims of terrorism, although the organization and functioning of these networks remain relatively vague. There are two types of proximity cells. First, those created by the Wilaya of Great Algiers, which has placed them at the disposal of local authorities. Second, those created by the Social Development Agency (ADS), which is a governmental organization.

Proximity Cells Pertaining to Local Organizations. These proximity cells do exist currently only at the level of the Wilaya of Algiers. They do not have autonomy, and suffer from the bureaucratic administration, a handicap that hinders their efficiency. Their initial mission is to provide multidisciplinary support to assist the population. Each proximity cell is composed of five to about twenty professionals from different disciplines: one or two medical doctors, psychologists, social workers, a sociologist, a jurist, a nurse, an educator, an architect, cultural and sport trainers. The majority of cell members are young professionals with little experience, who are hired as part-timers.

Social Development Agency's Proximity Cells. The Social Development Agency is a governmental institution which was created in July 1997. The principal mission of the ADS is to provide services that can contribute to the social reintegration of disadvantaged, distressed or marginalized people. The ADS is among others responsible for financial compensation for victims of terrorism. The following services may be offered by the proximity cells to the population:

- Providing information on social rights, environmental hygiene and disease prevention actions.
- Helping their clients gain access to public health, education, professional training, social protection and employment services and trying to create income-generating activities.
- Providing some psychological aid for persons in distress.
- Promoting cultural and sport activities.

There are currently twenty ADS-operated proximity cells in the entire country. The objective is to have one in each Wilaya (department) and to increase the number according to the need. The aim of these different professionals' presence is to be as close as possible to the citizen and to meet his multiple needs. The involvement of cultural and sport trainers in the cells indicates the special interest given to youth, the rationale of which is to revive sport and leisure activities. The presence of a social worker in a cell besides the doctor and the psychologist shows the importance given to socio-economic aspects associated to health needs.

Non-governmental Organizations and Associations

Since the Law of Association was issued in 1989, many NGOs and associations have appeared and became active in the health and social fields, such as women associations providing services to disadvantaged women and widows. Several associations provide support to the victims of terrorism, and other professional associations—medical, research etc.—are involved in providing services to individuals and families. However, the exact number, type of activities and capacity of these organizations need to be assessed to determine the potential area of networking and collaboration.

Analysis of the Potentials and Limitations of Available Resources

Algerian professionals have found themselves, overnight, obligated to be efficient in a task they have not been prepared for. Moreover, they have to act from within a system that is at least not inducive to action. Our analysis points to the disordered character of measures taken by public authorities in the management of tragedy consequences.

There is a great debate around the needs of victims of terrorism and the implications of the security situation on the society, but it has to do more with political agitation than with a will to design interventions to solve problems in a rational way. In some cases, the actions taken are clear examples of political opportunism and exploitation of others' grief. We mention several points to illustrate our observations. First, quarrels and conflicts between different associations of terrorism victims determine the help for traumatized persons. There are power conflicts between actors belonging to different parties and political manipulation is quite usual. This is often the case with women who lack experience about associations, have lost a husband, a brother or a son, and who are supported by different influencing groups. Associations of victims may want to mobilize people at the detriment of psychological and psychosocial help needed by the victims. Political will and interest is needed to mobilize resources and funds for victims, but it should be paired with professionalism and concern for human rights.

Second, there are concerns related to the training of psychologists and other health professionals. Although the tragedy is more than ten years old, it has no impact on the training of psychologists and other health professionals supposed to design interventions for victims of terrorism. Until now, few things have been done in this direction. Despite some initiatives taken by government institutions or non-governmental organizations, psychologists are still far from meeting the real and urgent needs.

Third, psychological and psychosocial interventions have been set up as networks of proximity cells. Although the basic concept of proximity cells is appropriate, their impact on the field is still limited. Almost all professionals employed in these proximity cells are young graduates who have little experience and have no prior training for the expected task. Thus, working continuously with persons who have experienced the most varied tragedies and who have gone through the most difficult traumas, constitutes a burden that affects even the most experienced and the best prepared health workers.

Fourth, we noticed that clinical psychologists have quickly realized the necessity for supervision and monitoring, not only to provide them a technical regular support in their activities, but also to support them and enable them to cope with the tragedies they encounter daily. Without this support, it seems quite dangerous to expose young professionals to repeated traumas, which will most likely disorganize them. We have been able to estimate the danger of this disorganization on the occasion of a training program that SARP has organized for a group of twelve psychologists from proximity cells. The situation experienced by some of them can itself be traumatic. They found themselves overwhelmed by feelings of pity, which made them lose the necessary professional distance (Bouatta, 2000). Although these structures of supervision and monitoring to support the professionals in coping with traumatic stories are still dysfunctional, it is a great advantage that they exist. Any mental health program for victims of terrorism must start from this reality of emotional stress experienced by professionals, without being engulfed by these stressful emotions.

SARP: EXPERIENCE AND STRATEGIES IN MENTAL HEALTH SERVICES

The Algerian Society of Research in Psychology (SARP) was created in December 1989 by a young research team of the Institute of Psychology and Educational Sciences at Algiers University. It has been set up as non-profit scientific association, with the objective of providing services in the fields of training, practice and clinical research. For the members of the team, these three dimensions are essential to the psychologists' profession. It was clear to the founders of SARP from the beginning that a healthy structure for the organization would be independence and freedom of initiatives. They insured independence by limiting their revenues to income of products and membership fees.

SARP's Mission and Objectives

SARP has been created to accomplish the following mission:

- Provide and develop prevention and psychological treatment for individuals and groups that demand or need such interventions.
- Contribute to the improvement of the training of psychologists and professionals by organizing regular specialized training, refresher courses and continuous education.
- Participating in research development of psychology and education.
- Participating in the production, printing and diffusion of all types of products necessary for training and practice of professionals in the fields of psychology and education.

Within SARP three internal functional structures have been created to carry out the activities needed to achieve its goals. Each one of these three structures has been directly put under the responsibility of a psychologist-researcher with relevant experience. The Prevention and Psychological Treatment Center (CPPP), the Training and Perfectioning Center (CFP) and Research, Publication and Diffusion Center (CERED). These three centers constitute the operational components through which the association's annual activity program is managed and translated into concrete operations. Each center must elaborate an action plan related to its sector of competence. This action plan is examined and endorsed by the administration council.

SARP's Principles and Strategy for Interventions for Victims of Trauma

The previous paragraphs do not leave an optimistic impression with regard to the way public authorities manage the implications of the tragedy in Algeria. This is why our hopes turn a lot more toward civil society and different non-government organizations that attempt to invest in the field. From its part, SARP has decided to engage in broadening and deepening its psychological and psychosocial interventions for victims of trauma. The SARP approach, in this domain, is guided by three principles.

(a) The first principle recommends the necessity for *multiplicity and variety of approaches, interventions and actors* that would undertake such a task. This implies the need for collaborative action through a network encompassing all associations and organizations working in the field of psychology, social work and health.

(b) The second principle advocates the encouragement of *interventions capable of evolving in time* by integrating new lessons drawn from the daily practice through monitoring and research.

(c) The third principle favors *sustainable and autonomous interventions that ensure long-term provision of services*, which are not dependent on the changing policies and interests of a particular donor or sponsor. The strategy of SARP in this respect is to pair the interventions with the creation of another activity, carried out by the same team, to make the interventions sustainable.

The SARP Intervention Model with TPO Partnership

The intervention model that SARP attempts to set up is a service that combines three complementary levels of action (de Jong, 1995).

The first level of intervention concerns a functional structure capable of carrying out research, initiating training, ensuring a minimum of supervision for professionals, and providing individual, family and group treatments. These activities are carried out by the Prevention and Psychological Treatment Center (CPPP), established in Dely Ibrahim (Arar, 2000). The CPPP is a reference source for all SARP activities that necessitate clinical help. The activities of the CPPP may be summarized in three axes as follows:

- Regarding psychological and psychosocial interventions, the CPPP provides specialized psychological and psychosocial services to victims of terrorism and to the general population. An average of 50 individual and group consultations per week are provided. Group treatments are currently reserved for children who have difficulties in school. Since July 1998, a social worker has developed interventions to assist victims of terrorism who need legal and social assistance. This structure is also a follow-up reference for the *Centre d'aide psychologique aux victimes* (psychological support center for victims) in Sidi Moussa, which was opened in April 2000.

- Regarding supervision, the CPPP ensures supervision for psychologists who work in the center, for psychologists who work in other institutions—especially those who develop interventions in areas that have been heavily affected by terrorism—and also for young psychologists who need to be prepared for interventions on site. In sum, about twenty psychologists benefit currently from the supervision services provided by the center.
- Regarding research, the CPPP is the place where data are collected for about ten research works from university researchers or students who prepare for a graduate degree.

The second level of intervention concerns interventions within existing organizations and networks that request SARP's help. These may be health-care institutions of any type, psychological and psychosocial help centers for victims of terrorism, associations of victims, or public institutions. The principles that guide this type of interventions are simple and are based on the needs of the following target groups:

- Young psychologists working in isolation and distress in several health-care institutions.
- Teams that wish to have an experienced clinical worker in order to analyze their difficulties and give another meaning to their project.
- Hospital services that are regularly confronted with emergency and trauma problems, and do not have psychologists in their teams.
- Associations of victims of terrorism who wish to consult SARP and refer victims who need assistance.
- Health-care institutions whose teams look for an experienced clinical worker to ensure supervision over their activities.
- Since a few months, SARP has begun to support several organizations by placing one or several trained and experienced psychologists at their service.

The third level of intervention concerns interventions on site, by setting up proximity cells in areas where there is an important expressed need. The first organization of this type designed in our program is the *Centre d'aide psychologique aux victimes* in Sidi Moussa, which is one of the most affected regions by terrorism. This psychological help center for victims has been functioning since April 2000. Its objectives are:

- To provide legal and social assistance to victims of trauma to help them assert their claims and attempt to benefit from support and compensation schemes that are provided by the government.
- To carry out preventive and screening activities in mental health, especially for school-age children.
- To provide psychological support to victims: individual, family and group follow-ups and educational-psychological workshops for school-age children, focusing on activities to stimulate again the desire for living and learning.
- To develop community approaches that attempt to renew social ties between community members.

Psychological Help and Psychosocial Interventions Program

A description of this program, by its diversity, gives an idea about the development of SARP activities. The program consists of brief psychological interventions, psychological treatment offered in the CPPP center in Dely Ibrahim, psychological interventions provided for institutions outside SARP, and psychosocial interventions provided by the *Centre d'aide psychologique aux victimes* in Sidi Moussa.

Brief Psychological Interventions. In the communities of Sidi Moussa and Dely Ibrahim brief psychological interventions have been developed on-site. Contact with the inhabitants has often taken place inside their homes and sometimes through local key persons who had been prepared by SARP. These interventions were aimed to screen the population to find persons at risk and refer them to the available services. They were delivered in the context of research on mental health needs of the population which we have carried out through the use of a questionnaire conceived by TPO, which was adapted by our team. The experience shows that, when these research tools are used by psychologists who have been trained beforehand, they make it possible to collect useful data for the research, but they also create the opportunity for interventions such as counseling, especially for persons who have been most affected by trauma.

The total number of persons who have benefited from such interventions was about 650 in the two communities until October 1999. These interventions have created a large demand for psychological support in both areas. The opening of the Sidi Moussa center later was greatly welcomed by the families there.

Psychological Treatment in SARP's Psychological Center. The number of consultations carried out during the first trimester of 1999 at the Prevention and Psychological Treatment Center (CPPP), was 1501 for 122 patients; that is, an average ratio of 11 consultations per patient. Initially, the center systematically separated victims of violence from other patients. But gradually, it turned out to be impossible to maintain this separation, for at least two reasons: First, therapists discovered the sequelae of Algeria's dramatic situation in patients who did not come initially to seek help for trauma or violence. Second, the impact of traumatic situations cannot be separated from the general mental health situation in a country that has experienced a multi-faceted tragedy which has permeated all aspects of daily life. At the prevention level, such a separation seems very delicate and unrealistic.

In the year 2000, the center provided 2,546 consultations for 301 patients. Of these patients, 60% were adults and 40% children. shows the type of presented problems according to the therapist's assessment (Table 4).

The center maintains a sliding scale fee system and exempts all victims of terrorism and their families from paying fees. On the whole, 20% of patients pay their consultations, 50% benefit from free-of-charge consultations, and 30% benefit from a reduction.

Psychological Interventions Provided for Institutions Outside SARP. This service of SARP has been initiated to help set up psychological

Table 4. Motive for Consultation (SARP, CPPP, 2000)

Motive		N	%
Anxiety	Generalized, panic, functional complaints	34	11
Depression		34	11
Neurosis	Phobia, somatization, obsessive, sexual problems	16	5
Psychosis		23	7
Posttraumatic	Somatization, adjustment, insomnia	13	4
Mental retardation		18	6
School difficulty		57	19
Relational problems	Marital, familial, adjustment	27	9
Behavior disorders	Delinquent, antisocial	28	9
Other	Anorexia, bulimia, drug abuse, sexual abuse, trichotillomani	37	12
Psychological testing		14	5
Total		301	

consultations within institutions that do not employ psychologists. The aims of these activities are two-fold:

- Developing particular psychological interventions that are adapted to the needs of the institution.
- Helping the establishment of a consultation which will be autonomously carried out by the institution itself in the future.

In this framework, SARP has set up a psychosomatic consultation service within the cardiology department of Beni Messous university hospital center. Three SARP psychologists provide two consultations per week. Two other interventions of the same type have started since June 1999, the first one focusing on associations of terrorism victims, the second one on women associations.

Psychosocial Interventions Provided by the Sidi Moussa Center. The *Centre d'aide psychologique aux victimes* in Sidi Moussa has been created in an area deeply affected by violence. This area witnessed two of the very first and largest scale massacres. In Ben Talha, more than 400 people were massacred in only one day. The effect of this massacre on the social structure and life in general has been great. In Rais, another village in Sidi Moussa, a second massacre took place, which was greatly publicized for the brutality of the killings and mutilations. Besides these massacres, and for ten long years, this area has been under the constant threat of assassinations, kidnappings, and intimidation. Although many families have escaped from Sidi Moussa, the majority remained in place, enduring threats and losses simply because they had no other place to go.

In the center treatment is provided free of charge for all clients, the majority of whom have lost one or more family members. Most of them are very poor and deprived of resources. They have lost their homes, land and work because they had to leave for safer areas, or because of the destruction of the infrastructure. Many of the families have lost the father or breadwinner. The majority of the clients are therefore women and children, of rural or semi-rural origin, many of whom are illiterate or have only limited education.

Since its start in April 2000, the center has received 113 individual patients, of which 46 were children/adolescents and 67 adults (44 women and 23 men). Usually the problem is presented as a family problem. Examples of the problems presented to the therapists are:

- Children: difficulties at school, aggressive behavior, behavior problems, nightmares related to the traumatic events.
- Adults: mood disorders, irritability, insomnia, fears, depression and multiple somatic pains and aches.

The clients usually are aware of the relation between their symptoms and the events they have been through during the crisis. The center adopts a wide variety of interventions both at the individual, group and family level. Children and adolescent groups usually employ an art therapy or psychodrama approach. Therapy groups for women allow them to support each other and exchange information and experience.

Until now, individual consultation is predominant. However, there is a need and tendency to use group and family interventions more to be able to deal with the size and quality of the problems presented.

In many cases, the therapists realize the need for social interventions. Since May 2000, a large proportion of the clients (248) have asked for social assistance and received social interventions. The problems presented to the social worker are:

- Administrative problems, usually presented by women with little education who have to deal with administrative and legal offices in order to receive assistance.
- Children who are dismissed from schools after having failed.
- Material needs and financial problems, such as the lack of jobs or homes. In these cases, the social worker orients and accompanies the clients to the appropriate organizations and associations.
- Undiagnosed or untreated medical illnesses. In these cases, the social worker refers the clients to hospitals or other organizations for treatment. She has developed an outreach service (home visits and networking) in which she visits families known to have problems like child abuse, and patients needing medical or therapeutic care (67 visits since May 2000).

The center is starting to develop its network of partners in the educational, health and legal systems. We realized that such a network is not only a complementary, but an integral part of the service. Currently, the center is compiling an inventory of associations and organizations that can be approached for awareness raising, training and collaboration.

Training and Supervision

The training activities of SARP target different types of personnel who already provide interventions or are likely to do so in the mental health domain in general, or in national programs that have been set up to provide psychological and psychosocial support to victims of terrorism. These target groups are essentially clinical psychologists, educational psychologists, school psychologists, psychiatrists, medical doctors and social workers. Some of the training activities specifically target psychologists who carry out interventions through TPO/SARP projects and through (future) partner organizations of SARP, especially proximity cells. These training activities are of manifold types.

Long-term Training

Theory and Clinic of Trauma. A long-period training program lasting for two years with 150 hours of training per year. It offers a certificate on theory and clinic of trauma. It is a graduate-level training offering 6 hours of weekly teaching. The program includes reading and discussions of research on trauma, discussion and follow-up of clinical cases, discussion and follow-up of on-site interventions, and closed seminars that last from three to four days on themes related to trauma. Currently, 23 people participate in this training, of which 21 are psychologists and 2 psychiatrists. Nine participants work directly on the SARP/TPO project, the remaining participants come from the following institutes: Health Care Center of Sidi Moussa, Headquarters of National Security, Social National Insurance, CHU (university medical centers), psychiatric hospital of Blida, and the 'Orientation Center for Youngsters in Moral Danger'.

Short-term Training Seminars. The short-term training seminars are three or four days long. In 1999–2000 there were two training seminars on supervision, three on family therapy, one on diagnosis of mental disorders for health professionals, four on CIDI (Composite International Diagnostic Interview), two on group therapy, two on networking and proximity work for psychologists, one on grief work with victims of violence and one on supervision over psychological work.

National Scientific Days on Violence and Trauma. Each year since 1998, SARP has organized a national scientific day which focuses on issues of assessment, treatment and latest advances in insights on violence and trauma. Each day gathers more than 300 persons, psychologists, medical doctors, psychiatrists, social workers, teachers, staff of Social Development Agency and other local public authorities. The purpose of this national scientific day is educating and sensitizing professionals in mental health about trauma and violence. It is also a good opportunity to make the TPO/SARP program more known in Algeria, and to promote the creation of a professional network, coordinated and established in different areas. The 2001 national day focused on the results of the epidemiological study conducted by SARP in order to share and exchange its insights with colleagues and partners.

Intervention On-site Training. This training combines screening, counseling and collection of epidemiological data. In 2000 fifty-six professionals from different disciplines who carry out interventions in various institutions (proximity cells, hospitals, universities, associations) and in different areas of the country, were trained during several short-term seminars (three days) in the use of questionnaire research and counseling practice.

Training of Professionals in the Public or Private Sectors.
Several training conventions have been established between SARP and other institutes:

- Training convention with the Social Development Agency: SARP has established a partnership with ADS to ensure a one-month training program cum practicum in France for a group of 23 psychologists. They are psychologists who carry out interventions in proximity cells belonging to ADS in different regions of Algeria (Governorship of Algiers, Oran, Constantine, Anaba and Setif). This training program deals with different topics: emergency interventions, social violence, exclusion, and violence in work settings. The agreement with ADS can be considered a great opportunity for SARP, as it shows clearly that Algerian public authorities begin to consider it as a serious and reliable partner.
- SOS Women in Distress Association: A scientific supervision and training convention has been signed with this association. The task here is to supervise and monitor the setting up of a structure which should provide women in difficult situations with psychological and psychosocial assistance, be it victims of terrorism, women facing material and social difficulties, or women taken care of several children alone. In addition to that, SARP's task is to evaluate the work of the psychologists in this association and to offer perfectioning training.

Supervision Practice

SARP's supervision practice has already been conceived and operates currently according to two complementary modes:

Supervision Groups Functioning within SARP

- There is a group of psychologists who implement interventions at the SARP center on a full or part-time basis. Currently, this group consists of 12 psychologists and three supervisors. Five psychologists from this group are able today to conduct supervision groups themselves.
- One psychologist-supervision group participates in the training of psychologists who prepare themselves for a certificate on theory and clinic of trauma. This group consists of 23 psychologists, 11 of whom are working in different institutes such as Algiers University.
- 'Orientation Center for Youngsters in Moral Danger', Social National Insurance, the health-care center of Sidi Moussa, several proximity cells and several university medical centers.

Supervision Groups Set Up Outside SARP. These are groups which are conducted in the quarters of SARP partners: currently SOS Women in Distress Association, Raped Women Help Center and ADS proximity cells specialized in helping victims of terrorism. The particularity of these supervisions is that they are aimed at team work and not at individual psychologists.

Supervision for Psychology Students in Algiers University. SARP supports graduate and postgraduate students preparing an MA thesis through:

- Providing supervisors from the SARP senior staff.
- Assisting the students in selecting thesis topics with emphasis on trauma, psychosocial and clinical areas.
- Providing adapted instruments for research (products of SARP).
- Assisting the students in statistical analysis.
- Providing literature, articles and documents on the subject.

Research, Documentation and Publications

SARP documentation center. In order to provide resources for professionals, researchers and students, SARP has started a documentation center for psychology and trauma.[1] The center also documents MA and PhD theses of psychology students. A team in SARP has been assigned the task of initiating the *Annuaire de psychology et éducation*, an index that collects all the works on psychology in Algeria and about Algeria.

SARP periodical review. In January 2000, the experience of SARP on trauma in Algeria was published in *Psychologie SARP* number 7 (230 pages). The next issue will be a special issue about the results of the epidemiological study.

Translation and publication. SARP has made a translation into Arabic of the WHO/UNHCR book *Mental health of refugees* (de Jong and Clarke, 1996). The aim of this translation is to popularize the elementary principles of mental health and support to persons at risk. Also, SARP is involved in the translation and adaptation of psychosocial and psychiatric instruments: CIDI 2.1, SCL-90-R, and questionnaires for Coping, Social Support, Trauma and Life events.

Research

Working groups. The aim of these working groups is to provide space and resources for researchers and students. Currently three working groups are active in SARP. The Clinical Psychology and Psychosomatics Workgroup focuses on

---

[1]The center currently includes issues of 18 reviews in psychology, more than 500 articles and 572 books in a variety of subjects related to clinical psychology (438), trauma (75) and occupational psychology (59).

studies in clinical psychology, students preparing theses, discussions and literature reviews. The Psychometry Workgroup focuses on translation and adaptation of psychological tests to be used in the local context. The Occupational Psychology Workgroup is involved in research and assessment of the psychological environment of working people in institutions and organizations.

Epidemiological survey. In collaboration with TPO, SARP has conducted a survey on the prevalence of distress and disorders in a sample of 650 adults in Algeria. The survey used translated and culturally adapted instruments and enabled SARP to objectively assess the mental health needs in its target areas.

Study on the cost-effectiveness of interventions. In order to assess the effectiveness of its interventions, and in collaboration with TPO, this study uses a cost-effectiveness model to study patient, therapist and treatment variables measuring changes after an intervention in a sample of 100 patients and 30 controls.

CONCLUSION

Algeria is essentially a rich country. Its terrain, culture, natural and human resources qualify it to be one of the most advanced countries in the third world. However, Algeria is witnessing one of the bloodiest civil and political conflicts. The rise and decline of fundamentalism has been associated with a severe fragmentary reaction of the infrastructure of the country and the social values and individual well-being of its inhabitants. The reactions at the different levels seem to form a vicious cycle in which loss and grief lead to vulnerability and more loss. Communities, families and individuals are entangled in the meshes of conflict and violence, and gravitate down the scale of well-being to a state of poverty, misery and depression.

Terrorism is not a temporary, time-limited phenomenon. Its effects extend—like an epidemic—in time and scope. The aftereffects are expected to last for many years to come and to extend to generations that have not been directly exposed to the crisis. Trauma and its impact have not been limited to those who suffered their direct impact. Even areas that were not directly exposed to the massacres have shown reactions at the social and individual levels.

The loss of resources, sense of insecurity and guilt-ridden grief characterize the psychological effects on the population. Both males and females of all age groups have shown measurable psychological distress in reaction.

The effect of the violence on the social structure and functioning of the Algerian society is immense: a lack of trust, feelings of hopelessness, and a decline in social cohesion and support threaten to become the long-term aftereffects of the crisis on the population.

Recently, mental health professionals have directed their attention to the impact of the tragedy. In analyzing the impact of the tragedy, the classical psychodynamic and individual-oriented interventions proved unsuccessful in the face of the size and nature of suffering and mental illness in the exposed communities. The complexity and extent of exposure and reactions call for the statement that interventions with communities affected by terrorism are not the responsibility of any single agency. There is a need for a concerted and collaborative effort from all concerned.

Actually, the reaction of the governmental and civil institutions to the impact of this tragedy has been disoriented and scattered, and suffered from problems of lack of resources and coordination. SARP, in collaboration with TPO, has launched a mental health program that attempts to deal with the consequences of trauma at the community, family and individual levels. Starting from its own resources concerning professionals, training, research and clinical interventions, and drawing upon the potential resources in the professional and public communities in Algeria, SARP has been able to initiate a model that is acceptable to other professionals and institutions that demand services. Both the change in conceptualization and modes of intervention, and the increasing demands pose a challenge to the professionals of SARP. On the one hand, they aim at expanding and disseminating the model through training and sensitization, and on the other hand, they realize the need to evaluate and monitor the interventions that were introduced and increase their efficacy.

ACKNOWLEDGEMENT. The authors are thankful to M. Boukhaf, M.A. University of Algiers, for translation of the original French text of this chapter.

REFERENCES

Aït Sidhoum, M. A. (1997). Le psychologue, le traumatisme, l'insécurité et la gestion de l'économie psychosomatique: L'expérience d'une consultation psychologique à Alger [The psychologist, the traumatism, the insecurity and the management of the psychosomatic economy: The experience of a psychological consultation in Algiers]. *Psychologie Clinique et Projective*, *3*, 109–125.
American Psychiatric Association. (1994). *Diagnostic and statistical manual of mental disorders* (4th ed.). Washington, DC: Author.
Arar, A. (2000). Quelles options pour l'organisation de l'aide psychologique [What options for the organization of the psychological help]. *Psychologie SARP*, *8*, 89–103.
Benyoub, R. (1999). *Annuaire politique de l'Algérie* [Political yearbook of Algeria]. Alger: ENAG.
Bouatta, C. (2000). Le psychologue face au traumatisme de l'autre: Une histoire à deux temps [The psychologist facing the traumatism of the other: A history at two times]. *Psychologie SARP*, *8*, 57–87.
De Jong, J. T. V. M. (1995). Prevention of the consequences of man-made or natural disaster at the (inter)national, the community, the family, and the individual level. In S. E. Hobfoll & M. W. De Vries (Eds), *Extreme stress and communities: Impact and intervention* (pp. 207–227). Boston: Kluwer.
De Jong, J. T. V. M., & Clarke, L. (Eds). (1996). *Mental health of refugees*. Geneva: World Health Organization.

Derogatis, L. R. (1977). *The SCL-90 manual*. Baltimore: John Hopkins University School of Medicine.
Freud, S. (1962). General theory on neuroses. In J. Strachey (Ed. and transl.), *The standard edition of the complete psychological works of Sigmund Freud* (Vol. 4). London: Hogarth Press. (Original work published in 1895).
Khaled, N. (2000). Recherche-action sur la santé mentale d'une population longtemps exposée aux événements traumatiques: Considérations méthodologiques et résultats de terrain [Action research on the mental health of a population exposed to the traumatic long-term events: Methodological considerations and field results]. *Psychologie SARP, 8*, 37–51.
Marty, P. (1990). *Psychosomatique de l'adulte* [Psychosomatics of the adult]. Paris: Presses Universitaires de France.
Ministère de la Santé et de la Population. (1998). *Statistiques 1997* [Statistics 1997]. Alger: Author.
Office National des Statistiques (ONS). (1999). *IV Récensement général de la population et de l'habitat 1998: Principaux résultats* [IV General census of the population and the habitat 1998: Main results]. Alger: Author.
Robins, L. N., & Regier, D. A. (1991). *Psychiatric disorders in America: The epidemiologic catchment area study*. New York: The Free Press.
Rouadjia, A. (1991). *Les frères et la mosquée* [The brothers and the mosque]. Alger: Bouchene.
Samai-Ouramdane, G. (1990). Le Front Islamique du Salut à travers son organe de presse Al-Munquid [The Islamic Salvation Front through its press release Al-Munquid]. *Peuples méditerranéens, 52*, 155–165.
Weissman, M. M., Bland, R. C., Canino, G. J., Faravelli, C., Greenwald, S., Hwu, H. G., Joyce, P. R., Karam, E. G., Lee, C. K., Lellouch, J., Lepine, J. P., Newman, S. C., Rubio-Stipec, M., Wells, J. E., Wickramaratne, P. J., Wittchen, H., & Yeh, E. K. (1996). Cross-national epidemiology of major depression and bipolar disorder. *JAMA, 276*(4), 293–299.
Wells, K. B., Stewart, A., Hays, R. D, Burnam, M. A., Rogers, W., Daniels, M., Berry, S., Greenfield, S., & Ware, J. (1989). The functioning and well-being of depressed patients: Results from the Medical Outcomes Study. *JAMA, 262*(7), 914–919.

10

How Can Participation of the Community and Traditional Healers Improve Primary Health Care in Kinshasa, Congo?

JAAK LE ROY

THE AIMS AND METHODS OF THE PROJECT

In 1994 Kinshasa, the capital of the Democratic Republic of Congo, had a population of more than 5 million people, of whom the large majority lived in poverty and unhealthy environmental conditions in old and new shanty towns. From day to day the urban population had to survive a chronic economic regress and to deal with rapid socio-cultural transitions.

The health care system and the whole public sector was undermined by the economical crisis and by political and administrative instability. This situation deteriorated during the following years and particularly after the onset of war in Congo. Sound epidemiological data which could demonstrate shifts in the general health situation of the population were lacking (Figure 1).

The objective of this project was to find models and ways to improve primary health care in Kinshasa and comparable urban contexts in sub-Saharan Africa which are confronted with severe economic and social dislocation (Devisch et al., 2001).[1] At the start of the project we put forward a set of premises, which were the starting point of our conceptual model and methodology.

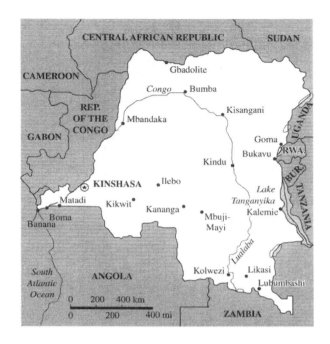
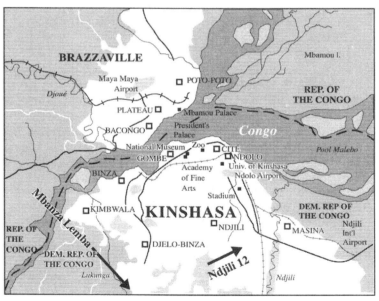

Figure 1. Maps of Congo and Kinshasa.

Firstly, we considered the health care system to be the totality of persons, institutions and activities who were perceived by the population as providers of health care and used as such. As well as the care offered in the public or private medical sector, this included all forms of treatment provided by traditional healers and faith healers. Health policies should open their perspective beyond the medical field and consider the role of all provisions of health care presenting which had a historically, culturally and practice-based evidence.

Secondly, the population should participate in the organisation of primary health care. As the users are directly confronted with issues such as quality, accessibility, equity and coverage, their experiences and insights are important sources of information. Moreover the participation of the community can form a constructive counterpower which is necessary to balance the power of corporate groups and health care institutions. The pragmatic influence of the community on the health care organisation is expressed by the users through their help seeking routes. But a more explicit and public use of this knowledge can provide tools and strategies which make the health care provision and organisation more effective as well as socio-culturally more relevant. The first and second premises were explicitly mentioned as important building blocks of the primary health care model decided at the Alma Ata conference in 1978 (WHO, 1978). As in most sub-Saharan African countries, this Alma Ata policy had been introduced by the Congolese government and formed the foundation of the public health care organisation. According to the spirit of the Alma Ata conference, both the integration of traditional forms of health care and organized community participation would guarantee the socio-cultural relevance of the primary health care model. Since 1978, however, the value and role of traditional care with regard to public primary health care had a very low priority on the agenda of health systems research and development in Africa (Akerele, 1990; Anyinam, 1987; Bannerman et al., 1983; Last & Chavunduka, 1986; WHO, 1976; Dozon, 1987; Green, 1988). Community participation had on the contrary been a central issue in some countries, but most often it had been reduced to the financial participation of the community and the management role of health committees in district health care services (Brunet-Jailly, 1997; Fassin, 2000; Grodos, 2000).

Thirdly, in order to improve parts of the health care system, an action-research methodology had to be used combining research and developmental

---

[1]The action-research project is part of the joint research project 'Choice, utilisation and satisfaction of healthcare in Kinshasa' sponsored by the European Commission; DG Research, IncoDev sector health systems (DGXII TS-CT94-0326). Three partners joined in this project: CERDAS, Institute for sociological studies, University Kinshasa, R. D. Congo (Prof. D. Lapika, Mr. Kyulu, Mr. Matula, Mr. Mulopo) Africa Research Center, Department of Anthropology, Catholic University Leuven, Belgium (Prof. R. Devisch co-ordinator of the project, Prof. F. De Boeck); RIAGG, Regional Community Mental Health Care Institute, Maastricht, Netherlands (Dr. J. Le Roy). Publications referring to this project are Devisch, 1995, 1996: Devisch et al. 2001. Le Roy, 1994, 1997, 2000b; Le Roy & N'situ, 1998).

action (Checkland & Holwell, 1998; Devisch et al., 2001; Grodos & Mercenier, 2000). This methodology enables the construction of models which can be tested in a real context. Action-research methods are also particularly valuable because they do not exclude, as in convential research methods, the non-quantifiable human processes which have an important influence on the functioning of social systems. Such methodology also has more chance of producing sustainable results, since the contextual resources and constraints are taken into account (Black, 1994). The constraints and resources which determine the help-seeking experiences of the population and the help-providing practices of care-providers are economic, historical, cultural, social, psychological and political (Augé, 1984; Bell & Chen, 1994; Good, 1994, 1997; Fassin, 1992, 1996; Feierman & Janzen, 1992; Heggenhouwen, 1991; Janzen, 1989; Janzen & Prins, 1979; Meyer & Geschiere, 1999; Rogler & Cortes, 1993; de Sardan, 1998).

The fourth premise of the project was that care for mental distress and illness should be part of primary health care policy. This premise accorded with the decision made by national governments at the Harare conference to consider treatment and prevention of mental health problems as one of the concerns of primary health care. Before defining adequate mental health policies, a better understanding of mental health problems and of current solutions was needed. It was also relevant to relate the mental health problems of the population to important socio-economic, political and cultural transitions and crises (Bibeau, 1997; Blue & Harpham, 1996; Canino et al., 1997; Corin E. et al., 1992; De Boeck, 1996; de Jong, 1987, 1994; Desjarlais et al., 1995; Douville, 1998; Kleinman, 1980; Le Roy, 2000a,b; Mauss, 1985; Werbner & Ranger, 1996; WHO, 1990).

These premises led to the construction of a set of hypotheses or conceptual model (Grodos, 2000, Grodos & Mercenier, 2000). The hypothesis was that the functioning of primary health care could be improved by innovative forms of community participation built on the knowledge of the users and on social dynamics in the community (Figure 2).

This chapter relates to the action-research project in Quartier XII of Ndjili, one of the empoverished shanty towns of Kinshasa, during the years 1994 to 1997. From 1998 onwards, this project has been continued by the local community with minimal external support.[2] The chapter follows and describes the

---

[2]In the team who was responsable for the design and implementation of the reported household study and intervention in Ndjili 12 were associated J. Le Roy (RIAGG Maastricht), A. N'situ (Psychiatric Clinic University CNPP, Kinshasa, R. D. Congo), J. de Jong et I. Komproe (Transcultural Psychosocial Organisation and Free University, Amsterdam, Netherlands), A. Matula (CERDAS Kinshasa). Assistants were D. Matumona and P. Ibanda. The exchange and discussion with D. Lapika, R. Devisch and members of the CERDAS and ARC teams who operated in other shanty towns was helpful in setting up the design and in assessing the experience in Ndjili 12. After the research the local project with the committee of Ndjili 12 has been further supported by RIAGG Maastricht and CNPP Kinshasa.

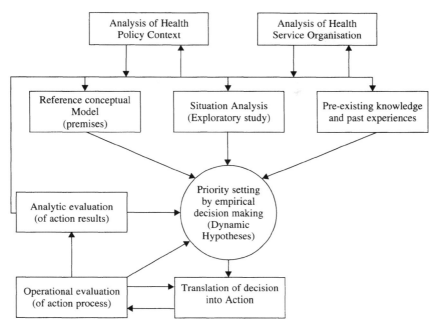

Figure 2. Methodological scheme for health systems research (adapted from Grodos and Mercenier, 2000).

different steps in this project. In line with the hypothesis, we first carried out a qualitative and quantitative study on the current help-seeking patterns of households, on mental distress and the diverse health care practices in Kinshasa today. This exploratory study enabled us to understand the apparently chaotic health care practices, and the effect of socio-cultural transitions on health care in general. This situation analysis and pre-existing knowledge from literature and past experiences enabled us to develop the dynamic hypotheses, priority setting and the translation of these decisions into action. The activities and some of the processes of intervention are described. Finally we discuss the results of the action and how they feed back to the original working hypothesis.

THE PERSPECTIVE AND HELP-SEEKING PRACTICE OF THE USER

Socio-Ecological Situation of Neighbourhoods

At the beginning of the project we carried out an overall appraisal of the situation in the neigbourhoods of Ndjili 12, built in the 1950s, and Mbanza-Lemba, constructed at the end of the 1970s (see Figure 1).

Quartier 12 Ndjili (17,000 inhabitants) was an area with much public and commercial activity. The population was considered socially and economically adapted to a 'modern' way of living and culturally heterogenous. However, traditional attitudes, beliefs and practices continued to play an important role in households and in the use of health care. The medical coverage was quite dense and we predicted that traditional medicine would have become very marginal as a result of 'modernisation'.

Mbanza Lemba (22,000 inhabitants) was considered a poorer shantytown, with harsh environmental conditions and a lack of public urbanisation planning. Traditional values, solidarity and a village-like environment, with some scope for small-scale agriculture, created social cohesion for its inhabitants. Medical services were scarce or too expensive at the nearby university clinic and private clinics.

The populations of these neighbourhoods in the 1990s assimilated and became more socially and culturally mixed than before owing to continuing migration from the villages to Kinshasa and to migration in Kinshasa itself as a result of economic regression.

General Socio-Economical Situation

The social situation of households in Kinshasa was analyzed in 1995–96 by De Herdt and Marysse (1997) and this confirmed the state of poverty and economic regress of the population. In 1996, GDP per head had fallen back to 100 USD, which was 200 USD below the survival minimum. Only 5% of the potentially active population was officially employed. In the period 1989–95 the regression in Zaire, measured in health indicators, had been gradual, from average to below average for S-Saharan Africa. This evolution had become irreversible. The analysis indicated that informal networks probably compensated to some extent for the regress, while 'the structure of the social tissue seems to be constantly redesigned in function of the most urgent problems, the most readily available solutions and the capability of 'political entrepreneurs' to reallocate problems and solutions to 'their' garbage can' (De Herdt & Marysee, 1997). They concluded that this capability of coping successfully was not only present at the household and individual level, but also among extra-household social networks at the neighborhood level.

It was clear that social vulnerability and disadvantage with regard to health care were more pronounced not only when the income was low but also when the resources and 'entrepreneurship' of the supportive network were lacking.

Social Transitions and Vulnerability

Help-seeking practices are the pathways, strategies, tactics and assumptions underlying multiple, parallel or successive therapeutic actions taken by the patient and family. We designed a half-structured questionnaire to investigate how patients and families sought and found treatment for their illnesses.[3] The analysis of the socio-demographic characteristics of the population in both neighbourhood samples revealed only minor differences. The population of Ndjili and Mbanza-Lemba was multi-ethnical and most of the households were composed of a nuclear family.

Overcrowded housing with an average of eight persons per house produced extremely precarious conditions and 80% of the families were very poor. Only 5% of the households had a regular income. The other 95% lived by informal petty trade and with intra-family or extra-family support. These social patterns rooted in the severe economic crisis had major consequences in the psycho-social life of the family. Every household in the sample was confronted with several structural challenges and tensions. Dependency of family solidarity and on outsiders (friends, neighbours, brothers or sisters in the prayer-group) was inevitable. It generated stress, envy, suspicion, and enhanced obligations in these relationships. A person with a better position and income carried the heavy burden of supporting an expanding network of people. The women were responsible for the education of the children, for the household, and in half of the cases for the income. This generated serious physical and psychological stress. The man, not providing a regular income, and confronted with woman and children who earned more than himself, felt threatened in his self-esteem as husband and father. However he was still supposed to take the important decisions, to exercize authority and to guarantee the functioning of family and social laws. Children and adolescents, particularly females helping their mother or older sister, were providing income on which the family and the child became dependent. School attendance and education suffered in such cases. Children who earned a good income were also experienced as a danger by the parents, particularly the fathers, because in their imagination and, in many cases also in reality, these children could not be ruled any longer by traditional authority.

---

[3]The core of the questionnaire is a combination of TPO's Help-seeking Behaviour and Explanatory Questionnaire with the Bradford Somatic Inventory (a questionnaire on somatisation) with an additional series of questions regarding the dynamics of family and social life. We used the questionnaire to study a random sample with 50 families in zone Ndjili (quartier XII) and 50 families in quartier Mbanza Lemba, and later to interview patients in treatment contexts. The qualitative and quantitative data were interpreted together with the anthropological and clinical findings of participant observation and in-depth interviews in these contexts. After pretesting and adaptation, it was applied between April–August '95 by two assistants who had been trained in interviewing families. For each interview 2–3 encounters with a family were necessary. The interview was carried out with the person in the family who had taken the most recent help-seeking step. No illnesses were excluded.

Nearly all young adults in the families of the sample had no regular income. They stayed longer in their elders' homes than before, which represented an additional burden for the parents instead of a support. Without income, they were unable to engage officially in marriage relationships. The latter were postponed and unofficial (traditionally irregular) sexual relationships developed. Pregnant unmarried girls often became an additional burden for the parents.

Types of Illness

The illness reported in the household survey was the one for which the family had undertaken the most recent help-seeking action. The sample included all ages and types of illness.

On the basis of a full description of the complaints, we divided the illnesses reported in the survey into five *categories*. The first category, called by us 'simple somatic illnesses' (41% of the sample of 100 households), was composed of the illnesses with one or two dominant features which according to bio-medicine were somatic and considered by the population and healers as a 'natural' disease. Typical examples are malaria and other infectious diseases. The second category (12%), was named, and was composed of 'somatic, chronic illnesses'. Examples are tuberculosis, chronic arthritis, diabetes, chronic respiratory diseases and AIDS. The third category (40%), called 'somatisation illnesses', was composed of illnesses with a specific cluster of multiple somatic features, referring to a particular part of the body, combined with a general feeling of illness in the whole body. The latter can be considered as culturally bound syndromes or culture-bound folk illnesses (Helman, 1990) with local names used by healers and sometimes by patients themselves. We also utilized the term 'somatisation', to indicate that these syndromes express a combined form of somatic and mental distress. In most of these culture-bound syndromes accounts of the illness express in different ways and with varying intensity depressive moods, emotions of sadness, worries, loss, aggressive impulses, fears and anxieties. The expressions of distress were either self-centered or concerning relationships with others. These syndromes can be related—not reduced—to the common mental disorders (depressive, anxiety and somatoform disorder) (Douville, 1998; Kirmayer, 1989, 1991, 1992; Kirmayer & Robbins, 1991; Kirmayer et al., 1994; Kleinman & Good, 1985; Mumford, 1994; Helman, 1990; Littlewood, 1991, 1998). The fourth category (5%), called 'psychotic illnesseses', is composed of illnesses with behavioral problems, which by the population and healers and in medicine are considered as major mental illnesses. They include the major psychiatric disorders like personality disorders with dissociative and psychotic symptoms, acute psychosis, schizophrenia, manic and melancholic mood disorders. The fifth category (2%), 'epileptic illnesses' is used for simple or repetitive convulsive and epileptic disorders.

Plural Help-Seeking

We have found that medical care is used by a very large majority (91%) of the help-seekers in the household sample, with a preference for private and clinical services. Half of the help-seekers combine for some reason (inefficacy, costs, causes) this medical intervention with health care based on traditional and faith-healing explanatory models. Patients of traditional healers and faith-healing churches, nearly always combine this care (in a preceeding or a following step) with medical treatment.

The help-seeking patterns of the whole population are characterized by an important plurality of steps and by an important heterogeneity, signifying the combination of heterogenous models of health care (bio-medical, traditional and faith care). The dominant pattern in the majority of the cases is that one starts with the medical care. When this is not successful a second or further trial of medical care is made or traditional or faith-healing is started. When more than three steps are needed the heterogeneity becomes highly prevalent (75%). The number of help-seeking steps is associated with the type of illness. Patients suffering from 'somatisation', 'psychotic' and 'epileptic' illnesses more frequently need multiple and heterogenous steps in comparison with patients with a simple or chronic somatic illness.

Satisfaction and Effectiveness

Satisfaction with a received treatment is the result of several factors of which some have been explored in the survey. We report here three factors: the 'fit' between the patient's and the care-provider's explanatory models, the effectiveness of the treatment and the cost.

Help-seekers as well as care-providers, make use of explanatory models for the causes of the illness. Explanatory models stem from different bodies of knowledge and are culturally sensitive (Kleinman, 1980, 1988; Kirmayer et al., 1994; Helman, 1990). Research on therapeutic relationships suggests that the effectiveness of a form of treatment is, amongst other factors, related to communication and a consensus between the explanatory models of care-seeker and care-provider (Helman, 1990; Kleinman, 1980). A shared belief that the illness is caused and explained by a particular mechanism enhances the chance of an effective treatment.

The household survey indicated a lack of attention given in the therapeutic relationship to good communication and consensus in the large majority of the cases, causing suspicion and dissatisfaction amongst the users. Problems of communication were reported in the three therapeutic systems.

The ineffectiveness of a treatment was the main reason for a user's stopping a treatment and switching to another. During the interviews, the help-seekers and families indicated that their first concern was the effectiveness of the treatment in terms of the removal of symptoms and general distress. Patients distinguished clearly between a partial recovery and a more general well-being. The latter was sought by all possible means. Patients became interested in the meaning of the illness only when interpersonal problems or sorcery were suspected, and when a first and second step had not given a good result.

We concluded that in particular the pathways of people suffering from culture-bound syndromes/somatisation illnesses were heterogenous, multiple, long and for nearly half of them ineffective, after at least two years of multiple treatment.

Satisfaction was also related to financial conditions. In general, if the family was not extremely poor, it could find primary treatment at an affordable price in the medical, and particularly in the sponsored public sector, and in the traditional sector. Generally the latter asked a symbolic payment or gift and some asked for the payment of their real expenses (herbal products). Faith-healers did not ask payment unless they used herbal or allopathic medicine. However, once a treatment lasted longer or when medical investigations, expensive medication or surgery were prescribed, the family always needed financial support from the extended family or social network. Families indicated that the price was not the decisive criterion for the choice. As a system of social security was only available for those families whose father had a regular job (5%), multiple care was always causing serious financial problems and increased interpersonal dependency.

MENTAL DISTRESS

Classification

We have indicated that the author had screened systematically the reports of the interviews, with regard to the complaints and narratives of somatic and mental distress presented by patients. The category 'somatisation' included all the syndromes, except the psychotic and epileptic disorders, through which various modes of psycho-social and mental distress were expressed. Amongst the most frequent culture-bound syndromes or 'somatisation illnesses' were distinguished: (1) 'pota libumu' or 'internal haemorrhoids' with pain in the intestinal tract and anal area; (2) 'stomach' with pain and burning in gastric and heart region; (3) 'lukika' 'headache', 'head', with pain and burning in the head; (4) 'vertebral column', 'impotence', 'back-ache' with pain in the low back area, mainly for males; (5) 'stérilité' of women with pain in the lower belly and infertility; (6) 'mpese', a dermatosis of the whole skin. In order to explore the level of mental distress, a culture-adapted screening instrument measuring levels of mental distress was part of the questionnaire used in the household survey.[4]

Prevalence and Etiology

When we focus on the adult population, our study indicates a high prevalence of mental distress. Forty percent of the adults were above the critical threshold of the BSI scale used. When we use the five illness categories in the adult sample, it is clear that 53% of the persons older than 15 have a 'somatisation illness' or culture-bound syndrome. The analysis suggests a significant relationship between a positive BSI score and the clinical classification of 'somatisation' or culture-bound syndrome. Mental distress is an important dimension of culture-bound syndromes. Detailed investigation of the different syndromes in this category in the qualitative part of the study has shown that the syndromes include and relate to different degrees of anxiety and emotional distress. The differences in level of distress and somatisation between the two neighbourhoods were not significant.

The prevalence of mental distress was particularly high for women older than 40 years. Living in large families and overcrowded housing made people vulnerable to mental distress and somatisation illness. The study also revealed the association of poverty and socio-cultural disruption of the household with mental distress. Families today in the urban context were more and more disrupted by inter- and intrapersonal tensions and conflicts.

The group of persons with mental distress had a higher prevalence of disturbing and emotionally distressing events in the six months prior to the onset

---

[4]In recent epidemiological surveys Mumford has used his Bradford Somatic Inventory in Pakistan, India, UK (1991, 1994, 1997). It was designed as a first stage screening instrument for common emotional and mental distress. The BSI is based on the clinical experience that most people suffering common mental disorders in non-western countries spontaneously express their illness experience and distress in somatic experiences, and not in psychological complaints. The BSI is not designed for and does not distinguishes major mental illnesses like psychotic disorders or epilepsy. The BSI proved to be an effective screening instrument with a sensitivity of 80% and a specificity of 70% of anxiety and depressive disorders (classified as neurotic, non-psychotic disorders) when related to other psychiatric instruments and interviews (ICD-10). It can serve as a research inventory and not as a standardised rating scale. It has to have a positive predictive value for common psychiatric morbidity of 60%. The cut-off score for the BSI-21 is 14. This cut-off score was not validated in Congo. It means that 60% of patients scoring above this threshold will turn out to have a psychiatric disorder (anxiety, depressive or somatoform disorder in the DSM-IV). The predictive value of psychiatric illness enhances when the score is higher than 14. In the BSI a number of typical symptoms of emotional distress like headache and fatigue have been left out because they are not differentiated from the emotional distress related to clear somatic, organic disorders.

of their illness, and in particular of death and loss of family members and of conflicts in the family. They also showed association of their suffering with these events. When the family members could not themselves resolve the family tensions they addressed themselves to traditional and faith healers. When the family did not agreed to seek help there, or when this care was ineffective, these tensions remain unchallenged and continue to produce emotional insecurity and anxiety.

Coping Strategies and Treatment

In order to copy with the severe emotional distress and the anxiety linked with these conflicts and losses, persons sought individually or with their nuclear family for new supportive social groups offering social and psychological support. However, the study of the help-seeking trajectories and faith healing practices provided evidence that when families and persons were seriously trapped in chronic culture-bound syndromes, mental distress and family conflicts, the support of these social groups was often not effective or sustainable. This vulnerable group of the population was then obliged to search further, and to become dependent on faith healers for the restoration of their disturbed mental and social equilibrium. The rapid growth of faith healing groups was a sign of the rise in the prevalence of serious psycho-social distress. Religious prayer groups and faith healing groups seemed to be very attractive to the mentally distressed. In the group of the non-mentally distressed persons 45% went to these groups to pray or to be healed, while in the group of the mentally distressed persons the frequency of participation reached 75%. Even when participation in the rituals of the faith healing or prayer group did not completely cure the symptoms, we found that many patients remained in this group because they were valued and integrated in a small community offering social support and emotional belonging to a substitute family.

The majority of the persons with complaints and syndromes that related to all types of mental distress (common minor and major illnesses) were dissatisfied with the result of their help-seeking itinerary. Half of the care-seekers with somatic illnesses were completely healed, but only a quarter of the mentally distressed. Some symptoms might have disappeared but often anxiety remained, or a general feeling persisted that the reconstruction of good relationships had not been achieved. In terms of health policy and coverage, these mentally distressed people can be considered as a health care category which is particularly vulnerable and excluded. These people are to some degree satisfactorily treated by healers but not at all by biomedical care. When traditional care is not considered acceptable or when it has been unsuccessful, a large proportion of the patients seek support and care in the numerous healing churches and prayer groups. A small number of them find their way to psychiatric care.

HEALTH CARE PROVISION

Medical Care

Current Situation. The D. R. of Congo (at that time Zaire) had adopted and ratified the primary health care model and strategies described in the Alma Ata convention. Primary health care needs were taken care of in the public services (health centers and general hospitals) organized in 340 districts in the rural as well as in the urban areas (*Zones de Santé*). However, particularly in the capital Kinshasa, numerous private health care centers and polyclinics, but also some state hospitals, and the medical services of private companies or NGOs were not integrated in the hierarchical organisation of the health system. In reality all the institutions were accessible for primary health care and actively competed with each other on the health market.

In 1994, the health care system was in a catastrophic situation and since then further deteriorated. Internationally isolated, Congo did not receive any more international financial support. The medical health system missed the necessary financial external resources they were dependent on, and all public, state-related infrastructures and services regressed rapidly.

Medical personnel lost all confidence in their own institutions and were demotivated by low salaries and the very precarious work conditions.

Underutilisation of Public Services. According to the doctors, this lack of confidence was transferred to the patients, accounting for the underutilisation of the services. Other reasons given by the medical sector for their underutilisation were the degraded infrastructure, the decrease of financial prospects of patients, the absence or loss of social security due to massive unemployment and riots in '91 and '93, and the bad quality and control of medical drugs.

Health authorities in Kinshasa explained that lowering the financial contribution to treatment costs (fees for treatment and drugs) had not reduced the level of underutilisation. They also could not understand why many ill people seemed to use traditional or faith healing, as well as medical care, for the same illness. Mental health care was available in the psychiatric university hospital. This clinic only utilized 10–20% of its capacity and several departments were closed. One public ambulatory mental health center and some private practices operated in the city.

The medical care-providers knew that some of their patients also visited traditional healers but they did not cooperate with these. Traditional and spiritual healers for their part sometimes sent their patients to a hospital for investigation or specific medical care.

Formal and Informal Privatisation. What we had seen in the help-seeking study was confirmed in the interviews with medical care-providers.

All primary care centres and all hospitals were directly accessible and competing with each other on the medical market. Although general guidelines with regard to the organisation of the primary, secondary and tertiary services existed, they were in practice not respected by help-seekers and providers. Many doctors and nurses combined a job in some medical institution with work in private practice. Apart from the health centres in the 20 health zones (districts) of the urban primary care network which were sponsored by the European Union or by some countries and church organisations, all other medical care was privatized. At the urban and national health policy level, the medical officers of the health zones tried to manage primary services and their urban network while at grassroots level the district organization was constantly undermined by the uncontrollable growth of privatized health provisions and by the uncontrollable autonomy of hospitals operating at the primary level. The health committees of the health zones were in the service of the district health officers. They did not really operate as a counterpower nor as an intermediary organisation between the community and the health care system. A large part of the population was not fully aware of the existence and the role of these health committees, which were officially representing the community. Another part of the population was critical towards these committees or the public primary services, which were identified with the corrupt and ruined state. When a person chose a medical care-provider he visited primarily someone in or near to his neighbourhood known for the quality of his care. Public health centres that were burocratic and too standardized in their approach easily lost their patients.

Traditional Healers

We summarize the findings from our in-depth interviews and participant observation with 60 traditional and 20 faith healers, which were relevant to the action-research project. Our research has built further on earlier anthropological and clinical research in Kinshasa and other sub-Saharan areas describing numerous forms of traditional healing. These were available from both initiated and self-made healers over the entire city (Bibeau et al., 1990; De Boeck, 1991; de Rosny, 1985; Devisch, 1990; Devisch & Mbonyinkebe, 1989; Fassin, 1992; Janzen, 1978; Lapika, 1984). Charismatic faith healing was offered by numerous Pentecostal congregations and hundreds of independent communities often designated as Churches of the Holy Spirit (Devisch, 1995, 1996; Le Roy, 1994, 1997, 2000a; Matula, 1993).

Explanatory Model. In the minds of those who provide such forms of healing, health and illness not only touch upon a state of disorder within one's own body but also concern relationships between members of the kinship group as well as between these persons and the world of ancestral and cult spirits. From their perspective, health and illness have to do with fields of force in and between persons, and a type of socially constituted, culture- and site-specific knowledge, dialogical discourse, practice and interaction.

According to the traditional healers we interviewed, an illness could be caused or sustained by a 'natural' cause (infection, nutrition, accident) and/or by a 'human' cause. Human causes for example were conflicts in the family, a transgression or neglect of transgenerational family codes, or conflict with other families, neighbours or colleagues.

Treatment. All the traditional healers cured the signs of the illness and the somatic disorder with a variety of herbal treatments. When the herbal treatment was not efficient, 'human' causes were suspected and explored. Some healers gave advice and counselled the patient or the whole family on managing their relational problems. When the healer was convinced that the family could not clarify and resolve their tensions themselves, he referred them to a healer-diviner (specialized in diagnosing and treating 'human' causes) or a faith healer. These specialists treated the signs of bodily and/or mental disturbance with herbal and ritual forms of treatment. These ritualized treatments were psychotherapeutic interventions aiming at reframing the relationships of the family according to social and solidarity obligations and rights, marriage rules, transgenerational kinship codes and the worship of ancestors. Successful interventions had always helped the family to rearrange and repair through words and actions previously conflicting relationships.

Illnesses Treated by Healers. Traditional healers as a group treated a variety of illnesses in five classifications: simple complaints (malaria, gastrointestinal or gynaecological infections, colds, for instance), chronic somatic complaints with a 'natural' cause (such as diabetes, arthritis, asthma), the culture-bound syndromes, major mental illness and epilepsy. Traditional healers of major mental illness and epilepsy were more rare and highly valued. Each healer was originally initiated into the treatment of one or two illnesses, but in Kinshasa many healers offered help for two to ten or more illnesses. The healers were convinced, on the basis of their experience, that medical care was effectively treating the two first groups of illnesses but was unable to solve the third, fourth and fifth groups. According to their belief, medical caregivers could eventually reduce some symptoms of these three categories but not the disturbance itself as it was rooted in a 'human' cause related to the actual family or ancestors.

Some of the culture-bound syndromes, as already mentioned, include emotional distress (general anxieties, depressive feelings, particular fears), together with identity and relational problems to varying degrees. However, the healers (both traditional and faith healers) and the population in general did not consider these forms of distress a mental health problem (a name reserved for psychotic illness) with its solution a task for the psychiatric service. The task of the psychiatric service was in this perspective restricted to pharmacological treatment of psychotic, behavioural and epileptic disorders and, only when not cured by the healers, also of the CBS. Only persons who were well informed about psychiatry through higher education or their profession would seek care for 'somatisation' illnesses in the psychiatric polyclinic or ambulatory centre. To summarize in a different way, traditional healers believed—and this belief is shared by the faith healers and the large majority of the population—that the psychotherapeutic and sociotherapeutic dimensions of the treatment of minor and major mental distress (and dealing with intrapersonal and interpersonal disorders) were the domain of healers and not of doctors.

Transformations of Traditional Practices. Traditional healing practices had undergone transformations which were the result of historical processes and socio-cultural disruption in African society. Most of the healers considered themselves as herbalists and had a tendency to deny or even reject the traditional explanatory models or the use of ritual objects and practices. While they indicated that 'human' aspects were causing illnesses they reduced their interventions to herbal treatment and to advice and counselling. It was as if using overtly their divinatory and psychotherapeutic capacities and referring to ancestral laws and codes, they transgressed the rules learned during their Christian education. The devaluation and banning of ritual practice had often taken place in the earlier generation of their parents in the villages, under the influence of colonization, and were later reinforced by identification with the 'modern' life of the 'white' in Kinshasa. The consequence of internalized repression by the coloniser through the generations was that the practices of most of the healers had become reduced to the somatic expression of the illness, and disconnected from its meaning.

The ethnographic approach revealed however the distinction and gap between the discourse of the healers about their practice and the practice itself. When one looked in greater detail at the patient-healer relationship and the content of the advice it became clear that the most experienced healers were referring to the reestablishment of social rules and restructuring of family equilibrium, but without referring to the ancestral spirits. In order to become accepted by the medical world and the health policy-makers, many healers themselves devalued the psychotherapeutic and sociotherapeutic dimensions of their art. This evolution explains why they lost the therapeutic power to treat patients with serious relational and social problems and why they referred them more and more to faith healers.

The consequence of these changes was that a person with a 'somatization' illness or culture-bound syndrome living in a family who through the abovementioned transformation had no access to good traditional healing, was obliged to continue to seek ineffective care in the bio-medical field or to address himself to a faith healing group. This logic also explained the high percentage of participation of households in prayer groups and healing churches. As no other psychosocial form of care was known, credible and acceptable, to the general population, seeking help in these groups became in fact a logical next step.

Faith Healers

Historical Background. The faith healer belongs to a tradition of spiritual healing going back to the Mpeve ya longo church groups of the Holy Spirit, created by the prophet Simon Kimbangu during Belgian colonization in the beginning of the 20th century. In support of ideological and religious beliefs, the Belgian coloniser had tried to eradicate practices which were considered contrary to the development of colonizing enterprize. Traditional health care was completely denied and given a folk medicine status. The ritual aspect with its practices of divination and centuries-old references to ancestral life was abolished by law, the symbols destroyed and the practizers persecuted. State and missionary organisations in the colony combined their efforts to destroy large areas of indigenous culture and beliefs.

Explanatory Model of Faith Healers. Healing groups conducted by prophets incorporated many beliefs and practices from Protestant and Catholic missionaries, while rejecting any form of traditional ritual or healing practice, and remaining strongly rooted in Congolese culture. They took up the task of healing people refering often to Biblical narratives of the prophets, but within this religious model, using the traditional beliefs and concepts concerning health and illness, body and mind, group and family. 'Divination with the ancestral spirits' was transformed into 'revelation through the Holy Spirit'; 'sorcery from the ancestral spirits' became 'sorcery from the (d)evil spirits'; 'healing through the power of the ancestors' became 'healing through the power of God'. Healing groups were and still are particularly attentive to the crises and conflicts that families and individuals have to confront in the modernization of their society.

Faith Healing in Charismatic Groups. Faith healing is a ritualized sociotherapeutic treatment in a group conducted by a faith healer and his cotherapists. The internal cohesion of the group is created by adhesion to the common rules and life-style and by identification as members (brothers, sisters) of this religious community. The organisation of daily life in the community and of the ritual sessions offer a clear supportive framework. The group is organized around the belief that the Holy Spirit provides healing and care through the faith healer and his therapeutic group. The good Spirit will expel the bad destructive forces which are considered to cause to the illness or the family disorder. The therapy is imagined as a common fight against these bad forces. The group is organized around a charismatic figure (the prophet) and provides anxious and ill patients and families with a secure basis and a protective shield. Some faith healers combine their faith healing practices with herbal treatment and sometimes with neuroleptic or other allopathic drugs.

Two thirds of the patients in these faith healing communities have a culture-bound syndrome and are more or less emotionally and mentally distressed. Former or actual experiences of their traumatized family group are reactivated in the group context. In the 'revelations' of the prophet, the illness gets meaning in terms of disturbances and conflicts in the network of the patient, or in relation to his personal behavior and moral attitudes. The illness is attributed to a mixture of causes from different belief-systems—traditional, medical, spiritual, moral and social—and an understanding of the whole is offered to the patient.

Involvement of Family. In the last phase of the treatment, the most important persons in the family network of the patient are invited by the prophet to attend a therapeutic meeting and family ritual. In the presence of the patient, a clear explanation is given by the prophet and the concerned family members are pressed to accept this 'interpretation' of the conflicts and actions by which they have provoked the evil. Using his symbolic and imaginary power and knowledge, the prophet-therapist indicates how a conflict should be resolved and how responsibilities should be taken up and by whom. This intervention re-unites the family, decentralizes the patient from his pathogenic nodal position and re-creates order in the family.

The Crisis of Public Health Care

Underutilization of public primary care was due to a combination of factors. The uncontrolled and chaotic development of private medical care, the autonomy of hospitals providing health care ranging from primary care to surgery, the low satisfaction of the users with regard to the quality of the patient-therapist relationship, and the results of the treatment. The economic and institutional crises of the country gradually destroyed the foundations and quality of the public health system. By analogy with other social sectors, a growing informal and privatized health care was replacing the official health system. Underpaid medical care-providers (doctors, nurses, pharmacists) who continued to work in their bankrupt medical institutions offered primary health care in private centres and clinics. Being easily accessible and appreciated, these informal forms of medical care further undermined the public organization of health care and enhanced the financial burden on families.

Medical health provision on the primary and secondary level was bio-medically oriented and disease-focused. Psycho-social and cultural dimensions and particularities of health problems were not addressed by medical personnel except in rare public primary health centres or by some private care-providers (doctors, nurses). Throughout the study it was confirmed that medical care-providers in the different types of services were unable to detect and treat social and mental distress. They stayed within their bio-medical paradigm when a patient presented a 'somatization' illness or a culture-bound syndrome. They confined themselves to diagnostic protocols and treatment, and did not take the time to listen. On the contrary, doctors and nurses responded to anxiety and somatization illnesses with massive prescription of painkillers, tranquillizers, and neuroleptics. The few specialized psychiatric services (the university psychiatric hospital, small departments of general hospitals and one mental health centre) were utilized by the population when a major mental disorder (psychosis and personality disorders) or when common mental disorder (depression, anxiety and somatoform disorders) has not been resolved by previous medical or traditional care-providers). In general, the population considered these services as an asylum for 'mad' persons with disruptive social behaviour and as providers of psychopharmacological treatment. As a specialized part of the medical network, they were not recognized by the population as services which could help mentally distressed people to solve their interpersonal distress and family disturbances. The analysis made clear that primary mental health care, and in particular a service with psychotherapeutic and sociotherapeutic aims, was much needed at community level. However, it should be created, made known and accepted by both the community and the bio-medical establishment.

The district-based primary health care system had a tradition of health care committees of users, with an advisory role in relation to the district health officer. These health care committees, often composed of formally educated persons with some links to health care, public administration or education, usually minimized the existence and frequent utilization of traditional health care by the population. In the minds of health care professionals and health committee members, traditional care, which they or their family members themselves used when necessary, was disconnected from and irrelevant to public medical care. As traditional therapists were not organized, those health professionals who would have liked to inform themselves about traditional treatment and eventually cooperate, did not know how to address them as a group.

Transformations in Community-Based Traditional Care and Faith Healing

The situation in Kinshasa showed that the transformation of traditional knowledge and practice was a continuing process. The divide was deepening between the somatically oriented herbalist dimension of the treatment on one side and the social, relational, emotional and psychological dimensions on the other side.

The latter was mainly located in faith healing practices. The consequence of these processes was a probable loss of quality and effectiveness in these treatments. As patients, and in particular those with culture-bound syndromes and mental illnesses, needed and sought well-being involving the whole person and his/her relationships, they were obliged to reconnect what had fallen apart through their long plural and heterogenous help-seeking itinerary. The paradoxical development of traditional healing had two sides. On the one hand, to become more accepted as a form of medicine by policy-makers, the health system and the urban population, the majority of the healers promoted the biological part of their art and devalued, reduced, hid, denied or forgot the sociodynamic and psychotherapeutic part. On the other hand, the faith healers regularly attacked the traditional healers as sorcerers because 'they deal with the ancestral spirits and sorcery'. At the same time they had taken over from the traditional healers the despized and discarded knowledge and practices (with regard to traditional kinship and ancestral codes) and had transformed them within a socially acceptable mould (a Christian logic of good and bad). As a result of these processes faith healing communities and to some the degree also the prayer groups, linked with the official churches, attracted a large proportion of the mentally and socially distressed population in the poor shanty towns of Kinshasa because they combined a transformed version of traditional healing with moral education, psychosocial support, sociotherapeutic treatment, herbal and sometimes allopathic medication.

Traditional healers in Kinshasa, as well as faith healers, worked and lived in the community and were fully integrated in their neighbourhoods. They shared the same poverty and sociocultural environment as their patients. They considered their healing practices as services to the community. Their health care could be considered in organisational terms as a form of private practice with community-oriented goals while also providing limited sources of income. The larger faith healing groups were often formally organized as non-governmental religious organisations, while traditional healers had no formal status as health care providers.

We concluded that traditional healing was a valuable form of health care for the community, in particular for a number of frequent and specific syndromes. Its integration in a system of primary health care contained the risk of a further dilution of its therapeutic armamentarium and effectiveness. In order to preserve its accessibility and quality for the population, traditional medicine was in need of a strategy which would learn from and to some extent counteract current transformations.

In terms of public health policy, the study also showed that traditional healing was not well known or no longer trusted by a larger part of the 'modernized' population in Kinshasa. Official recognition of this community-based form of medicine had been promised by earlier governments since the 1970s but had been continually postponed. In the household study the interviewees, except those who were radically against traditional healers, said that the utilization of traditional healers suffered from a serious lack of quality guarantees and good information on indication criteria and specialization. They also wished that between the worlds of healers and doctors there should be greater cooperation when this was necessary for the benefit of the patient. Many felt that medical care-providers were often not sufficiently qualified either, and that some should have referred them to colleagues or healers earlier.

THE COMMUNITY ACTION PROJECT

The exploratory study of the practical experiences of care-users and providers at grass-roots level in the community, made it clear that Kinshasa's health care was determined by an ongoing process of economic regression and social transformation, where both users and providers responded to the crisis with their own resources and beliefs. Dynamic interdependences were demonstrated in the above paragraphs between the social and cultural context, the health care provision, the illnesses, and the strategies of the help seekers and health-providers. The study had revealed, besides the serious shortcomings, important reservoirs of local knowledge, health care practices and social dynamics. The hypothesis was that the quality of primary health care could be improved by innovative forms of community participation built on the knowledge of the users and on the social dynamics and resources in the community.[5] The practice of such community participation could lead to the development of strategies and practices that are both effective and socioculturally relevant. This refers to what in Figure 2 is indicated as 'priority setting by empirical decision making'.

This priority setting had to take into account a number of aims and conditions indicated by the situation analysis and the conceptual model.

Responsibility and ownership. The people who carry a certain responsibility in the local context are involved from the outset in formulating the action.

---

[5]The exploratory study provided also important insights into mental health problems and cues for working on a model to improve mental health care. Such a project would go beyond the action project in the neighbourhood and would only have a chance to be realized if particular contextual, financial and professional conditions could be fulfilled. As this was not the case, we decided at that moment to make mental health care the central topic of a future project. The core concept of this project will be the creation of a culturally-sensitive mental health care provision which is anchored and cooperates within a community-based network of care. We also assumed that the improvement of traditional health care and community participation was indirectly beneficial for community-based mental health treatment and that the action-research would produce relevant analysis for the future mental health project.

Researchers and actors negotiate and take a collective decision with regard to the structure, aims and resources of the intervention. They are committed throughout the process to sustain the experience and to participate in the analysis and modifications. In an action-research which is not primarily requested by the participants, the researcher will have to create the conditions through which a common desire for such a collective project of research and change can emerge and develop. This common desire is necessary since intervention provokes tensions, anxiety and resistance. Changes in a social system also question the local balance of social, political and economic power and can produce conflicts for the researchers and actors in their relationships with the groups to which they belong.

Aims of community intervention. The setting should take into account the existing plurality and heterogeneity of health practices. It would aim at developing links that respond to the needs of the population and enhance the quality, accessibility and equity of health care. Links between population and care-providers on the one hand and between the different care-providers on the other hand. Although supported and sponsored by the research project it should have the capacity to become self-supportive.

Setting and boundary of the community intervention. We had seen that resources of traditional healing and healers were available in the community but also that the quality of their care decreased when they applied their art to biological interventions. We also knew that bio-medically oriented health care officers, clinicians and researchers tended to reduce healing to herbal treatment and considered that the efficacy of traditional healing had to be tested empirically before it deserved respect. When such an action-research project had been initiated in the realm of a medical institution (medical faculty, district health system, ministry of health, medical NGO) both healers and the community would automatically enter into the above collusive logic, based on a bio-medical paradigm. We concluded that an innovative development of both community participation and involvement of traditional healing was only possible when a new setting was created and owned by the community and the healers themselves.

This setting could only come into being and develop further by an action in a social space with defined boundaries. Neighbourhoods in the shantytowns of Kinshasa are social environments which offer a balance of similarity and diversity, a sense of a localized identity and of belonging to a social whole. Often a neighbourhood identity is shaped by some particular factor, a historical event, or a characteristic of the population, its origin, or geographical unity. As we have seen in the preliminary study, neighbourhoods are not closed worlds with fixed populations, but constantly moving social unities in which all kinds of sub-groups (different age, gender, ethnic origin, religious background, political opinion) live together. According to our model, the new setting should have roots in and connections with all these diverse sub-groups. Moreover the people participating in this setting should not be there as elected representatives of the population, installed by the local administration or sent by the sub-groups, but as persons respected in the neighbourhood and socially involved.

We chose Ndjili 12 for the action-research, mainly because we were well informed on the health situation in this neighbourhood and because our research assistant was able, on the basis of his social networks in Ndjili 12, to select twenty people to an introductory conference with the researchers. This conference was held in one of the meeting rooms of a central community building. In the following paragraphs we describe how this conference became the starting point of a new setting, a neigbourhood committee, which went on to design and manage a number of specific actions with local care-providers and with the primary health authority of the health zone (district) of Ndjili. The final 'priority setting' and 'translation of the decision into action' (see Figure 2) was jointly made by the research group and community.

CONTENT AND PROCESSES OF THE ACTION

First Phase: Creation of the Setting and First Meeting

Creating a community-based new setting in a neighbourhood, independent of the medical organization, did not imply a refusal of the policy and organization of the district primary care system. On the contrary we made the assumption that the relationship between the community and the district organisation could be improved and that the community initiatives would have a constructive impact on the health district policy. At a regular board meeting, before the start of the intervention, we informed the complete board of medical health district officers and representatives of many public health centers of Kinshasa, about the premizes and strategy of our action-research project. The Medical Inspector-General of Kinshasa was informed separately and gave his support. He and other health authorities also participated later at evaluation meetings on the project.

The first action was the conference in Ndjili 12. At the beginning of this very informative and stimulating meeting a number of influential inhabitants had clearly expressed their viewpoints on the health care situation. The examples given by them confirmed findings of the preliminary household study. Some of them explicitly denied the utilisation of traditional and faith healing practices. The representations of the women, who had informal leadership positions (market, social club) in the neighbourhood, together with a local youth leader opened the debate. The 'officials' confirmed the existing underutilisation of the official structures, especially because of high costs and geographical location. The participants pointed to solutions for better or cheaper medical care in the neighbourhood. However, all stressed the point that old or new structures had to respond to the real demands and needs of the inhabitants of the neighbourhood. The collaboration between different types of health care was considered as an opportunity for traditional or faith healing to be validated by biomedicine, which in such a setting would be functioning as censor and guarantor. The common viewpoint expressed in the meeting was that the accessibility and quality of local care could be improved by comprehensive information of the population, with forms of cooperation and by strategies to guarantee the level of quality and cost.

We pointed out that in the beginning the team of researchers were considered to be representatives of medical institutions or sponsoring bodies. The information we gave at the start but also during the meeting regarding our institutional background, financial potential, aims and roles as researchers was helpful in avoiding a massive idealisation of our role and dependence by the community on the researchers and their imagined power. We also noticed that the dialogue had permitted contributors to speak openly about traditional treatment but that hesitation remained with regard to faith healing. Several referred to personal experiences with effective traditional healing while only one person mentioned participating in the activities of faith healing groups. The latter seemed to raise much more controversial feelings and opinions in the audience than traditional healing. The existence of faith healing as a form of religious practice was not questioned but there was no agreement to consider these practices to be forms of health care.

One month after, the majority of the participants in the first meeting and some newcomers met with the team of researchers. The project of the action-research had been discussed favourably in the neighbourhood during various informal meetings. A committee of 15 inhabitants was constituted and it was agreed that new members could join later if they agreed to participate in weekly meetings and administrative or other tasks. Three researchers (one Congolese and one Belgian psychiatrist, with one Congolese anthropologist) would be involved in the committee work and take part in the meetings of the committee. They would participate as researchers and the Congolese psychiatrist would also serve as regular consultant for the committee with regard to the relationships with medical authorities and internal organisational matters. It was agreed that the small budget would be used for administrative expenses and that small bonuses would be paid for certain tasks after discussion in the committee. Management of the budget and expenses would be by the secretary of the Committee and the Congolese psychiatrist, representing the research team.

Phase Two: Implementation and Processing the Activities

The committee discussed and agreed with the original model and discussion. Priorities were set and translated into a plan of actions. The committee and researchers agreed on an intervention with four specific objectives:

1. The inhabitants would be informed about the available types of traditional healing (types of illnesses and healers, and their organisation).
2. Guarantees for the quality of this form of treatment would be sought. This strategy would enable inhabitants to use this provision better.
3. Conditions would be created for the different care-providers to transform their difficult relationships into some form of co-operation.
4. The committee, on behalf of the users and the community, would take the role of mediator and creator of connections between care-seekers and care-providers, between medical and non-medical care-providers, and between population, care-providers and health district/local authorities.

After two years an assessment of the results would be undertaken by the committee and the researchers (in Figure 2: 'analytic evaluation of action results'). The committee and the researchers would then consider with the district health authorities if and how the action could be integrated in the primary health care policy and structure. The particularity of action-research is that the objectives and precise actions during a project are decided as a result of a continuing assessment of the objectives and results of a previous phase (in Figure 2: 'operational evaluation of action process').

Start of the Committee Work—Information and Network with Traditional Healers. The group chose this first activity after having settled its own structure. Members defined themselves as the Research Committee for the improvement of primary health care in Ndjili12. They also decided on the creation of a social fund amongst the members, with a monthly small contribution. They considered that a regular payment would stimulate the cohesion of their group and reinforce solidarity between the participants. This fund would be used to support families of members during critical periods by paying, for example, high medical or funeral costs. Eventually the fund would also be used to invest in socio-economical activities. The researchers also decided to contribute personally to this fund. Through this personal financial commitment, the committee members transformed the setting into a real group, becoming owners of the project and rooting it in a network of social relationships.

The 15 members of the committee formed small teams who made a survey of all the care-providers in the neighbourhood. They explained the aims of the project and collected information about the types of illness that the healer treated. Forty-two persons who practiced regularly or occasionally traditional treatment were interviewed. These healers were also invited to participate in open meetings which the committee organized in the neighbourhood, allowing healers, committee members, patients and inhabitants to meet and discuss. After this survey, the committee members informed the inhabitants of the neighbourhood at meetings in the church, in the market or through other social networks about this survey, the role of the committee and the aim of the project.

Quality and Organization of their Practices. At meetings with the healers, the committee members expressed the doubts of the population regarding the quality and effectiveness of their treatment. The development of a method to assess their effectiveness was questioned. The healers on their side asked the committee and the researchers to provide them with some official recognition, which would protect them from complaints from families regarding malpractice or from control by the public authorities. A major request from several healers was that the committee would take the lead in organizing a network of traditional healers, research facilities for them to practice and guarantee them a minimal income. After intensive debates regarding the ethical, financial, organisational, political and practical aspects of this request, the researchers and committee further clarified the role of the committee. The committee members, who understood very well the background of the requests made, felt forced into a position which was contradictory to the original definition of their role. In line with the chosen model, they were representatives of the users and mediators between community, public organizations and care-providers. The committee decided to help the healers to find solutions relevant to these issues and to refer inhabitants of the neighbourhood to them. But they also urged them to organize their practice and their cooperative network themselves. The healers also proposed that as a method of assessing their effectiveness, the committee should visit their clients randomly (provided that the latter would agree and that their privacy would be guaranteed) to register the illness, type of treatment, effectiveness, fees and general satisfaction. It was agreed that one person on the committee (the youngest member) would interview patients chosen randomly from the healers' lists of patients. A simple questionnaire, assessing different aspects of the treatment and constructed to that end by the researchers and the healers, was used during the interviews. Results would be anonymous and discussed in the committee. With this assessment method therapeutic secrecy and autonomy could be respected while the conditions were created to discuss quality issues critically. It was assumed that the healers would take the responsibility themselves concerning the quality and organization of their treatment. The first result of the implementation of this proposal was that a group of eight healers emerged who had a regular practice and good results. The other healers did not participate in the assessment for various reasons. Several of them saw patients occasionally. Others did not want to participate because their request for formal recognition or monthly payment had not been fulfilled. Some did not respond without any particular motivation. The second result was that amongst all the illnesses reported by the healers, a set of ten syndromes could be identified which were frequently mentioned and considered as belonging to the specific field of traditional medicine. This list corresponded well with the list of syndromes and illnesses reported in the household survey, as detailed above.

Contacts of Traditional and Medical Care-Providers. First a census of the local health centres and clinics was made in the neigbourhood. Four had been listed and visited by members of the committee. The physicians and nurses at these centres were asked, amongst other questions, whether according to them, the ten syndromes were efficiently treated by traditional healers. Meetings were organized, as a next step, with the group of healers and local medical care-providers to discuss these findings and elaborate possibilities for cooperation. The nurses of the four clinics all agreed to participate in a meeting and expressed their interest in collaborating without obligation or constraints with the healers and the committee.

The medical care-givers engaged themselves to inform their patients, if necessary, about the possibilities of traditional care and indicate names of healers. Although this did not result in clear referrals the healers found it important that the medical caregivers were now well informed.

The absence of referrals was explained by the healers as the incapacity of the physicians and nurses at the centres to accept their own limitations. The committee members noticed that the medical care-providers agreed 'off the record' on the successes of traditional healing but that officially referring a patient would be interpreted as disowning or depreciating their professional identity and group. Referral could only be carried out in a tacit and indirect way. Traditional healers on the other hand while attacking the superior attitude of the physicians, continued to seek recognition for their results from the medical group. In a repetitive pattern they reinforced their own 'inferiority' and the 'superiority' of the others.

The cohesion between healers improved, the number of patients and their self-confidence grew and healers referred more patients between themselves. The complaints about low fees (compared to the cost of collecting or buying herbal products) and irregularity in payment by patients remained. The self-organization of the healers with the support of the committee had preserved the particular setting, secrets and practice of each healer, and his effectiveness in healing the bodily and social distress of patients. There was also discussion during the meetings of healers, community and researchers on the extent to which psychotherapeutic and sociotherapeutic aspects of the patient-healer relationships were important for the population. The committee members on their side could more easily and confidently advise and help those who sought these healers. As a parallel process during the project the committee utilized the funds collected to support some families in great need.

The Evaluation of the Results and the Process
Community information

The Committee reported that two years after the start of the project a number of the inhabitants, in particular key persons and leaders in the community, were well-informed about the Committee's objectives and actions. They also knew that help seekers could ask for information from a committee member about qualified healers or be directed to one of them. An independent survey amongst key persons in the community confirmed this evaluation. The Committee recognized that it had not established a regular relation with faith healing groups, because several committee members did not believe that illnesses could be cured by faith healers who 'only used water and praying'. Some also felt that it was contrary to their community role, to their own religious convictions and to the pluriform orientation of the project to engage as a committee with religious groups and to refer patients to these groups.

Organisation and quality control of the traditional healers

With regard to the organisation of the traditional healers, it was clear that a form of auto-selection had taken place and that a core group of 8–10 healers had come to the fore. The element of control by the community seemed to be the most determinant factor in this selection. It is likely that the more competitive and efficient practitioners had continued to collaborate with the committee. The healers said they had derived much benefit from the action. Being known in the neighbourhood as qualified and serious healers, they now exercized their art more openly. Their clientele had increased and felt more confident. This growth of their clientele, in spite of the rather low fees, allowed them to pass from a casual to a more professional practice and to increase their incomes.

Specialisation of traditional practices

With regard to quality, they reported among themselves a tendency towards specialization. At the start of the project, like most of the healers in Kinshasa, they had claimed to be capable of treating a minimum of at least five illnesses. After the quality assessment had been introduced, it was noticed that the healers had limited their practice to one or two specific illnesses. As a result of the project, a collaboration between traditional healers had been instituted spontaneously. As a consequence of the return of the specialisation which traditional care-providers had lost progressively in town, a straightforward collaboration with mutual recognition was established. They no longer hesitated to refer patients between themselves. The patients benefited from these referrals in terms of efficiency and time. Finally the committee noted that this collaboration led to persistent pressure by the traditional healers to create a centre or a common space for the exercize of their art.

Links between medical and traditional care-providers

The dialogue between the medical and traditional care-providers had made a start. The four clinics of the district and one other had been associated for six months with the activities of the committee but only two answered invitations and participated in the meetings of the committee regularly. A slow evolution was noticed with regard to public recognition by local physicians of the value of traditional healing for some illnesses. Collaboration however did not follow in spite of all their undertakings. The creation of a space for dialogue between care-providers in the neighbourhood was described by all as a very positive contribution with as yet unexplored potential.

Networks created by the committee

The committee succeeded in creating cohesion and collaboration between people belonging to very different local networks (state, church, independent). Progressively a new network of solidarity has been established, represented materially by the creation of a social fund and a system of internal support for members within the group, as well as by the organisation of communal meals and other social activities. The group developed the capacity to become a self-managing structure, able to operate with a very small budget. The committee directed patients to the different care-providers and decided to give advice to people in adjacent neighbourhoods on developing a similar structure.

Contacts with the health and administrative authorities of the district took place at an official meeting where the project was described, and met with appreciation. The committee was asked by the district health officer to send representatives to the official health committee of the district. From 1998 the committee had to slow down the work and reduce their activities as a result of the war in Congo and political turmoil which caused the migration or death (by violence or illness) of several members and healers in 1998 and 1999.

COMMENTS AND DISCUSSION

The action-research had chosen the option of setting up and monitoring and evaluating a pilot intervention at grassroots level in a neighbourhood of the Ndjili health district with community representatives and local care-providers. The three core objectives, devised and managed by a local committee, were to provide a better link between the population of the neighbourhood and local care-providers, to promote links between local care-providers, and to participate in improving health care policy at the local district level. This community intervention appeared to be relevant and sustainable and provided information about the applicability of this model to the local and comparable contexts. The decision of the research team, based on a conceptual model and a situation analysis, to first establish conditions which enabled the community to create a new structure in the neighbourhood was a crucial factor. A second point of equal importance was that the community and the researchers took time and used dialogue to come to a common understanding and agreement on the model. The model included a clear vision of the role of the committee and its connections with the other partners in the action. The actions raised new questions which enabled us to develop the model further. Some of these questions are indicated in the final paragraph.

The Results and the Hypothesis of Change

The results of the intervention confirm that an innovative type of community participation to improve the quality and access of locally provided health care was possible. The innovative dimension of this participation was three-fold. Firstly it provided a structure and defined conditions enabling the participation of different social and cultural sub-groups in the community. This structure was autonomous, self-managing and not owned by health or state authorities. Secondly this structure (the committee) chose to create and develop links between users, community representatives, traditional healers, medical care-providers and health authorities. It aimed to achieve a better quality, accessibility and equity of care for the inhabitants. Thirdly these links were created and developed gradually through dialogue and common activities and rules. Fourthly the dialogue and contracted actions utilized the local resources of users and care-providers as much as possible without forcing the latter to participate. This produced strategies to improve the local health care organization, the access to traditional practices, to improve quality control, specialization, and referral between traditional healers, and to establish contacts between medical and traditional care-providers with the district health care system. It was found that such processes of change need long periods of time, and that they are slowed down, but not destroyed, by social and political turbulence.

The action-research also initiated unexpected results. The financial fund, created and managed by the committee members, continued to function as a binding and supportive factor. Some committee members took the initiative with other inhabitants to create a local system of food provision at affordable prices. The researchers and traditional healers developed mutual confidence and could study the etiologies, treatment logics and in particular the social and psychological dimensions of certain culture-bound syndromes.

Social Dynamics and Community Participation

We have shown in the above paragraphs that the creation and development of a group structure in the neighbourhood was essential in order to make community participation operational and functional. The formation and development of the committee was a strategy which built on constructive social dynamics of solidarity and collective responsibility, present in the Congolese society, and which challenges the processes of fragmentation and social regress.

Constructive Social Dynamics. If one analyses what happens at grassroots level, it is possible to distinguish a process of 'informalization' (de Villers, 1996). In these process Western models, concepts or norms are reshaped according to sociocultural norms and values. This leads to the transformation of social institutions and actions by more informal and personalized African codes of practice (Chabal & Daloz, 2000; Devisch, 1996; de Villers, 1996). The latter have often been created as social tactics of people who have been dominated and oppressed, in order to preserve a limited but familiar space of freedom and identity (de Certeau, 1984). A clear example in the project was the creation of a social fund by the group of key-persons in the community and the opening ritual of committee meetings. By creating the fund the committee members added to their western structure (a committee with a president, treasurer and secretary and a membership) a practice which is rooted in the traditional registering of solidarity and gift-countergift. This combination of attitudes and habits which draw from a singular fusion of 'modern' and 'traditional' conventions is also operative when the committee members start their meeting by praying and asking God wisdom and support. This invocation of the Christian God (Nzaambi) who had replaced the invocation of the ancestral spirits (Nzaambi Phungu) is also practiced by the traditional healers at the onset of a treatment session with a patient. We also see this 'African' convention of gift-countergift when the committee negotiates with the traditional healers with regard to their mutual role in the project.

The conclusion drawn from our experience is that action-researchers or public health officers who want to introduce innovative and culturally-sensitive changes in the African public health system have necessarily to take into account this 'informalisation' and fusion of multiple conventions. They have to build on these social dynamics and search in informal ways for connections with the formal, 'modern' types of organisation (for example at district and national level).

Challenges and Boundaries. When we look at the strategies of help-seekers, care-providers and community we notice that the organisational issues of health care were related to issues of meaning and power. Users, care-providers and community key persons were all from social groups which tried to guarantee the survival of their systems of meaning and power. In our example we saw that the distribution of the power to heal and to give meaning to illness was distributed between the medical providers and the traditional and faith healing one. We also noticed, in the example of the treatment of the mental illness and culture-bound syndromes, that this distribution could shift as a result of social, cultural and economic factors.

Consequently, a project which intends to produce change will influence the balance of power on different levels and raise tensions or conflicts in and between social or corporate groups. The evolution and results of an action-research or development project have to be linked with these dynamics and the conductors of such a project have to be able to understand and manage them. Experience with conscious and unconscious processes in groups and institutions is necessary (Le Roy, 1994; Le Roy & N'situ, 1998; Rouchy, 1995, 1998) and part of the work of the researchers with the committee was to help them to analyse and deal with the dynamics in which they were involved. This analysis primarily concerned the anxieties and insecurities raised by the project in the participants. In fact every person involved had to put at risk his own identity and the safety of belonging to his own professional and social groups. Every committee member, researcher, healer or nurse had to surmount the doubts and criticisms of his or her own defining group because the project tried to create links and dialogue between persons belonging to professional and social groups separated by different ideologies. This explains for example the resistance to engage in practical collaboration between doctors and healers, between healers themselves, between the community members and faith healers, or between traditional and faith healers. As the work between committee and healers has shown, it was only when the anxieties and doubts had been resolved that parties performed in practice what they had previously agreed in words. Similarly, as long as the committee was beset by doubts and fears about the faith healers, it was unable to open a dialogue with them.

The evolution of the project revealed areas where community participation and collaboration raise particular fears and conflicts. These problems need further detailed study and understanding. The faith healers and their churches are perceived as very united, strong social bodies which have developed on the fringe of public community life. By their independence and capacity to heal illnesses which involve interpersonal and intergenerational problems the faith healers are endowed with important imaginary and symbolic powers. The work of the committee with the faith healing churches will probably be possible once the members personally and as a group feel ready to relate with these real and imagined power dynamics.

The research team was anchored in a more global research project and had meetings with other researchers and other teams involved in that project. There were regular contacts with the medical officers and the inspection. These contacts were necessary not only to assess developments but also to contain members' own fears and doubts. The fact that the main researchers were psychiatrists or psychotherapists facilitated the project. We were conscious owing to our own anthropologically-informed training and by the study with the healers, that many patients who were seeking treatment with healers suffered serious personal emotional distress. We also thought that the loss or denial of the psychotherapeutic and sociotherapeutic capacities of the traditional healers had to be challenged. We had also indicated to the community and healers why we found that healers had to find their own ways to legitimate (or not) their quality and organisation, and why dependency or counterdependency in relation to the medical profession had to be avoided. However we also indicated that they should enjoy the same working conditions as medical care-providers in the community, enabling them to practize their valuable care within a public health system.

REFERENCES

Akerele, O. (1990). Traditional medicine and primary health care: A time for re-assessment and re-dedication. *Curare, 13*, 67–73.
Anyinam, C. (1987). Availability, accessibility, acceptability and adaptability: Four attributes of African ethno-medicine. *Social Science and Medicine, 25*, 803–811.
Augé, M. (1994). Order biologique, ordre social: La maladie, forme élementaire de l'événement [Biological ordre, social order: Illness, elementary from of the event]. In M. Augé, & C. Herzlich (Eds.), *Le sens du mal: Anthropologie, historie, sociologie de la maladie* (pp. 35–92). Paris: Editions des Archives Contemporaines. (Original work published 1984).
Bannerman, R. H., Burton, J., & Ch'en, W.-C. (Eds.). (1983). *Traditional medicine and health care coverage: A reader for health administrators and practitioners.* Geneva: World Health Organization.
Bell, D., & Chen, L. (1994). Responding to health transitions: From research to action. In L. C. Chen, A. Kleinman, & N. C. Ware (Eds.), *Health and social change in international perspective* (pp. 491–502). Boston: Harvard University Press.
Bibeau, G. (1997). Cultural psychiatry in a creolizing world: Questions for a new research agenda. *Transcultural Psychiatry, 34*(1), 9–41.
Bibeau, G., & Buganza, M. H. (1990). *Traditional medicine in Zaire: Present and potential contribution to health services* (2nd ed.). Ottawa, Canada: International Development Research Centre.
Blue, I., & Harpham, T. (1996). Urbanisation and mental health in developing countries. *Current Issues in Public Health, 2*, 181–185.
Black, N. (1994). Why we need qualitative research. *Journal of Epidemiology and Community Health, 48*, 425–426.
Brunet-Jailly, J. (1997). *Innover dans les systèmes de santé: Expériences d'Afrique de l'Ouest* [Innovating in health systems: Experiences of West-Africa]. Paris: Karthala.
Canino, G., Lewis-Fernandez, R., & Bravo, M. (1997). Methodological challenges in cross-cultural mental research. *Transcultural Psychiatry, 34*(2), 163–184.
Chabal, P., & Daloz, J.-P. (1999). *Africa works: Disorder as political instrument.* Oxford, England: James Currey.
Chavunduka, G. L. (1994). *Traditional medicine in modern Zimbabwe.* Harare, Zimbabwe: University of Zimbabwe Publications.
Checkland, P., & Holwell, S. (1998). Action research: Its nature and validity. *Systemic Practice and Action Research, 11*(1), 10–21.
Corin, E., Uchoa, E., Bibeau, G., Koumare, B., Coulibaly, B., Coulibaly, M., Mounkoro, P., & Sissobo, M. (1992). La place de la culture dans la psychiatrie africaine d'aujourd'hui [The place of culture in African psychiatry today]. *Psychopathologie Africaine, 24*(2), 149–181.
De Boeck, F. (1991). Therapeutic efficacy and consensus among the Aluund of Southwest Zaire. *Africa, 61*, 159–185.
De Boeck, F. (1996). Postcolonialism, power and identity: Local and global perspectives from Zaire. In R. P. Werbner, & T. O. Ranger (Eds.), *Postcolonical identities in Africa* (pp. 75–106). London: Zed Books.
De Certeau, M. (1984). *The practice of everyday life.* Berkeley, CA: University of California Press.
De Jong, J. T. V. M. (1987). *A descent into African psychiatry.* Amsterdam: Royal Tropical Institute.

De Jong, J. T. V. M. (1994). Prevention of the consequences of man-made or natural disaster at the (inter)national, the community, the family and the individual level. In S. E. Hobfoll, & M. W. De Vries (Eds.), *Extreme stress and communities: Impact and intervention* (pp. 207–227). Boston: Kluwer.

De Herdt, T., & Marysse, S. (1997). Against all odds: Coping with regress in Kinshasa, Zaïre. *The European Journal of Development Research, 9*, 209–230.

De Rosny, E. (1985). *Healers in the night.* Maryknoll, NY: Orbis Books.

De Villers, G. (Ed.). (1996). *Phénomènes informels et dynamiques culturelles en Afrique* [Informal phenomena and cultural dynamics in Africa]. Brussels, Belgium: Institut Africain-CEDAF.

Desjarlais, R., Eisenberg, L., Good, B., & Kleinman, A. (1995). *World mental health: Problems and priorities in low-income countries.* Oxford, England: Oxford University Press.

Devisch, R. (1990). The therapist and the source of healing among the Yaka of Zaire. *Culture, Medecine and Psychiatry, 14*(2), 213–236.

Devisch, R. (1995). Frenzy, violence, and ethical renewal in Kinshasa. *Public Culture, 7*, 593–629.

Devisch, R. (1996). 'Pillaging Jesus': Healing churches and the villagisation of Kinshasa. *Africa, 66*, 555–586.

Devisch, R., Lapika, D., Le Roy, J., & Crossman, P. A. (2001). Community-action intervention to improve medical care services in Kinshasa, Congo: Mediating the realms of healers and physicians. In N. Higginbotham, R. Briceno-Leon, 7 & N. Johnsons (Eds.), *Applying health social science: Best practice in the developing world.* London: Zed Books.

Devisch, R., & Mbonyinkebe Sehabire. (1997). Medical anthropology and traditional care. In P. G. Janssens, M. Kivits, & J. Vuylsteke (Eds.), *Health in Central Africa since 1885: Past, present and future* (Vol. 1, pp. 47–64). Brussels: King Baudouin Foundation.

Douville, O. (1998). L'identité/alterité, fractures et montages [Identity/alterity, breakages and construction]. In R. Kaes (Ed.), *Difference culturelle et souffrances de l'identité* (pp. 21–44). Paris: Dunod.

Dozon, J. (1987). Ce que valoriser la médecine traditionnelle veut dire [What appraisal of traditional medicine expresses]. *Politique Africaine, 28*, 9–20.

Fassin, D. (1992). *Pouvoir et maladie en Afrique* [Power and disease in Africa]. Paris: Presses Universitaires de France.

Fassin, D. (1996). *L'espace politique de la santé* [The political space of health]. Paris: Presses Universitaires de France.

Fassin, D. (2000). *Les enjeux politiques de la santé* [The political issues of health]. Paris: Karthala.

Feierman, S., & Janzen, J. M. (Eds.). (1992). *The social basis of health in Africa.* Berkeley, CA: University of California Press.

Good, B. (1994). *Medecine, rationality and experience.* Cambridge, England: Cambridge University Press.

Good, B. (1997). Studying mental illness in context: Local, global or universal? *Ethos, 25*(2), 230–248.

Green, E. (1988). Can collaborative programs between biomedical and African indigenous health practitioners succeed? *Social Science and Medicine, 27*, 1125–1130.

Grodos, D. (2000). *Le district sanitaire urbain en Afrique subsaharienne: Enjeux, pratiques et politiques* [The urban health district in sub-saharan Africa: Issues, practices and policies]. Louvain, Belgium: Catholic University of Louvain.

Grodos, D., & Mercenier, P. (2000). *Health systems research: A clearer methodology for more effective action.* Antwerp, Belgium: Institute of Tropical Medecine.

Heggenhougen, H. K. (1991). Perception of health-care options and therapy-seeking behaviour. In J. Cleland & A. Hill (Eds.), *The health transition: Methods and measures* (pp. 85–98). Canberra, Australia: Health Transition Centre, The Australian University.

Helman, C. G. (1990). *Culture, health and illness.* London: Wright.

Janzen, J. M. (1978). *The quest for therapy: Medical pluralism in Lower Zaire.* Berkeley, CA: University of California Press.

Janzen, J. M. (1989). Health, religion and medicine in Central and Southern African traditions. In L.E. Sullivan (Ed.), *Healing and restoring: health and medicine in the world's religious traditions* (pp. 152–170). New York: MacMillan.

Janzen, J. M., & Prins, G. (Eds.). (1979). Causality and classification in African medicine and health [Special issue]. *Social Science and Medicine, 15B*(3), 169–437.
Kirmayer, L. J. (1989). Cultural variations in the response to psychiatric disorders and emotional distress. *Social Science and Medicine, 29*(3), 327–339.
Kirmayer, L. J. (1992). Cross-cultural measures of functional somatic symptoms [Review]. *Transcultural Psychiatric Research Review, 29*, 37–44.
Kirmayer, L. J. (1993). Healing and the invention of metaphor: The effectiveness of symbols revisited. *Culture, Medecine and Psychiatry, 17*(2), 161–195.
Kirmayer, L. J., & Robbins, J. M. (1991). Functional somatic syndromes. In L. J. Kirmayer, & J. M. Robbins (Eds.), *Current concepts of somatization: Research and clinical perspectives* (pp. 79–106). Washington, DC: American Psychiatric Press.
Kirmayer, L. J., Young, A., & Robbins, J. M. (1994). Symptom attribution in cultural perspective. *Canadian Journal of Psychiatry, 39*(10), 584–595.
Kleinman, A. (1980). *Patients and healers in the context of culture: An exploration of the borderland between anthropology, medicine and psychiatry.* Berkeley, CA: University of California Press.
Kleinman, A. (1988). *The illness narratives.* New York: Basic Books.
Kleinman, A., & Good, B. (Eds.). (1985). *Culture and depression: Studies in anthropology and cross-cultural psychiatry of affect and disorder.* Berkeley, CA: University of California Press.
Lapika Dimomfu. (1984). *L'art de guérir chez les Kongo du Zaïre: Discours magique ou science médicale?* [The art of healing of the Kongo in Zaire: Magical or medical discourse?]. Brussels, Belgium: CEDAF-Institut Africain.
Last, M., & Chavunduka, G. L. (Eds.). (1986). *The professionalisation of African medicine.* Manchester, England: Manchester University Press.
Le Roy, J. (1994a). Processus thérapeutiques groupaux dans les églises de guérison à Kinshasa [The therapeutic group processes in the healing churches of Kinshasa]. *Connexions, 63*, 101–124.
Le Roy, J. (1997). Migrations, ruptures et reconstructions identitaires dans la modernité d'une capitale africaine, Kinshasa [Migrations, ruptures and identity reconstruction in an African capital's modernity, Kinshasa]. *Revue PTAH (Psychanalyse, Traversees, Anthropologie et Histoire), 1997*, 1–2.
Le Roy, J. (2000a). Group analysis and culture. In D. Brown, & L. Zinkin (Eds.), *The psyche and the social world* (pp. 180–201). London: Jessica Kingsley. (Original work published 1994).
Le Roy, J. (2000b). Mental health and social development: Policies and research. In J. Le Roy, & K. Sen, *Health systems and social development: An alternative paradigm in health systems research* (pp. 47–54). Luxemburg, Luxemburg: European Communities.
Le Roy, J., & N'situ, A. (1998). Le groupe, opérateur de changement et de recherche: recherche-action communautaire pour l'amélioration des soins de santé dans un quartier de Kinshasa [The group, operator of change and research: Community action-research to improve health care in a neighbourhood of Kinshasa]. *Connexions, 1998-1*, 79–107.
Littlewood, R. (1991). Against pathology: The new psychiatry and its critics. *British Journal of Psychiatry, 159*, 696–702.
Littlewood, R. (1998). *The butterfly and the serpent: Essays in psychiatry, race and religion.* London: Free Association Books.
Matula, A. (1993). *Queté de santé et thérapie dans les églises Mpeve ya Nlongo* [The quest for health and therapy in the churches of Mpeve ya Nlongo]. Kinshasa, Congo: Université de Kinshasa.
Mauss, M. (1985). Essai sur le don: Forme et raison de l'échange dans les sociétés archaiques. [The gift: The form and reason for exchange in archaic societies]. In M. Mauss, *Sociologie et anthroplogie.* Paris: Quadrige (Original work published 1950).
Meyer, B., & Geschiere, P. (Eds.). (1999). *Globalisation and identity.* Oxford, England: Blackwell.
Mbonyinkebe Sehabire. (1989). *Au coeur de la vie en ville: Le tradipraticien Yaka à Kinshasa* [In the heart of town: The Yaka traditional healer in Kinshasa]. Unpublished doctoral dissertation, Catholic University of Louvain, Louvain, Belgium.

Mumford, D. B. (1991). The Bradford Somatic Inventory: A multi-ethnic inventory of somatic symptoms reported by anxious and depressed patients in Britain and the Indo-Pakistan subcontinent. *British Journal of Psychiatry, 158*, 379–386.

Mumford, D. B. (1994). Can 'functional' somatic symptoms associated with anxiety and with depression be differentiated? *International Journal of Methods in Psychiatric Research, 3*, 133–141.

Mumford, D. B. (1997). Stress and psychiatric disorder in rural Punjab: A community survey. *British Journal of Psychiatry, 170*, 473–478.

Olivier de Sardan, J. P. (1998). *Anthropologie et développement: Essai en socio-anthropologie du changement social* [Anthropology and development: Essay in socio-anthropology of social change]. Paris: Karthala.

Rogler, L. H., & Cortes, D. E. (1993). Help-seeking pathways: A unifying concept in mental health care. *American Journal of Psychiatry, 150*(4), 554–561.

Rouchy, J. C. (1995). Identification and groups of belonging. *Group Analysis, 28*, 129–142.

Rouchy, J. C. (1998). *Le groupe, espace analytique: Clinique et théorie* [The group, the analytic space: Clinical work and theory]. Toulouse, France: Eres.

Werbner, R. P. & Ranger, T. O. (Eds.). (1996). *Postcolonial identities in Africa*. London: Zed Books.

World Health Organization. (1976). *Traditional medicine and its role in the development of health services in Africa*. Brazzaville: WHO Regional Office for Africa. World Health Organization, Regional Committee for Africa, 26th Session, Kampala 8–15 Sept. 1976.

World Health Organization. (1978). *The promotion and development of traditional medicine*. Geneva: World Health Organization.

World Health Organization. (1990). *The introduction of a mental health component into primary health care*. Geneva: World Health Organization.

Author Index

Aarts, PG, 69, 81
Abas, M, 81
Aber, JL, 19, 86
Aboud, F, 354, 366
Abramson, H, 36, 81
Abu Hein, F, 20, 81, 323, 334
Abu-Nasr, J, 18, 81
Adamolekum, B, 53, 81, 193, 202
Ager, A, 48, 81
Ahearn, FL, 53, 81, 82, 152
Aiello, P, 315
Ait Sidhoum, MA, 381, 403
Akerele, O, 54, 81, 407, 437
Al-Ajeel, M, 87
Al-Asfour, A, 87
Allen, T, 15, 81, 366
Allodi, F, 60, 81
Andersen, RM, 48, 81
Andrews, B, 6, 82
Angell, RH, 85
Anyinam, C, 407, 437
Arad, R, 33, 89
Arar, A, 393, 403
Araya, M, 354, 366
Arcel, LT, 202
Ardrey, R, 221, 255
Armenian, HK, 252, 255
Arroyo, W, 21, 81
Arunakirnathan, T, 234, 255, 255
Atchison, M, 10, 87
Augé, M, 408, 437
Avedon, JF, 314

Bagilishya, D, 35, 82
Baker, A, 16, 19, 81
Bandura, A, 255
Bannerman, RH, 407, 437
Baron, N, 6, 73, 75, 82, 170, 202, 250, 255
Bastian, G, 315
Becker, G, 39, 82
Bell, D, 408, 437
Ben, R, 30, 83, 85, 152, 279, 397
Bennett, TL, 30, 83, 279
Bennett-Johnson, S, 279
Benyoub, R, 372, 403
Berry, JW, 27, 82, 151, 152, 280
Besch, K, 269, 271, 279
Beutler, L, 279
Beyene, Y, 39, 82
Bhattarai, R, 90, 281
Bibeau, G, 408, 418, 437
Black, N, 213, 408, 437
Bland, RC, 385, 404
Blank, AS, 41, 82
Bleich, A, 10, 88
Blendon, RJ, 10, 87, 202
Blue, I, 9, 82, 408, 437
Boehlein, JK, 94, 104, 152, 262, 279
Boothby, N, 19, 82
Bornemann, T, 6, 84, 86, 154, 158, 202, 203
Bouatta, C, 392, 403
Bracken, PJ, 151, 152
Bravo, M, 437

Breslau, N, 32, 82
Brewin, CR, 6, 82
Broadhead, JC, 81
Brody, EB, 152, 159, 168
Bromet, EJ, 10, 61, 82, 85
Bronfenbrener, U, 82
Brown, AM, 233, 257, 439
Brunet-Jailly, J, 408, 437
Bryman, A, 48, 82
Buganza, MH, 437
Burnam, MA, 404
Burton, J, 437
Bush, KD, 252, 255

Canino, GJ, 385, 404, 408, 437
Cardeña, E, 53, 77, 90, 280, 281
Celentano, DD, 16, 89
Ch'en, W-C, 437
Chabal, P, 435, 437
Chambless, DL, 262, 279
Chandler, DP, 104, 108, 110, 129, 130, 152
Chang, JC, 6, 82
Chaulet, P, 44, 86
Chavunduka, GL, 407, 437, 439
Checkland, P, 408, 437
Chen, L, 408, 437
Cheng, ATA, 6, 82
Chi-Yung Chung, R, 85
Choi, S, 115, 153
Choulean, A, 115, 152
Clarke, GN, 85

Clarke, L, 69, 85, 132, 152, 241, 256, 267, 277, 279, 401, 403
Clifford, T, 306, 314
Cohen, RE, 2, 53, 82
Cohon, JD, 2, 82
Collins, S, 115, 152, 154
Cooper, B, 233, 257
Corcoran, JDT, 10, 82
Corin, E, 408, 437
Corradi, J, 82, 88
Cortes, DE, 47, 88, 408, 440
Coulibaly, B and M, 437
Craig, G, 82, 276, 279
Creed, F, 273, 279
Crescenzi, A, 292, 314
Crits-Christoph, P, 279
Crossman, PA, 438
Cutrona, CE, 34, 82

D'Zurilla, T, 273, 279
Daloz, J-P, 435, 437
Damian, S, 241, 255
Daniel, EV, 227, 228, 256, 404
Danieli, Y, 69, 90
Daniels, M, 404
Dasen, PR, 27, 82
Davenport, P, 109, 152
Davidson, JRT, 10, 82, 89
Davis, GC, 32, 82
Dawes, A, 19, 82
De Boeck, F, 418, 437
De Certeau, M, 435, 437
De Girolamo, G, 3, 4, 46, 82, 87, 104
De Herdt, T, 410, 438
De Jong, JTVM, 6, 7, 10, 11, 17, 28, 35, 37, 40, 41, 47, 49, 51, 53, 54, 59, 68, 69, 71, 73, 75, 77, 78, 82, 83, 84, 87, 89, 90, 94, 122, 132, 147, 152, 154, 166, 167, 183, 202, 203, 236, 241, 256, 267, 273, 274, 275, 276, 277, 279, 280, 281, 314, 340, 366, 393, 401, 403, 407, 408, 437, 438

De Rosny, E, 418, 438
De Silva, KM, 210, 256
De Villers, G, 435, 438
Delvert, J, 108, 152
Deng, FM, 2, 82
Derogatis, LR, 383, 404
Desjarlais, R, 3, 4, 12, 13, 83, 102, 152, 168, 169, 170, 176, 181, 190, 191, 202, 408, 438
Devisch, R, 405, 407, 408, 418, 435, 438
Dickason, D, 88
Dohrenwend, BP, 34, 83, 84
Dönden, Y, 314
Donelan, B, 82, 84
Donelan, K, 10, 87, 202
Douville, O, 408, 412, 438
Dozon, J, 407, 438
Dunkel-Schetter, C, 30, 83, 86
Dyregrov, A, 19, 83

Ebihara, M, 108, 152
Egan, G, 267, 273, 280
Eisenberg, L, 3, 83, 152, 202, 271, 273, 280, 438
Eisenbruch, M, 6, 53, 83, 89, 94, 100, 101, 105, 106, 119, 121, 122, 133, 151, 152, 153, 154, 155, 229, 256
Ekblad, S, 6, 84, 86, 87, 202, 203
El Masri, M, 6, 10, 11, 83
El-Sarraj, E, 10, 81, 84, 321, 322, 323, 324, 335
Elias, C, 10, 87, 202
Elioto, J, 164, 203
Endale, Y, 337, 366
Epstein, M, 315
Erikson, EH, 221, 256
Erikson, KT, 228, 256
Eth, S, 17, 18, 21, 81, 84
Evers, HD, 114, 153

Fairbank, JA, 32, 68, 69, 73, 82, 84, 86, 90
Fairbanks, LA, 87

Faravelli, C, 404
Farias, P, 13, 84
Fassin, D, 408, 418, 438
Feierman, S, 408, 438
Feinstein, A, 82
Figley, CR, 84, 153, 202, 203
Finkler, K, 35, 84
Fisher, L, 10, 86
Flanzbaum, H, 38, 84
Fleck, J, 152
Flinterman, C, 90
Foa, EB, 10, 82
Folkman, S, 30, 34, 84, 86, 271, 280
Fowlie, A, 82, 276, 279
Frank, JB and JD, 274, 275, 280
Frankel, M, 10, 87, 202
Frankl, VE, 247, 256
Freed, W, 87
Freud, S, 31, 53, 84, 385, 404
Frey-Wouters, E, 82, 84
Friedman, MJ, 10, 59, 68, 82, 84, 86, 89, 153, 262, 280
Fromm, E, 216, 217, 256
Fukuyama, F, 29, 84

Garfield, 145
Garreton, M, 82, 88
Gask, L, 273, 274, 280
Gath, D, 273, 280
Geertz, C, 114, 153
Geevathasan, MG, 235, 256
Geffray, C, 14, 84
Geiller, JE, 152
Gerrity, ET, 82, 86, 153, 262, 280
Gersons, BPR, 153, 202, 203
Geschiere, P, 408, 439
Gibbs, S, 151, 153
Giel, R, 16, 84
Goff, B, 88
Goffman, E, 76, 84
Goldberg, D, 28, 84, 273, 274, 280
Good, B, 3, 40, 83, 86, 87, 107, 152, 202, 271, 273, 280, 408, 412, 438, 439

Author Index

Goodhand, J, 230, 256
Goodwin, J, 17, 18, 84
Goody, J, 37, 84
Grant, M, 277, 280
Green, A, 28, 84
Green, BL, 35, 68
Green, E, 407, 438
Greenfield, S, 404
Greenwald, S, 404
Greiger, W, 205, 256
Greve, HS, 109, 153
Grodos, D, 408, 409, 438
Groenjian, AK, 7, 88
Grünfeld, F, 90
Gunawardena, RALH, 219, 256
Guragain, G, 260, 280
Guthrie, E, 273, 279

Haas, P, 62, 85
Habershaim, N, 89
Haggerty, BJ, 87
Halpern, E, 16, 85
Hancock, G, 339, 366
Handelman, LH, 153
Hanewald, G, 89, 166, 203
Harpham, T, 9, 82, 408, 437
Harrell-Bond, B, 85, 202
Harries, A, 44, 86
Hays, RD, 404
Healy, J, 152
Heggenhougen, HK, 438
Helman, CG, 243, 256, 412, 413, 438
Helzer, JE, 10, 85
Hema, N, 155
Hendin, HA, 62, 85
Hermanns, JMA, 7, 87
Hetherly, V, 278, 280
Him, C, 88
Hirsch, H, 256
Hobfoll, SE, 28, 30, 34, 73, 82, 83, 85, 89, 90, 403, 438
Holwell, S, 408, 437
Hough, RL, 32, 86
House, JS, 34, 85
Hubbard, J, 21, 85
Hudelson, PM, 48, 85

Hughes, M, 10, 85
Hume, D, 230, 256
Hutt, M, 260, 280
Huxley, P, 28, 84
Hwu, HG, 404

Ihezue, UH, 233, 256
Irish, DP, 37, 85
Ivey, AE and M, 274, 280

Jablensky, A, 6, 202
Jackson, DA, 37, 88
Jalbert, R, 107, 154
Janoff-Bulman, R, 32, 85
Jansson, B, 6, 202
Janzen, JM, 408, 418, 438, 439
Jaranson, J, 10, 84
Jareg, E, 225, 256
Jayawardena, K, 219, 256
Jensen, PS, 18
Jensen, SB, 6, 75, 82
Jeyanthy, K, 227, 256
Jeyaraja Tambiah, S, 85
Jha, R, 279
Johnson, B, 279
Jordan, K, 32, 86, 317
Joseph, S, 202, 237
Joyce, PR, 404
Jurugo, E, 202

Kadiragamar, L, 215, 256
Kagawa-Singer, M, 61, 85
Kagitcibasi, 115
Kall, K, 155
Kalton, GW, 233, 257
Kaplan, CD, 48, 85, 314
Kaplan, HI, 66, 85, 196, 202
Karam, EG, 404
Katon, W, 87
Keane, TM, 10, 82, 84, 86, 89
Keehn, RJ, 10, 85
Kelly, PK, 315
Ken, P, 39, 82
Kessler, RC, 10, 33, 47, 85
Ketzer, E, 83, 314
Khaled, N, 6, 11, 83, 382, 404
Khulamo-Sakatukwa, G, 81

Kiernan, B, 95, 152, 153
Kim, U, 153
Kinney, R, 88
Kinzie, JD, 21, 22, 85, 88, 94, 141, 143, 152, 153, 262, 279
Kirmayer, LJ, 10, 86, 105, 153, 412, 413, 439
Kleber, RJ, 153, 202, 203
Kleinman, A, 3, 39, 40, 83, 86, 87, 120, 152, 153, 202, 262, 271, 273, 274, 280, 308, 314, 408, 412, 413, 437, 438, 439
Kolb, LL, 31, 60, 86
Komproe, IH, 6, 10, 11, 53, 77, 83, 87, 89, 90, 166, 203, 280, 281, 314, 407
Korf, DJ, 48, 85, 86
Kortmann, F, 354, 366
Koumare, B, 437
Krueger, RA, 49, 86
Krystal, H, 31, 32, 86
Kulka, RA, 32, 86

Lakshmman, N, 256
Lanham, K, 88
Lapika, D, 407, 418, 438, 439
Last, M, 2, 146, 158, 189, 206, 407, 439
Laufer, RS, 31, 86
Laungani, P, 37, 87
Launier, R, 34, 86
Lavelle, J, 10, 87, 202
Lawrence, P, 89, 243, 256
Lazarus, RS, 30, 34, 86, 271, 280
Le Roy, J, 407, 408, 418, 436, 438, 439
Ledoux, JE, 32, 86
Lee, CK, 404
Lellouch, J, 404
Lepine, JP, 404
Levi, L, 6, 202
Lewer, N, 230, 256
Lewinsohn, P, 88
Lewis-Fernandez, R, 437
Lipson, JG, 151, 153

Lira, E, 15, 88
Littlewood, R, 83, 412, 439
Litz, BT, 10, 86
Lobel, ML, 86
Loksham, C, 279
Lopez, AD, 8, 9, 87
Loshani, NA, 227, 256
Lundquist, KF, 37, 85

Machel, G, 14, 86
Macksoud, MS, 19, 86
Maher, D, 44, 86
Mahjoub, A, 16, 86
Makaju, R, 11, 89, 90, 274, 280, 281
Malone, K, 152
Malpass, RS, 262, 280
Mandlhate, C, 83
Manogaran, C, 223, 256
Manson, S, 85
Marmar, CR, 32, 86
Marsella, AJ, 6, 46, 82, 84, 86, 87, 153, 154, 158, 164, 178, 202, 203, 262, 265, 280
Martel, G, 108, 153
Martin, SF, 12, 86, 177, 178, 197, 202
Marty, P, 381, 404
Marx, B, 10, 86
Marysse, S, 410, 438
Masten, AS, 85
Matthews, KL, 278, 280
Matula, A, 407, 418, 439
Mauss, M, 408, 439
Mayou, R, 273, 280
Mbape, P, 81
Mbonyinkebe Sehabire, 438, 439
McCurry, S, 279
McEvoy, L, 10, 85
McFarlane, AC, 3, 4, 32, 46, 82, 87, 88, 90, 104, 155, 165, 174, 202, 203
McInnes, K, 46, 87
McSharry, S, 88
Mehta, HC, 130, 153
Meichenbaum, D, 54, 87, 99

Mendelsohn, M, 89
Mercenier, P, 408, 409, 438
Mesfin, A, 6, 10, 11, 83
Meyer, B, 408, 439
Mghir, R, 21, 87
Mikulincer, M, 33, 89
Mollica, R, 10, 46, 60, 62, 87, 94, 107, 154, 202
Monaco, V, 10, 86
Moon, JH, 151, 154
Moosa, F, 89
Mounkoro, P, 437
Mrazek, PJ, 87
Muecke, MA, 150, 154
Müller, M, 87
Multipassi, LR, 31, 60, 86
Mumford, DB, 412, 415, 440
Murray, C, 8, 9, 87
Murthy, RS, 36, 37, 87
Mwiti, GK, 59, 84
Mynors-Wallis, L, 273, 280
Myslewic, E, 154

Nadarajah, K, 233, 257
Nader, KO, 16, 17, 18, 19, 87, 88
Nehru, J, 222, 256
Nelsen, VJ, 37, 85
Nelson, CB, 10, 85
Nepote, 113, 154
Newel, K, 28, 87
Newman, SC, 404
Nikapota, A, 241, 256
Nixon, A, 318, 335
Northood, AK, 85
Novick, P, 87

Obeyesekere, G, 34, 209, 210, 257
O'Dowd, 274, 280
Ojendal, J, 108, 154
Olivier de Sardan, JP, 440
Orley, J, 84, 86, 87, 154, 158, 170, 202, 203
Osmond, H, 24, 89
Ovesen, J, 108, 154

Paardekoper, BP, 7, 20, 57, 76, 87

Pagani, F, 252, 257
Palihawadana, M, 216, 257
Pankhurst, R, 339, 347, 366
Papay, P, 10, 87
Parameshwaran, SV, 256
Parkes, CM, 37, 87
Pearl, JH, 151, 154, 257
Pennebaker, JW, 47, 87
Perera, J, 233, 257
Peveler, R, 273, 280
Phuntsok, K, 313, 314
Pitman, RK, 31, 32, 87, 88, 104
Piyadasa, L, 212, 257
Ponchaud, F, 96, 154
Poole, C, 46, 87
Poortinga, YH, 27, 82, 262, 280
Pope, KS, 279
Porée-Maspero, E, 108, 154
Poudyal, BN, 53, 77, 90, 279, 281
Prabaharan, S, 230, 257
Pradhan, H, 279
Prasain, D, 90, 259, 279, 280, 281
Prins, G, 408, 439
Punamäki, RL, 10, 16, 20, 84, 88, 322
Pynoos, RS, 7, 16, 17, 18, 19, 81, 84, 87, 88

Qouta, S, 20, 35, 76, 81, 88, 321, 322, 323, 335

Rafalowicz, E, 10, 87
Rangaraj, AG, 157, 202
Ranger, TO, 408, 437, 440
Rapgay, L, 315
Raphael, B, 59, 84, 88, 195
Rappaport, J, 28, 88
Rasiah, S, 233, 257
Raskin, A, 87
Rath, B, 85
Raundalen, M, 19, 83
Realmoto, GM, 85
Regier, DA, 385, 404
Regmi, S, 11, 89, 279, 280
Renol, KK, 155

Reppesgard, HO, 227, 257
Robbins, JM, 412, 439
Robins, LN, 10, 85, 385, 404
Rogers, W, 404
Rogler, LH, 47, 88, 408, 440
Romanski, L, 32, 86
Ronen, T, 21, 88
Rosenbaum, M, 21, 88
Rosenbeck, R, 236, 257
Rosenblatt, PC, 37, 88
Rouadjia, A, 370, 404
Rouchy, JC, 436, 440
Rubio-Stipec, M, 404
Ruiz, HA, 226, 257
Rupesinghe, K, 4, 90
Russell, DW, 34, 82

Sack, WH, 22, 41, 85, 88
Sadock, BJ, 66, 85, 196, 202
Salimovich, S, 15, 88
Salmi, S, 10, 84, 335
Saltarelli, D, 252, 255
Samai-Ouramdane, G, 368, 404
Samarisinghe, D, 256
Sanderson, WC, 279
Sarason, SB, 73, 83, 85, 88
Sartorius, N, 38, 83, 90, 202
Sasikanthan, A, 234, 255
Sassi, L, 150, 154
Saul, J, 69, 90
Schindler, R, 151, 154
Schlenger, WE, 32, 86
Schnurr, PP, 84
Schreiber, S, 151, 154
Schriever, SH, 154
Sciarone, P, 4, 90
Scurfield, RM, 83, 86, 153, 262, 280
Seeley, J, 88
Segall, MH, 27, 82
Seligman, MEP, 162, 168, 203
Sell, H, 273, 280
Selye, H, 30, 88
Sen, A, 3, 88, 439
Shalev, AY, 10, 30, 32, 69, 88, 90
Shanfield, SB, 278, 280

Shapiro, F, 80, 81, 89, 275, 280
Sharma, B, 11, 43, 53, 77, 83, 89, 90, 259, 264, 274, 279, 280, 281
Sharma, GK, 43, 53, 77
Sharp, TW, 91
Sharpe, M, 13, 153, 273, 280
Shaw, J, 18, 85
Shawcross, W, 95, 154
Shepard, M, 233, 257
Shisana, O, 16, 89
Shoham, V, 279
Shrestha, NM, 11, 40, 89, 261, 267, 280
Siegler, M, 24, 89
Sieswerda, S, 12, 89, 166, 203
Silove, D, 69, 90
Silver, RC, 38, 91
Simek-Morgan, L, 274, 280
Siriwardene, R, 253, 257
Sissobo, M, 437
Sivachandran, S, 218, 257
Sivarajini, G, 227, 256
Sivashankar, R, 233, 234, 255, 256
Sivayokan, S, 106, 154, 230, 241, 243, 245, 257
Solomon, SD, 9, 48
Solomon, Z, 21, 33, 89
Somasundaram, DJ, 6, 10, 11, 53, 83, 89, 106, 122, 133, 147, 149, 154, 155, 224, 225, 227, 229, 230, 232, 233, 234, 235, 239, 241, 242, 243, 245, 255, 256, 257
Sonnega, A, 10, 85
Soomers, R, 155
Sovandara, S C, 155
Spencer, J, 210, 256, 257
Spinaci, S, 44, 86
Staub, E, 217, 257
Steinberg, AM, 7, 88
Sterk, C, 48, 85
Sterkenburg, JJ, 72, 89
Stewart, A, 404
Straker, G, 20, 89

Straus, A, 89
Strelzer, J, 34, 90
Sue, S, 279
Suleiman, R, 16, 88
Sultan, A, 82
Summerfield, D, 10, 38, 63, 84, 89, 151, 152, 166, 203, 335
Susman, JR, 47, 87
Svang, TOR, 10, 87, 202

Tardy, CH, 34, 89
Taussig, M, 151, 154
Taylor, S, 85, 275, 277, 280
Tedeschi, RD, 33, 89
Terr, L, 17, 33, 89
Thabet, A, 18, 81, 89, 322, 335
Thambiah, SJ, 216, 223, 257
Thapa, S, 53, 77, 90, 274, 280, 281
Theodore, L, 164, 203
Thion, S, 108, 113, 154
Thoits, PA, 34, 89
Thomas, L, 37, 89
Thomassen, L, 133, 154, 155
Toole, MJ, 13, 90
Topgay, S, 315
Tor, S, 46, 87
Trankell, I, 108, 154
Trawick, M, 218, 257
Tredoux, C, 82
Triandis, H, 115, 153
Tricket, EJ, 38, 90
Tseng, W-S, 34, 90
Tsultrim, L, 306, 314
Tudin, P, 89
Tylor, CE, 90

Uchoa, E, 437
Ugalde, A, 252, 258
Upton, P, 82
Ursano, RJ, 10, 69, 88, 90
Üstün, TB, 38, 90
Uyangoda, J, 215, 258

Valentine, JD, 6, 82
Van Boven, T, 77, 78, 90
Van de Goor, L, 4, 90

Van de Put, WACM, 6, 10, 11, 53, 83, 89, 108, 122, 154, 155
Van der Kolk, BA, 32, 33, 87, 88, 90, 155, 176, 195, 196, 202, 203
Van der Veer, G, 146, 155, 168, 203
Van Etten, M, 275, 277, 280
Van Ommeren, MH, 6, 10, 11, 12, 41, 43, 51, 53, 69, 77, 83, 89, 90, 259, 261, 262, 264, 274, 279, 280, 281, 314
Van Schaik, MM, 35, 37, 62, 83
Van Walt van Praag, MC, 315
Vecchiato, N, 354, 366
Ventura, MMF, 21, 90
Vickery, M, 95, 96, 155
Vines, A, 14, 90
Vitachi, T, 212, 258
Von Buchwald, U, 169, 203
Vostanis, P, 18, 89, 335

Waldman, RJ, 13, 90
Walsh, RP, 37, 88
Ware, J, 404, 437
Warfe, PG, 59, 84
Weine, S, 69, 90
Weinstein, E, 15, 88
Weisaeth, L, 32, 87, 88, 90, 155, 202, 203
Weiss, DS, 32, 86
Weiss, M, 271, 274
Weiss Fagen, P, 82, 88
Weissman, MM, 385, 404
Wells, JE, 404
Wells, KB, 385
Werbner, RP, 408, 437, 440
Westendrop, I, 90
Westermeyer, J, 2, 10, 13, 60, 91
Wickramaratne, PJ, 404
Wijeyasekara, A, 252, 258
Willetts, D, 339, 366
Williams, C, 91
Williams, DA, 279
Williams, HA, 16, 91

Williams, R, 202
Wilson, JP, 59, 84, 86, 88, 91, 151, 155
Wilson, KB, 15
Wing, JK, 202
Wittchen, H, 404
Woody, SR, 279
Wortmann, CB, 38, 91
Wyslewiec, 96, 154

Xagoraris, A, 32, 86

Yeh, EK, 404
Yehuda, R, 46, 87, 165, 202
Yesavage, JA, 10, 91
Yip, R, 13, 91
Yoon, G, 115, 153
Young, A, 439
Young, B, 37, 87
Yule, W, 202

Zivcic, I, 22, 91
Zwi, A, 252, 258

Subject Index

Action research, 48, 127, 130, 408
Acute stress disorder, 10, 340
Adolescents, 14, 16, 17, 18, 21, 22, 23, 29, 50, 75, 77, 86, 88–90, 235–237, 277, 355, 356, 363, 397, 411
Advocacy, 60, 69, 71, 200, 224, 326
Affective disorder, 147, 261
Aid dependence: *see* Dependency
Alcohol abuse, 98, 140, 171, 247
Algeria, 11, 15, 23, 24, 35, 42, 58, 79, 367–403
   children, 378, 397
   families, 378
   fundamentalism, 369–373
   modern history, 367–373
   rape, 379
   social structure, 375
   terrorism, 370–373
   women, 379
Amnesty International, 237, 279, 319
Angola, 3, 5, 21, 22, 24, 29, 90
Anxiety disorder, 104, 105, 148, 261, 323, 396
Arms control, 70
Awareness, 327

Basic psychiatry, 125, 150
Behavioral therapy, 79, 329
Bhutanese refugees in Nepal, 11, 12, 43, 259
   refugee camps, 265
Bio-medical paradigm, 423, 426
Body-oriented techniques, 140
Breathing exercises, 248
Buddhism, 215, 306, 310
Burial rites: *see* Funeral rituals

Cambodia, 53, 93–152
   culture, 123–124
   education, 129
   health care expenditure, 122
   health status, 121
   modern history, 95, 96, 129
Cambodian refugees, 10
Capacity building, 74, 75
Case management, 127, 141, 266, 270
Caste, 217
Categories of distress, 262
Child soldiers, 12, 18, 35, 56, 67, 68, 78, 224, 225, 246
Children, 7, 14, 166
   abandoned, 2, 14, 76
   attrition, 13
   continuous traumatic stress, 15
   coping skills, 73
   development, 15
   family support, 16
   psychosocial consequences of war, 16
   recreational activities, 198
   traumatic stress symptoms
      among adolescents, 18
      among children of early school age, 16
      among preschool children, 16
      among school-age children, 17
China, 44, 283, 284, 295
Christianity, 39, 207, 211, 218, 219
CIDI 2.1, 41, 62, 100, 102, 340, 384, 399, 401
Code of conduct, 111, 112, 117
Cognitive therapy, 79, 276, 329
Collective massacres, 377, 379
Collective trauma, 106, 208, 229, 242
   Sri Lanka, 229

Combat-related guilt, 62
Commitment
  long-term, 61
Community
  building, 127, 199, 201
  campaigns, 72
  development, 28
  empowerment, 28, 48, 58, 73
  involvement, 48
  meetings, 50
  mobilization, 28
  psychology, 28
Community action project [Congo], 425
  aims, 426
  phases, 427
  setting, 426
Community awareness
  about mental health problems, 127, 176, 201
  education, 201
Community-based rehabilitation program, 266
Community concern
  assessment of, 48–51
Community Crisis Intervention Team [Sudan], 195, 196, 200, 201
Community education, 185, 188
Community health workers
  Sri Lanka, 240
Community level
  and trauma prevention interventions, 65, 71–76, 77, 78
Community mediation, 177, 279
Community participation, 407, 408, 425, 426, 436
  challenges, 435
Community workers, 126
Community workshop, 188
  curriculum, 190
Compensation, 77, 78, 90, 171, 278, 349, 356, 379, 390
Composite International Diagnostic Interview: *see* CIDI 2.1
Conflict management, 113
Conflict mediation, 201
Conflict resolution, 69, 70, 73, 114
Conflicts
  internal, political and ethnic, 4, 199
Congo, 3, 14, 29, 405–440
Conservation of Resources (COR), 30

Conspiracy of silence, 38, 60
Coping strategies, 24, 34, 37, 40, 49, 76, 89, 109, 229, 250, 251, 310, 311, 312, 339–342, 346, 350, 361–363
  indigenous, 37, 73, 97, 101, 107, 110, 251
Coping Style Scale, 340
Cost-effectiveness, 44, 53, 63, 65, 333, 402
  as selection criterion for programs, 63
  study TPO, 63
Counseling skills, 75, 137, 145, 146, 265, 267, 268, 305
Counseling, 37, 78, 144, 294, 299, 303, 308, 329
  family, 328
  Nepal, 267, 271
  Sri Lanka, 241
Counselors
  Nepal, 275, 278
  training of, 146
Crisis intervention, 57, 66, 71, 77, 149, 176, 177, 196, 200, 305
Cultural sensitivity
  as selection criterion for programs, 61
Culture change, 171
Culture, 34, 61
Culture-bound syndromes, 51, 412, 414, 415, 416, 419, 424, 434, 435
Curative groups, 197
CVICT, 43, 44, 259–279

Dalai Lama, 216, 283–285, 290, 295, 311
DALY, 8
Declaration of Alma Ata, 407
Declaration of the Rights of the Child, 14
Dependency, 163, 168, 359–366
  gap, 55, 56
  in refugee camps, 76, 162
  syndrome, 50, 58, 76
Depressive disorder, 8, 10, 11, 17, 22, 47, 52, 415
DESNOS, 246, 340
Disability, 9, 190
  as selection criterion for programs, 46
Disaster preparedness training, 71
Dissociative disorder, 53, 86, 261, 262
Domestic violence, 35, 98, 113, 140
Donor policies, 56, 57
DSM-IV, 40, 340, 350, 384, 415
Dysfunctional families, 98

Subject Index

Early identification, 65, 77
Early/rapid interventions, 46, 47, 66, 77
EMDR, 80, 275, 276, 277
Emotional coping, 311
Emotional distress, 41, 164, 165
Emotional support, 34, 186, 195, 271, 274, 275, 277
Empowerment, 7, 25, 28, 29, 58, 65, 71, 73, 74, 88, 176, 325, 328, 330, 331, 366
  women, 330
Energy psychology, 275
Epidemiology, 10
  as selection criterion for programs, 45, 46
Epilepsy, 53, 54, 192, 194
  prevalence, 148, 187, 193
Eritrea, 5, 14, 338, 339
Ethical acceptability, 60–65
  as selection criterion for programs, 60
  informed consent, 61
  long-term commitment, 61
Ethiopia, 337–366
  children, 337, 354
  culture, 347
  internally displaced, 337–366
  men, 352, 353
Expatriates: *see* International staff
Explanatory models 39, 128, 138, 139, 151, 180, 278, 308, 309, 413, 418, 420
Exposure therapy, 79, 274, 276, 278
Expressive therapy, 249
Eye Movement Desensitization and Reprocessing: *see* EMDR

Faith healers [Congo], 416, 421–425
Families, 28, 30, 36
  extended, 109, 166, 169
Family
  breakdown, 158
  building, 78
  leaders, 120
  reunion, 76
  support, 16
  therapy, 78, 79, 245, 246, 247, 271, 399
  tracing, 76
Feasibility: *see* Cost-effectiveness
FIS, 367, 370, 371, 372, 375
Focus groups, 340
Food for Work program, 344, 352, 353

Forum for Protection of Human Rights, 260
Fundamentalism, 369–373
Funeral rituals, 38, 62, 242

Gaza, 18, 35
Gaza Community Mental Health Programme: *see* GCMHP
Gaza Strip, 317–336
  human rights, 319
  modern history, 317
Gazans: *see* Palestinians
GCMHP, 319, 321–336
Gender, 6, 13, 16, 30, 33, 50, 65, 179, 263, 323, 353, 363, 426
Global Burden of Disease, 8, 87, 102
Global Severity Index, 3
Government policies, 59, 60
Grief, bereavement, 37, 39, 73
Group rape, 35
Group therapy, 79, 141, 149, 245, 247, 399
Groups, 201
  Alcoholics Anonymous [Uganda], 197
  self-help groups, 197
Guiding principles for public mental health programs, 26–34

Harvard Trauma Questionnaire, 290, 291
Healers: *see* Traditional healers
Healing rituals, 101, 173, 174, 175
Health Staff Interview, 59
Health workers
  attitude of, 122, 148
  motivation, 150
Health-seeking behavior, 135
Help-seeking behavior, 242, 264, 296, 326, 409, 410, 413
  as selection criterion for programs, 46
Hierarchy, 110, 130, 134, 145, 310
High Commissariat of Human Rights, 68
High-risk groups
  children, 13
  elderly, 13
  families, 12
  women, 12
Hinduism, 209, 211, 216
Hopkins Symptom CheckList (HSCL), 291, 292, 340
Hospitalization, 48, 194

Human resources, 54, 101
Human rights, 6, 59, 278

ICD-10, 15, 40, 236, 261, 262, 415
Idioms of distress, 101, 106, 132
Illness categories, 262, 414, 415
Illness experience, 271
Imprisonment, 104
Income generation project, 72, 195
India, 283–316
Indigenous coping strategies: *see* Coping strategies
Individual level
  and trauma prevention interventions, 65, 67, 76, 78
Individual therapy, 79
Insecurity, 161, 163
Institute for Defense and Disarmament Studies, 27
Institutionalization, 80, 217
Integration of refugees, 161
Internally displaced persons, 2
  regions of origin, 4, 5
International Monetary Fund, 3
International staff, 177, 178, 185, 346, 359, 365
Intifada, 317
Iraq, 5, 19, 215, 233
Islam, 39, 62, 218, 368, 371
Israel, 3, 15, 20, 21, 88, 317–322, 332

Karma (Buddhism), 115, 116
Key informant interviews, 340
Khmer Rouge, 94–97
Kuwait, 19

Lamas [Tibet], 296, 301
Landmines, 70, 104, 146
Leadership, 172
Learned helplessness: *see* Dependency syndromes
Lebanon, 18, 19
Life Events and Social History Interview, 340
Life stressors, 32–33
Local authorities, 120, 134
Local resources, 117, 151
  mapping of, 137, 139
Long-term exile, 157

Long-term exile (*cont.*)
  secondary consequences, 170
LTTE, 205, 208, 213, 214, 221, 224, 229, 238

Major depressive disorder, 8, 12, 105, 301, 384, 385
Making merit (Buddhism), 116, 117
Manual, 240, 241, 248, 267, 299
Media, 70, 73
Medication: *see* Pharmacotherapy
Meditation, 119, 133, 140, 248, 249, 306, 307, 312
Mediums, 119, 144, 145; *see also* Traditional healers
Mental distress, 414
Mental health care professionals, 23, 59
  and cultural sensitivity, 61
Mental health clinics, 147, 151
  mobile [Sudan], 193
Mental health services
  decentralisation, 29
Mental health workers
  burnout, 251, 255
Mentally retarded people, 194
Mexico, 13
Migration
  cross-border, 3
  internal displacement, 3
  cross-continental, 3
MIM-Study, 11, 42, 62
Monitoring, 200
Monks (Buddhist), 117
Morbidity, 10, 11, 32, 42, 47, 51, 52, 168, 291, 415
Mourning, 35
  rituals, 73
Mozambique, 3, 14, 19, 56, 62
MSF, 7, 87
Muslims: *see* Islam
Mutual support, 107, 120, 144

Namibia, 62
Nepal, 3, 11, 12, 15, 35, 41, 43, 55, 77, 89, 90, 259–282
  modern history, 259
Network building, 78
Neurosis, 246, 396
NORAD, 223, 253
Nurses, 290

Subject Index

Occupational therapy, 238, 246, 250, 329
Ongoing trauma, 54
ONS, 367, 388
Order, 110, 134
Organized violence, 50, 159, 207, 212, 320, 323, 329, 372

Pain, medically unexplained, 274
Palestine, 3, 15, 19, 20, 233, 317, 319, 325, 328, 333, 334
Palestinian Authority, 319, 320
Palestinians, 5, 16, 317–336
  adolescents, 322
  children, 322,329
  ex-political prisoners, 321
  drug addicts, 329
  families, 322
  torture survivors, 329
  women, 322, 329, 330
Panic disorder, 10, 12, 384
Paranoia, 148, 221, 323
Participant observation, 49
Peace building, 199
Peace keeping forces, 70
PEACE, 62
Persecution of perpetrators, 70
Pharmacotherapy, 78, 80, 149, 245, 249, 329
  and sustainability, 58
Phenomenological narratives, 49
Physiotherapy, 269, 270, 329
Play therapy, 249, 246, 249, 329
Policy makers: see Government policies
Political acceptability
  as selection criterion for programs, 59
Poverty, 101, 139, 168
Prayers, 173, 175, 296, 301, 416
Prevalence, 10, 11, 21, 22, 42, 45, 46, 47, 51, 52, 53, 54, 64, 65, 68, 69, 86, 89, 104, 105, 113, 121, 162, 187, 191–193, 232, 234, 262, 265, 321, 339, 402, 415, 416
  as selection criterion for programs, 45
Prevention of trauma, 27
  interventions, 65–71
  primary, 65, 68–77
  secondary, 65, 77–80
  tertiary, 65, 66, 80
Preventive groups, 197
Preventive interventions, 67
  indicated, 67

Preventive interventions (cont.)
  primary, 65, 68–77
  secondary, 65, 77–80
  selective, 67
  tertiary, 65, 66, 80
  universal, 67
Primary Health Care, 24, 28
Primary prevention, 65, 68–77
Problem management, 271, 273
Problem resolving, 298, 309, 311
  problem-solving, 201
Psychiatric disorders
  seriousness, 52
  treatability as selection criterion for programs, 53
Psychiatric nurses, 177, 180
  supervision, 185
  training, 183
Psychodynamic therapy, 80
Psycho-education, 127, 135, 139, 246
Psychosis, 10, 52, 132, 148, 192, 245, 297, 307, 308, 324, 349, 396, 412, 423
Psychosocial counselors, 79, 177, 179
  burnout, 188
  selection, 179
  supervision, 182
  training, 181
  curriculum, 182
Psychosomatic disorder, 323
Psychotherapy, 54, 79, 80, 140, 141, 144, 203, 225, 238, 245, 247, 249, 267, 271, 274, 276, 290, 299, 329, 331, 386
Psychotropic drugs: see Pharmacotherapy
PTSD/PTSS, 164, 166, 261, 262, 264, 265, 290, 340, 348
  children, 22, 23
  complex, 54
  malignant, 236
  prevalence, 11, 12
  relationship with co-morbid disorders, 47
  and stressors, 32
Public education, 72
Public health services
  underutilisation [Congo], 417, 422
Public mental health
  approach, 23, 24
  criteria for selection of priorities, 45–65
  objectives, 44, 45
  programs, 24

Public mental health (*cont.*)
  progams (*cont.*)
    guiding policy principles, 24
    guiding service delivery principles, 25

QUALY, 8

Rape, 35
Rapid appraisal methods, 50
Rapid interventions, 46, 47, 66, 77
Reattribution through Education, 274
Rebel attacks, 169; *see also* Insecurity
Reconciliation, 199
Recurrent psychosis, 301
Red Cross, 3, 85, 202
Referral, 199
Refugee camps, 77
  settlement sites, 161
  transit camps, 161
Refugee care
  dependency, 168
  emergency phase, 7
  long-term, 168
  short-term, 169
Refugees
  economic, 4
  environmental, 4
  long-term, 157, 159
  number of, 2
  regions of origin, 4, 5
  training of, 76
Rehabilitation, 66, 80, 250
Reincarnation (Buddhism), 115
Relationships, 111, 114, 115
Relaxation techniques, 79, 140, 149, 239, 245, 247, 248, 273, 274
Religion, 215, 416
Religious festivals, 243
Reparation, 68, 71, 77, 78
Repatriation, 159
Repetition of words, 248
Research, 200, 333, 401
  focus groups, 49, 101, 162
  key informant interviews, 49, 101, 162
  multiflex snowball sampling, 48
  participant observation, 49, 162
  participatory action research, 100, 127, 130
  phenomenological narratives, 49, 101

Research (*cont.*)
  qualitative, 48
  sondeo method, 49
  translation of questionnaires, 292
Responsibilities
  family, 169
Rituals of misfortune, 243
Rituals, 296, 419
Role expectations, 145
Role models, 114, 126, 145
Rural development, 71

Sampling
  multiflex snowball, 48
SARP, 58, 373, 392
  intervention model, 393
  mission, 392
  objectives, 392
  principles, 393
Schizophrenia, 8, 13, 51, 64, 91, 106, 148, 170, 191, 192, 194, 301, 308, 412
SCL-90-R, 3, 401
Secondary prevention, 65, 77–80
Secondary traumatization, 76
Security measures, 70, 76
Selection criteria for interventions, 45–65
Self
  Cambodian concept of the, 114
  Western concept of the, 114
Self-help groups, 7, 78, 109, 127, 141, 144, 197
Self-reliance of refugees, 161, 162, 169
Separation from family, 103
Sequential trauma, 150
Service utilization, 48
  mission, 325
  objectives, 326
  services, 324
Sick-role, 63
Sinhalese, 205
  Buddhist identity, 219
Sleeping disorders, 98, 107
Social capital, 29, 30, 36
Social change, 124
Social cohesion, 114
Social integration, 108
Social networks, 35, 109, 114
Social phobia, 384
Social rehabilitation, 151

Subject Index

Social responsibility, 114
Social roles, 111
Social support, 328
   definition, 34, 35
Society
   community, 27
   levels of, 26
   society-at-large, 27
   structure of [Cambodia], 114
Society-at-large
   and trauma prevention interventions, 65, 68–71, 77, 80
Somatic pain, 264, 272
Somatization, 230, 232, 412, 414
Sondeo method, 49
South Africa, 19, 20
Specific Phobic Disorder, 384
Spiritual beliefs, 247, 354, 355
Spiritual healing, 311, 421
Spiritual world: *see* Supernatural world
Sri Lanka, 73, 205–258
   adolescents, 220, 235
   children, 233, 234, 246, 249
   child soldiers, 224, 235
   collective trauma, 229
   education, 223
   history, 205–211
   internally displaced, 227, 239
   modern history, 211–214
   myths, 221
   refugees, 226
   stress factors, 231
   women, 218, 232, 233, 246
Stress
   cumulative, 168
   definition of, 30
   theories on, 30
Structural Adjustment Programs, 3
Sudan, 3, 73
Sudanese People's Liberation Army (SPLA), 159
Sudanese refugees in Uganda, 12, 57, 62, 157–201
Suicide, 62, 105, 107, 158, 170, 196, 215
   prevention, 196
   taboo, 62
   underreporting, 62
Supernatural world, 115, 116
Supervision, 267, 269, 398, 400, 401

Support networks, 76, 195
Supportive therapy, 329
Survey, 341
   epidemiological, 402
Survival capacities, 63
Survivor guilt, 62
Sustainability, 305, 313, 362, 363, 364
   and donors, 56
   and human resources, 54
   as selection criterion for programs, 54
Symptom Check List (SCR-90), 340
Symptom management, 274

Tamils, 205
   diaspora, 222, 226
   Tamil identity, 220
   women, 233
TBA: *see* Traditional birth attendants
Teachers, 120; *see also* Community workers
Teaching manual on community mental health, 132
   problems with translation, 133
   training, 133
Terrorism, 370–373
   collective massacres, 377, 379
   victims, 374, 388
Terrorists
   traumatized, 386
Tertiary prevention, 65, 66, 80
Thailand, 62
Thought Field Therapy, 80
Tibet
   culture, 292, 296, 305–312
   medicine, 301
      and mental health, 305, 306
   modern history, 284–287
Tibetan refugees in India, 44, 283–316
Torture survivors, 289, 320
   complaints, 264
   Nepal, 260, 261, 262, 263
   services, 265, 270
TOT: *see* Training
TPO, 28, 55, 63
   intervention program, 44
   selection of priorities, 45
   theoretical model, 30–34
   working method, 44
Traditional birth attendants, 118, 119
Traditional coping: *see* Coping strategies

Traditional healers, 29, 54, 62, 73, 76, 98, 107, 113, 116–119, 172, 174, 194, 242, 247, 296, 301, 326, 354, 405, 418–420, 423, 424, 429, 430
   links with medical care providers, 431, 432
   organisation, 432
   quality control, 432
   as trauma therapists, 124, 151
Traditional healing methods, 117, 173, 242, 245
Traditional helping methods, 172, 190; *see also* Local resources
Traditional taxonomy of mental disorder, 125, 132
Training
   Algeria, 398
   community health workers, 267, 268
   Ethiopia, 356
   health assistants, 267
   India, 299, 330, 331, 332
   medical staff, 122, 148
   medical students, 241
   for mental health care professionals, 59
   midwives, 241
   native counselors, 277
   Nepal, 267
   nurses, 241
   for refugees, 58
   Sri Lanka, 240
   teachers, 279
   TOT, 61, 74, 75, 240, 299, 300
   TOTOT, 74, 75
Train-the-Trainer: *see* Training, TOT
Traumatic events, 100, 101, 166
Traumatic stress, 4
   appraisal, 33, 35
   contextual approach to, 31
   coping behavior, 34, 37
   demographic characteristics, 33
   event characteristics, 33, 35
   protective factors, 7, 166
   resources, social support, 34, 35
   risk factors, 6
   theories on, 30, 32

Traumatic stress (*cont.*)
   traumatic event-related characteristics, 33
Traumatization
   and time, 42
   collective, 106
   sequential, 42
Treatability of disorders
   as selection criterion for programs, 53
TRRO, 253

U.S. Committee for Refugees (USCR), 2, 5
Uganda, 11, 12, 19, 20, 157–201
UNDP, 338
UNHCR, 2, 59, 68, 69, 90, 132, 159, 160, 161, 162, 168, 169, 180, 190, 191, 195, 200, 226, 240, 241, 266, 267, 277, 401
UNICEF, 3, 12, 68, 90, 241, 252, 253, 337, 338, 345
Universal Declaration of Human Rights, 6
UNTAC, 112, 121
USA, 21, 22
Utilization of public health services, 122
   Cambodia, 148, 150

Vietnam, 62
Village associations [Cambodia], 120
Violence, 8
Visual therapy, 329
Vocational skills training, 29, 72
Voluntary repatriation, 70
Vulnerable groups, 134, 169

War, 3, 8
War tribunals, 70
Western psychology, 275, 290, 308
Western taxonomy, 339
WHO, 8, 68, 215
World Bank, 3, 8

Yoga, 245, 247–249, 266, 274
Youth: *see also* Adolescents
   activities, 198, 201
   clubs, 198
   pregnancy, 171

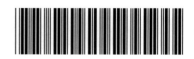